2004
YEAR BOOK OF
ANESTHESIOLOGY AND
PAIN MANAGEMENT™

The 2004 Year Book Series

Year Book of Allergy, Asthma, and Clinical Immunology™: Drs Rosenwasser, Boguniewicz, Milgrom, Routes, and Spahn

Year Book of Anesthesiology and Pain Management™: Drs Chestnut, Abram, Black, Lang, Roizen, Trankina, and Wood

Year Book of Cardiology®: Drs Gersh, Cheitlin, Graham, Kaplan, Sundt, and Waldo

Year Book of Critical Care Medicine®: Drs Dellinger, Parrillo, Balk, Bekes, Dries, and Roberts

Year Book of Dentistry®: Drs Zakariasen, Boghosian, Burgess, Hatcher, Horswell, McIntyre, and Zakariasen

Year Book of Dermatology and Dermatologic Surgery™: Drs Thiers and Lang

Year Book of Diagnostic Radiology®: Drs Osborn, Birdwell, Dalinka, Gardiner, Groskin, Levy, Maynard, and Oestreich

Year Book of Emergency Medicine®: Drs Burdick, Cone, Cydulka, Hamilton, Handly, and Quintana

Year Book of Endocrinology®: Drs Mazzaferri, Becker, Kannan, Kennedy, Kreisberg, Meikle, Molitch, Osei, Poehlman, and Rogol

Year Book of Family Practice®: Drs Bowman, Apgar, Dexter, Miser, Neill, and Scherger

Year Book of Gastroenterology™: Drs Lichtenstein, Dempsey, Ginsberg, Katzka, Kochman, Morris, Nunes, Reddy, Rosato, and Stein

Year Book of Hand Surgery®: Drs Berger and Ladd

Year Book of Medicine®: Drs Barkin, Frishman, Klahr, Loehrer, Mazzaferri, Phillips, Pillinger, and Snydman

Year Book of Neonatal and Perinatal Medicine®: Drs Fanaroff, Maisels, and Stevenson

Year Book of Neurology and Neurosurgery®: Drs Gibbs and Verma

Year Book of Nuclear Medicine®: Drs Coleman, Blaufox, Royal, Strauss, and Zubal

Year Book of Obstetrics, Gynecology, and Women's Health®: Drs Mishell, Kirschbaum, and Miller

Year Book of Oncology®: Drs Loehrer, Arceci, Glatstein, Gordon, Morrow, Schiller, and Thigpen

Year Book of Ophthalmology®: Drs Rapuano, Cohen, Eagle, Grossman, Myers, Nelson, Penne, Regillo, Sergott, Shields, and Tipperman

Year Book of Orthopedics®: Drs Morrey, Beauchamp, Peterson, Swiontkowski, Trigg, and Yaszemski

Year Book of Otolaryngology-Head and Neck Surgery®: Drs Paparella, Keefe, and Otto

Year Book of Pathology and Laboratory Medicine®: Drs Raab, Grzybicki, Bejarano, Bissell, and Stanley

Year Book of Pediatrics®: Dr Stockman

Year Book of Plastic and Aesthetic Surgery™: Drs Miller, Bartlett, Garner, McKinney, Ruberg, Salisbury, and Smith

Year Book of Psychiatry and Applied Mental Health®: Drs Talbott, Ballenger, Frances, Jensen, Markowitz, Meltzer, and Simpson

Year Book of Pulmonary Disease®: Drs Phillips, Barker, Blanchard, Dunlap, Lewis, and Maurer

Year Book of Rheumatology, Arthritis, and Musculoskeletal Disease™: Drs Panush, Hadler, Hellmann, Hochberg, Lahita, and Seibold

Year Book of Sports Medicine®: Drs Shephard, Alexander, Cantu, Nieman, Sanborn, and Shrier

Year Book of Surgery®: Drs Copeland, Bland, Cerfolio, Daly, Eberlein, Howard, Luce, Mozingo, and Seeger

Year Book of Urology®: Drs Andriole and Coplen

Year Book of Vascular Surgery®: Dr Moneta

2004

The Year Book of ANESTHESIOLOGY AND PAIN MANAGEMENT™

Editor-in-Chief
David H. Chestnut, MD

Associate Editors
Stephen E. Abram, MD
Susan Black, MD
John D. Lang, Jr, MD
Michael F. Roizen, MD
Mark F. Trankina, MD
Margaret Wood, MD, FRCA

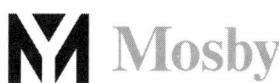 Mosby

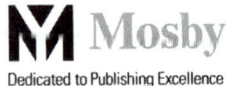
Mosby
Dedicated to Publishing Excellence

Vice President, Continuity Publishing: Timothy M. Griswold
Developmental Editor: Ali Gavenda
Senior Manager, Continuity Production: Idelle L. Winer
Issue Manager: Jason Gonulsen
Senior Illustrations and Permissions Coordinator: Chidi M. Nwaseki

2004 EDITION

Printed in the United States of America
Composition by Thomas Technology Solutions, Inc.
Printing/binding by Sheridan Books, Inc.

Editorial Office:
Elsevier
300 East
170 South Independence Mall West
Philadelphia, PA 19106-3399

International Standard Serial Number: 1073-5437
International Standard Book Number: 0-323-02080-1

Editorial Board

Table of Contents

Journals Represented

Mosby and its editors survey approximately 500 journals for its abstract and commentary publications. From these journals, the editors select the articles to be abstracted. Journals represented in this YEAR BOOK are listed below.

Academic Medicine
Acta Anaesthesiologica Scandinavica
Acta Neurologica Scandinavica
Acta Obstetricia et Gynecologica Scandinavica
American Journal of Cardiology
American Journal of Medicine
American Journal of Obstetrics and Gynecology
American Journal of Psychiatry
American Journal of Respiratory and Critical Care Medicine
American Journal of Surgery
American Surgeon
Anaesthesia
Anaesthesia and Intensive Care
Anesthesia and Analgesia
Anesthesiology
Annals of Internal Medicine
Annals of Thoracic Surgery
Annals of the Royal College of Surgeons of England
Archives of Internal Medicine
Archives of Surgery
Arteriosclerosis, Thrombosis, and Vascular Biology
British Journal of Anaesthesia
British Journal of Obstetrics and Gynaecology
British Journal of Surgery
British Medical Journal
Canadian Journal of Anesthesia
Canadian Journal of Surgery
Chest
Circulation
Clinical Journal of Pain
Clinical Pharmacology and Therapeutics
Critical Care Medicine
European Journal of Pain
European Journal of Vascular and Endovascular Surgery
Gastrointestinal Endoscopy
Infection Control and Hospital Epidemiology
Intensive Care Medicine
International Journal of Gynaecology and Obstetrics
International Journal of Obstetric Anesthesia
Journal of Bone and Joint Surgery (American Volume)
Journal of Bone and Joint Surgery (British Volume)
Journal of Cardiothoracic and Vascular Anesthesia
Journal of Clinical Anesthesia
Journal of Developmental and Behavioral Pediatrics
Journal of Maternal-Fetal and Neonatal Medicine
Journal of Neurosurgery
Journal of Neurosurgery: Spine

Journal of Pediatric Surgery
Journal of Pharmacology and Experimental Therapeutics
Journal of Spinal Disorders & Techniques
Journal of Thoracic and Cardiovascular Surgery
Journal of the American Medical Association
Lancet
Nature Medicine
Neurology
Neurosurgery
New England Journal of Medicine
Otolaryngology-Head and Neck Surgery
Pain
Pediatrics
Preventive Medicine
Proceedings of the National Academy of Sciences
Radiology
Regional Anesthesia and Pain Medicine
Scandinavian Cardiovascular Journal
Southern Medical Journal
Spine
Stroke
Surgery
Thorax
Transfusion

STANDARD ABBREVIATIONS

The following terms are abbreviated in this edition: acquired immunodeficiency syndrome (AIDS), cardiopulmonary resuscitation (CPR), central nervous system (CNS), cerebrospinal fluid (CSF), computed tomography (CT), deoxyribonucleic acid (DNA), electrocardiography (ECG), health maintenance organization (HMO), human immunodeficiency virus (HIV), intensive care unit (ICU), intramuscular (IM), intravenous (IV), magnetic resonance (MR) imaging (MRI), ribonucleic acid (RNA), ultrasound (US), and ultraviolet (UV).

NOTE

The YEAR BOOK OF ANESTHESIOLOGY AND PAIN MANAGEMENT™ is a literature survey service providing abstracts of articles published in the professional literature. Every effort is made to ensure the accuracy of the information presented in these pages. Neither the editors nor the publisher of the YEAR BOOK OF ANESTHESIOLOGY AND PAIN MANAGEMENT™ can be responsible for errors in the original materials. The editors' comments are their own opinions. Mention of specific products within this publication does not constitute endorsement.

To facilitate the use of the YEAR BOOK OF ANESTHESIOLOGY AND PAIN MANAGEMENT™ as a reference tool, all illustrations and tables included in this publication are now identified as they appear in the original article. This change is meant to help the reader recognize that any illustration or table appearing in the YEAR BOOK OF ANESTHESIOLOGY AND PAIN MANAGEMENT™ may be only one of many in the original article. For this reason, figure and table numbers will often appear to be out of sequence within the YEAR BOOK OF ANESTHESIOLOGY AND PAIN MANAGEMENT™.

Introduction

It is an honor and a privilege for me to continue my service as Editor-in-Chief of the 2004 YEAR BOOK OF ANESTHESIOLOGY AND PAIN MANAGEMENT.

Last year I identified 2003 as a year of transition for academic departments of anesthesiology. Specifically, I called attention to evidence of renewed academic activity in a number of academic departments of anesthesiology across the country. During the last year, I have been encouraged by the continued growth in the depth and breadth of anesthesia-related scholarly activity. However, while some university departments of anesthesiology are flourishing, others continue to struggle to meet escalating service demands. It is troubling that the leadership of some academic health centers have apparently made a decision to place a singular emphasis on clinical service at the expense of teaching and research.

This edition of the YEAR BOOK again includes a number of studies that focus on the following areas of interest to anesthesiologists: 1) preanesthetic assessment; 2) preanesthetic risk assessment, stratification, and reduction; 3) process and quality improvement; 4) outcomes analysis; and 5) the economics of operating room management and anesthesia care. Of interest, several studies specifically discuss economic and personal health issues for anesthesiologists. As in the past, many of the selected studies focus on the subspecialties of anesthesiology.

Readers will note the addition of 3 new chapters to the 2004 edition of the YEAR BOOK. Specifically, we have added chapters that focus on the following areas of interest to anesthesiologists: 1) geriatric medicine issues; 2) cardiopulmonary resuscitation; and 3) medical education and simulation.

I am grateful for the careful selections and thoughtful commentary provided by my 6 fellow editors. It is a privilege for me to work with such a distinguished group. I am sorry to tell you that this will be the last YEAR BOOK for 3 of these editors. Specifically, Drs John Lang, Mark Trankina, and Margaret Wood have resigned from the Editorial Board so that they can devote more time to other professional and personal responsibilities. Drs Lang and Trankina have each served on the Editorial Board for 3 years, and Dr Wood has served for a decade! I should like to thank each of them for their faithful service. I am pleased to tell you that I have recruited 3 outstanding successors, and I know that you will enjoy reading their selections and comments in the 2005 YEAR BOOK.

I hope that you enjoy reading our selections and accompanying comments as much as we have enjoyed preparing them for you.

David H. Chestnut, MD

1 Studies of Outcomes, Risks, Costs, and Benefits

Comparing Clinical Productivity of Anesthesiology Groups
Abouleish AE, Prough DS, Whitten CW, et al (Univ of Texas, Galveston; Univ of Texas, Dallas; East Texas Anesthesiology Associates; et al)
Anesthesiology 97:608-615, 2002   1–1

Background.—Measurements of the clinical productivity of medical groups have been used in the management of business operations and distribution of compensation through comparison with other groups with similar characteristics. Both academic and private practice anesthesiology groups have an interest in comparing clinical productivity, but most current comparisons rely on "per full-time equivalent (FTE)" measurements. The problem with FTE measurements is that they do not account for differences in staffing ratios (concurrencies) and therefore lead to inaccurate conclusions regarding the clinical productivity of anesthesiology groups.

In addition, there are a number of independent factors that affect clinical productivity, such as the speed of surgery, the type of surgery, and scheduling efficiency. It has been proposed that measurements based on "per operating room site," "per case," and "billed American Society of Anesthesiologists (ASA) units per hour of care" would allow meaningful comparisons of clinical productivity despite differing concurrencies. Whether these measurements would allow meaningful comparisons among multiple groups was investigated.

Methods.—Annual totals of total ASA (tASA) units, 15-minute time units, and the number of cases billed were collected from 11 private practice and 9 academic anesthesiology groups in 12 states. Also collected from these groups were data on the average number of daily anesthetizing sites (OR sites) staffed and the average number of anesthesiologists required to staff the sites. All anesthesia care billed with ASA units was included, with the exception of obstetric care. Clinical services not billed in ASA units were not included in the study. Productivity measurements were calculated, and the median and range for all groups and for private practice and academic groups were determined.

Results.—The productivity measurements that are influenced by duration of surgery were significantly different between the 2 groups. Private practice groups had shorter duration (median, 1.5 hours billed) than the academic groups (median, 2.6 hours billed). The tASA/OR site measurements were similar between groups, but the academic groups worked significantly longer hours billed per OR site per day (median, 6 hours vs 7.8 hours) to obtain the same level of tASA/OR site. There was a significant correlation between the hourly billing productivity and duration of surgery.

Conclusion.—It appears that the alternative method of comparing departmental productivity between anesthesiology groups presented here provides a meaningful comparison. In this study, measurements based on "per OR site," "per case," and "billed ASA units per hour of care," rather than "per FTE" measurements, showed that private practice groups provided care for cases of shorter duration than did academic groups.

▶ This is an extremely important article, in many aspects, as follows: (1) You can compare clinical productivity assessments, (2) You can rate efficiency among providers and the article gives you a technique for doing so, and (3) The billing units correlate strongly with case time; shorter cases are consistently associated with more billing units per time period. The ASA and its members may have to correct our billing unit system. This article would be stronger were it to include a clinical productivity assessment comparison among pain therapy areas, preoperative areas, and ICU areas to see if those could be evaluated.

M. F. Roizen, MD

The Effects of Surgical Case Duration and Type of Surgery on Hourly Clinical Productivity of Anesthesiologists
Abouleish AE, Prough DS, Whitten CW, et al (Univ of Texas, Galveston; Univ of Texas, Dallas)
Anesth Analg 97:833-838, 2003   1–2

Introduction.—The hourly clinical productivity (total ASA units per hour of anesthesia care; tASA/h) for anesthesiology groups is determined by surgical duration (hours per case; h/case) and type of surgery (ASA base units per case; base/case). Previous studies have shown that longer-than-average surgical duration has a negative effect on hourly clinical productivity. Base/case will vary within an individual practice when cases are grouped by the surgeon's primary specialty. The effect of surgical duration and type of surgery on hourly clinical productivity was evaluated when anesthesia care is provided for different surgical services.

Methods.—Data for the year 1999 were collected from the billing database of an academic anesthesiology department. Care performed outside the operating room was excluded, as was any care not billed with ASA units. Items examined included anesthesia codes billed, minutes of anesthesia care, faculty surgeon name, date of procedure, and operating room number. For each service, tASA/h was calculated by dividing the sum of base/case and (4 × h/case) by h/case.

Results.—During the study period, 12,769 cases were performed by 19 different surgical services. The mean base/case was 6.1 U, with a range of 4.0 U for orthopedic services to 16.0 U for cardiothoracic services. The mean h/case was 2.9 hours, with a range of 0.9 hours for otolaryngology/pediatric services to 5.4 hours for orthopedic spine services. The mean tASA/h was 6.35 U/h, with a range of 5.10 U/h for plastic surgery to 9.71 U/h for otolaryngology pediatric services. The top 3 services in terms of tASA/h (otolaryngology pediatric, pain management, and ophthalmology) had the shortest mean surgical duration. Because of longer h/case, services with high base/case did not necessarily have high tASA/h.

Conclusion.—Anesthesiology groups must be able to predict revenue and clinical productivity, and reliance on the base/case of a service to identify which surgical service will optimize billed units is inadequate. Both base/case and surgical duration data must be considered to accurately predict clinical and billing productivity.

▶ If you are in management of a group or think you want to be, this article is must reading. If you don't enjoy reading it, don't accept a leadership role in a group if that role is also responsible for financial performance. This article may be a great article to help differentiate those who might think they want to be involved in management of a group, and those who really want to do it when they know what it entails.

M. F. Roizen, MD

Use of Odds Ratios on Anaesthesia Related Studies
Ho KM, Marshall RJ, Walters S (Univ of Auckland, New Zealand)
Anaesth Intensive Care 31:392-395, 2003   1–3

Introduction.—Odds ratios are increasingly being reported in the anesthetic literature with the use of statistical techniques such as logistic regression and meta-analysis. The odds of an outcome is the number of patients who experience an outcome divided by the number of patients who do not. The odds ratio is the ratio of 2 odds of 2 distinct groups, usually treatment and placebo groups. Relative risk is a ratio of the risk in one group to the risk in another group. The odds ratio is usually a good approximation of relative risk, but it cannot be interpreted as equivalent. The use of odds ratio and its relationship to relative risk and the incidence of outcome were investigated.

Methods.—The OVID MEDLINE database was searched for articles published in 8 anesthetic journals between January 1, 1997 and April 31, 2002. Studies of interest reported odds ratio or "odds" in their abstract or text. Most articles concerned exposures that increased the likelihood of the outcome of interest and reported odds ratios greater than 1.0. Four studies reported odds ratios less than 1.0, indicating a decreased likelihood.

Results.—Eighty-seven original research articles and 60 meta-analyses reported odds or odds ratios. Relative risk could be estimated in 69 research articles (79%), only 2 of which reported relative risks in addition to the odds ratios. The median absolute difference between the reported odds ratios and the estimated relative risks was 1.8. Bias of an odds ratio represents the systematic overestimation or underestimation of the corresponding relative risk if they are interpreted as equivalent, and this is defined as odds ratio/relative risk. Bias increases when the incidence of outcome is high.

Discussion.—Many of the studies reviewed could have estimated relative risk, but few did. In some circumstances, reporting an odds ratio alone without relative risk might misrepresent the magnitude of the treatment effect. Odds ratio is still a valid measure of treatment effect, provided it is not viewed as an approximation or equivalent to relative risk. Relative risk should be reported as well, especially when the incidence of outcome is not rare or when the odds ratio is significantly smaller or larger than 1.

▶ Both odds ratio and risk are terms used to describe probability. The odds of an outcome is the number of patients who experience an outcome divided by the number of patients who do not. Its ratio is the ratio of 2 odds of distinct groups; for example, placebo and a treatment group. The risk of an outcome happening is the number of those who experience an outcome divided by the total number of people at risk.

In a 2 × 2 table of exposure versus nonexposure, and outcome versus nonoutcome, if the outcome positive who are exposed are labeled A, and the outcome negative who are exposed are labeled C, and the outcome (−) who are not exposed are labeled D, then the odds ratio is simply A divided by B over or divided by C divided by D. The relative risk on the other hand is A divided by (A + C), divided by B over (B + D). The odds ratio and the relative risk become close to one another when the outcome (−) groups, both C and D are much greater than the outcome (+) groups A and B.

This is an important article for what it shows and the fact that in many studies, both odds ratio and relative risk should be reported when the outcome-negative groups are not large.

M. F. Roizen, MD

Are Anaesthetists Prone to Suicide? A Review of Rates and Risk Factors
Swanson SP, Roberts LJ, Chapman MD (Sir Charles Gairdner Hosp, Perth, Western Australia)
Anaesth Intensive Care 31:434-445, 2003   1–4

Background.—The literature was reviewed to examine the rate of suicide among anesthesiologists.

Study Design.—The Medline 1966 to 2002 database was searched for English-language publications pertaining to this subject.

Findings.—In the general population of the United States, the reported suicide incidence is 12.3/100,000. Men have a higher rate of completed suicide than women in the general population, but not among physicians. Rates of suicide are higher among physicians than in the general population. Specific data available about the suicide rate of anesthesiologists are limited, but recent evidence suggests that anesthesiologists have a higher suicide rate than other physicians. Their rate of drug-related suicide is even higher, with half of all suicides involving anesthetic agents. Depression is a major risk factor for suicide among physicians, as it is for the general population. Suicidal verbalization and prior suicide attempts are strong risk factors. Substance abuse is also a major risk factor, with physicians more likely to abuse prescription medications. Profession-specific risk factors for suicide include censure by medical boards, medical litigation, and medical board surveillance.

Conclusions.—The prevalence of suicide is low among anesthesiologists. All medical professionals should seek appropriate medical management for depression and suicidal ideation and should not attempt to self-medicate or self-treat. Professionals have a responsibility to assist colleagues, but counseling should be provided by professional counselors. Outright confrontation should be avoided, especially in cases of substance abuse.

▶ This article by Swanson and colleagues is an in-depth article on suicide in anesthesiologists, but really deals with suicide for any physician. It finds that the actual prevalence of suicide among anesthesiologists remains very low; therefore, screening procedures would be difficult and would carry the risk of unacceptably high false-positive rates. Two special characteristics are brought out by the study: (1) that none of us should attempt to counsel a potential suicide victim unless we have expertise in the field and (2) that one-on-one confrontation with someone suspected of abusing drugs is not to be advised and immediate therapy is needed because confrontation carries an unacceptably high risk of suicide in the drug user.

M. F. Roizen, MD

Developing Priority Criteria for General Surgery: Results From the Western Canada Waiting List Project
Taylor MC, and the Steering Committee of the Western Canada Waiting List Project (Univ of Manitoba, Winnipeg, Canada; et al)
Can J Surg 45:351-357, 2002   1–5

Background.—All publicly funded national health services are forced to address the issue of waiting lists for health care services. Waiting lists are a source of public distress and political consternation, mainly because they involve extended suffering; disability; and, on occasion, death for patients on these lists. This situation is further exacerbated by the common public perception that these waiting lists may not be fair. There is increasing evidence that patients' chances of receiving needed services in a timely manner, solely on the basis of clinical urgency, are uncertain.

A recent report used the term "chaotic" to describe the management of waiting lists in Canada, and similar concerns underlie the participation of doctors in New Zealand in development of point-count priority criteria for assessing urgency for a variety of clinical conditions. To address these concerns, the Western Canada Waiting List Project (WCWL) was created as a federally funded partnership of 19 government and health care provider and research organizations. The goal of the WCWL was to develop tools for improving the management of waiting lists.

Methods.—The WCWL general surgery panel was 1 of 5 panels constituted under this project. The panel developed and tested a set of standardized clinical criteria for determining priorities among patients awaiting all types of elective general surgery. These criteria were applied to 561 patients in 3 western provinces of Canada. The set of criteria weights that collectively best predicted clinicians' overall urgency ratings were determined with regression analysis.

Results.—The priority criteria accounted for nearly two thirds of the observed variance in clinicians' urgency ratings for a mixed group of patients. The panel then refined the criteria and weights on the basis of empiric findings and clinical judgment. These revised criteria included a rating of the pain at its worst; the usual intensity of other forms of suffering; the usual frequency of painful episodes or suffering; the degree of impairment in usual activities due to surgical condition; and recent history of major complications or additional significant physical examination or test results. The interrater and test-retest reliability of criteria items appeared to be good on the basis of clinicians' ratings of 6 videotaped, standardized patient interviews.

Conclusion.—The criteria developed by the WCWL were considered to be easy to use and reflective of expert surgical opinion regarding clinical urgency. Further development and testing of the tool are warranted.

▶ Waiting lists for healthcare services are common in all publicly funded national health services. So if we go to that system in the United States, we should be aware of the consequences. But many countries have them and the waiting lists are considered chaotic, often based on the power of the surgeon and the availability he/she has rather than the urgency of the patient condition. This project looks at setting national priorities based on general accepted criteria of urgency that involve intensity of pain, intensity of other forms of suffering, frequency of painful episodes, usual degree of impairment and role functioning, impairment in social functioning, and history of major complications of the condition. Based on these criteria, the panel seems to be able to agree on a rational system for what condition should get priority on waiting lists. I guess my overall comment is I only hope that we can use our resources efficiently enough and motivate people to healthy choices well enough so we can reduce health care cost by the 35% or so that would result, and thereby not have to deal with waiting lists.

M. F. Roizen, MD

Robotics in General Surgery: Personal Experience in a Large Community Hospital

Giulianotti PC, Coratti A, Angelini M, et al (Misericordia Hosp, Grosseto, Italy)
Arch Surg 138:777-784, 2003   1–6

Background.—Few accounts of robot-assisted, minimally invasive surgery are available. This approach is currently limited by restricted movement, inability to perform high-precision sutures, unnatural positions required for the surgeon, and flat vision. Many issues remain to be resolved before it is widely used in a clinical setting. The experience of the Department of General Surgery, Misericordia Hospital, Grosseto, Italy, was reported.

Methods.—The da Vinci Surgical System was used to perform minimally invasive procedures of various types in 193 patients between October 2000 and November 2002.

Results.—The 207 robotic surgical operations included 179 single procedures and 14 double ones in the areas of abdominal, thoracic, and vascular surgery. For cholecystectomy, operative times, once the learning curve was completed, were similar between robotic and laparoscopic procedures; the conversion rates were 3.5% for the robotic procedure and 1.9% for the laparoscopic approach. For fundoplication, mean operative times and conversion rates were comparable between the robotic and laparoscopic procedures. Morbidity rate was 4.8% for robotic and 11.4% for laparoscopic procedures. The robot successfully performed thoracic esophageal dissection in 5 cases of esophagectomy. For subtotal gastrectomy, mean operative times were similar between robotic and open approaches. Morbidity rate was 30.0% for robotic total gastrectomy and mortality rate was 0.0%. Morbidity rate for robotic subtotal gastrectomy was 9.1% and mortality rate was 9.1%. For open procedures, the morbidity rate for total gastrectomy was 12.5% and the mortality rate was 25%; the morbidity rate for subtotal gastrectomy was 7.8% and the mortality rate was 0.0%. Robotic pancreatoduodenectomy required more time than open surgery. For the robotic group, the morbidity and mortality rates were 37.5% and 12.5%, respectively. For the open surgery group, the morbidity and mortality rates were 32.1% and 5.6%, respectively. Other surgeries performed by the robot included hepatobiliary, colorectal, thoracic, adrenal, splenic, gynecologic, and vascular procedures.

Conclusions.—The da Vinci system proved safe, sturdy, and relatively simple to use on a daily basis. Malfunctions were rare. Conversion was required in only 1.0% of cases overall. It took very little time to perform suturing, tie knots, and fully control the robotic functions, but full training in open and laparoscopic surgery is required for advanced procedures. Morbidity and mortality rates and postoperative stays with robotic procedures were similar to those of laparoscopic procedures. The learning curve for major, complex operations could not be evaluated, and the patient benefits could not be measured. Standards must be set for case selection, patient and port positioning, cart installation, and mechanical arm setting on the operating field. The experience reported documents robotic surgery as a feasible, safe, and easily managed option in a large community hospital, but new operative strategies and modifications of the pattern of port placement are also required. Further experience is needed.

▶ This is an interesting but descriptive article on the clinical experience of the da Vinci Surgical System for general surgery. Anesthesiologists in academic teaching hospitals are becoming increasingly familiar with robotic technology and have assisted in the system set-up. This report, however, comes from a community hospital in Italy and shows that in situations outside the university system, the methodology may be effective. However, whether robotic surgery becomes the standard of care remains to be seen in the distant future.

M. Wood, MD, FRCA

Surgical Advancement Influences Perioperative Care: A Comparison of Two Surgical Techniques for Sagittal Craniosynostosis Repair
Ririe DG, David LR, Glazier SS, et al (Wake Forest Univ, Winston-Salem, NC)
Anesth Analg 97:699-703, 2003   1 7

Background.—Although new advances have occurred in craniofacial surgery, the more limited methods used to achieve good cosmetic outcomes have proved less effective than initially believed. Spring-mediated craniofacial reshaping, a 2-stage procedure, was recently reported. A trial of this technique for sagittal synostosis was presented.

Methods and Findings.—The records of 8 children undergoing cranial vault reconstruction (CVR) and 9 undergoing spring-mediated cranial expansion (SME) for sagittal craniosynostosis were reviewed. Anesthesia times for the 2 techniques were comparable, at 4 hours 24 minutes for CVR and at 4 hours 27 minutes for SME (combined time for both procedures). Surgical times were 3 hours 25 minutes and 2 hours 21 minutes, respectively (combined times). The mean length of stay for the CVR group was 4.1 days, and for the SME group, it was 3.1 days. Blood loss was 48 mL in the SME group and 291 mL in the CVR group, a significant difference. All 8 patients undergoing CVR required blood, whereas none of those undergoing SME required it.

Conclusion.—Spring-mediated craniofacial reshaping significantly reduces blood loss and the need for blood transfusion in patients with sagittal craniosynostosis. This reduction, along with decreased invasive monitoring, may negate the theoretical risk of 2 anesthetics.

▶ This is a small study of a new and apparently less invasive treatment for craniosynostosis. A total of only 17 patients were studied. However, as these procedures are relatively uncommon, even in centers with a busy pediatric neurosurgery practice, these small studies are common. SME, which involves 2 procedures, is hoped to have similar long-term results as cranial vault remodeling. The new technique involves inserting springs into the cranium to accomplish the remodeling and then removing them several months later.

From these data, even with requiring 2 procedures, the newer technique is associated with shorter operating room time, less blood loss, and shorter combined hospital stay and ICU time. In addition, invasive monitoring appears to not be indicated for the placement or removal of the springs, while it is considered necessary by most anesthesiologists for CVR procedures. If SME does prove to have similar long-term results to CVR, it is likely to be associated with less morbidity and hospital cost and should, as these authors suggest, alter our anesthetic management of these patients.

S. Black, MD

Retrospective Evaluation of Unanticipated Admissions and Readmissions After Same Day Surgery and Associated Costs

Coley KC, Williams BA, DaPos SV, et al (Univ of Pittsburgh, Pa)
J Clin Anesth 14:349-353, 2002   1–8

Background.—The use of ambulatory surgery in the United States has increased steadily in the last decade. There were an estimated 31.5 million surgical and nonsurgical procedures performed in 20.8 million ambulatory surgery visits in 1996. Currently nearly two thirds (65%) of all surgical procedures are performed in the ambulatory setting. Improvements in technology and cost-containment initiatives have been cited as incentives for this shift toward outpatient care. However, there is increasing concern regarding unanticipated patient morbidity, unplanned hospital visits, admissions after ambulatory surgery, and additional costs in association with ambulatory surgery. The purpose of this study was to determine the rate of unanticipated admissions and readmissions and to characterize the associated reasons and costs.

Methods.—The setting for this retrospective study was a university teaching hospital. The study enrolled any patients undergoing same-day surgery over 12 months. The main outcome measures were all nonelective return visits to the hospital within 30 days and the reason for return.

Results.—A total of 20,817 patients were identified as undergoing same-day surgery at the study institution in 1999. Of these patients, 1195 (5.7%) returned to the hospital within 30 days or were admitted directly after surgery. Of these unanticipated admissions and readmissions, 313 (1.5%) were admissions immediately after the original same-day surgery. The mean age of the patients was 51 years; just over half (52%) were women and most (85%) were white. The most commonly reported reason for return was pain, which was cited by 38% of patients who had an unanticipated return to hospital. The general surgery service had the highest rate of unanticipated admissions or readmissions (3.2%), followed by otolaryngology (3.1%) and urology (2.9%). Of the 120 patients who returned with unanticipated admissions and readmissions for pain, 46 (38%) had orthopedic procedures as their index same-day surgery. The mean charges for patients with unanticipated admissions and readmissions due to pain were $1869 ± $4553 per visit, compared with charges of $12,000 ± $36,866 for non–pain-related admissions.

Conclusion.—About 1.5% of patients undergoing ambulatory surgery returned within 30 days due to problems directly related to the original surgical procedure. Pain was the reason for more than one third of these return visits, which involved significant costs. It would appear prudent to focus not only on pain in the hospital during ambulatory surgery but also on anticipation of pain-related issues after surgery.

▶ This study cites the relatively high importance of pain therapy and pain education if patients are to avoid readmission. This is an excellent retrospective review and one of the best in its completeness and variety of same-day surgery patients evaluated.

M. F. Roizen, MD

Impact of Hospital-Related Factors on Outcome After Treatment of Cerebral Aneurysms
Berman MF, Solomon RA, Mayer SA, et al (Columbia Univ, New York; Univ of California, San Francisco)
Stroke 34:2200-2207, 2003
1–9

Background.—Authorities continue to debate the effects of hospital volume and surgical experience on cerebral aneurysm outcomes. The mortality

TABLE 1.—Demographics and Form of Presentation at First Admission for Treatment

		By Diagnosis	
	All Admissions, n	Unruptured Aneurysms	Subarachnoid Hemorrhage
Admissions, n	5963	2200 (36.9)	3763 (63.1)
Unique patients, n	5598	2010	3588
Mean age, y	52.4 ± 13.6	52.5 ± 13.0	52.4 ± 13.9
Female, n (%)	3940 (70.4)	1474 (73.3)	2466 (68.7)‡
Race-ethnicity, n (%)			
Caucasian (67.9)*	3153 (62.5)§	1229 (69.3)	1924 (58.8)§
Black (15.9)*	935 (18.5)§	247 (13.9)	688 (21.0)§
Asian (5.6)*	106 (2.1)§	24 (1.4)	82 (2.5)†
Other (10.6)*	851 (16.9)§	273 (15.4)	578 (17.7)†
Unknown...	553	237	316
Hispanic (15.1)*	489 (10.7)§	165 (10.1)	324 (11.1)
Non-Hispanic (84.9)*	4081 (89.3)	1474 (89.9)	2607 (88.9)
Unknown ethnicity	1028	371	657

Note: Data are N (%) or mean ± standard deviation as appropriate. Demographic composition of patients at first presentation for treatment of cerebral aneurysm (clipping, wrapping, or endovascular therapy). Racial and ethnic composition of all admissions at first presentation varied significantly from what would be predicted from census data. Form of presentation (unruptured vs ruptured) also varied significantly with sex and race. Patients with unknown race or ethnicity were not included in corresponding analysis.
*Percentage of New York State population.
†$P < .05$.
‡$P < .001$.
§$P < .0001$.
(Courtesy of Berman MF, Solomon RA, Mayer SA, et al: Impact of hospital-related factors on outcome after treatment of cerebral aneurysms. *Stroke* 34:2200-2207, 2003. Reproduced with permission of *Stroke.* Copyright 2003 American Heart Association.)

TABLE 2.—Overall Outcome After Clipping or Endovascular Therapy for Treatment of Cerebral Aneurysm

	All Admissions (Including Unruptured Aneurysms With Prior SAH)	By Diagnosis	
		Unruptured Aneurysms (Excluding Unruptured Aneurysms With Prior SAH)	SAH
Admissions, n (%)	5656	1792 (31.7)	3645 (64.4)
Procedures (clipping or endovascular therapy), n (%)	5687	1796 (31.6)	3672 (64.6)
Adverse outcomes, n (%)	2509 (44.4)	382 (21.3)	2087 (57.3)*
In-hospital deaths, n (%)	559 (9.9)	44 (2.5)	511 (14.0)*
Admissions involving endovascular therapy, n (%)	739 (13.1)	361 (20.1)	331 (9.1)*
Length of stay (95% CI), d	12.6 (12.3-12.9)	6.2 (6.0-6.5)	19.9 (19.4-20.4)*
Total hospital charges (95% CI), $	45 000 (44 000-46 100)	24 800 (24 000-25 600)	66 300 (64 700-68 000)*

Note: Differences in outcome for treatment of unruptured versus ruptured aneurysms. Statistical comparisons are between patients with subarachnoid hemorrhage (SAH) and patients with unruptured aneurysms without prior SAH.

*P < .0001.

(Courtesy of Berman MF, Solomon RA, Mayer SA, et al: Impact of hospital-related factors on outcome after treatment of cerebral aneurysms. *Stroke* 34:2200-2207, 2003. Reproduced with permission of *Stroke.* Copyright 2003 American Heart Association.)

TABLE 3. Effect of Hospital-Related Variables on Outcome and Resource Utilization

	Unruptured Aneurysms			Ruptured Aneurysms		
	OR	95% CI	P	OR	95% CI	P
Adverse outcome						
Procedural experience	0.89	0.84-0.94	<0.0001	0.94	0.89-0.99	0.03
Percent embolization	0.83	0.71-0.98	0.026			
In-hospital death						
Procedural experience	0.94	0.90-0.98	0.002	0.95	0.92-0.98	0.005
Length of stay (reduction)						
Procedural experience	0.95	0.94-0.96	<0.0001			
Percent embolization	0.93	0.90-0.96	<0.0001			
Total charges (increase in overall charges)						
Percent embolization				1.07	1.01-1.15	0.034
Neurosurgical residency				1.26	1.06-1.50	0.009

Note: Table shows multivariate analysis combining hospital related variables. Model was corrected for age, sex, race, and ethnicity. Only variables achieving statistical significance were retained in the final model. Effects of procedural experience are expressed in terms of each additional 10 cases performed per year; effect of embolization is expressed per additional 10% cases done by embolization.

(Courtesy of Berman MF, Solomon RA, Mayer SA, et al: Impact of hospital-related factors on outcome after treatment of cerebral aneurysms. *Stroke* 34:2200-2207, 2003. Reproduced with permission of *Stroke*. Copyright 2003 American Heart Association.)

and morbidity after treatment of cerebral aneurysms were investigated with the use of New York State discharge data.

Methods.—All discharges of patients with a principal diagnosis of subarachnoid hemorrhage (SAH) or unruptured cerebral aneurysm (UCA) in New York State from 1995 through 2000 were identified (Table 1). Data on 2200 admissions for attempted treatment of UCA and on 3763 admissions for attempted treatment of SAH were analyzed. Treatment consisted of aneurysm clipping, wrapping, or endovascular coiling. In-hospital death or discharge to a rehabilitation or long-term care facility was considered an adverse outcome.

Findings.—Half of all procedures were performed at the 10 highest volume hospitals. Overall, hospital volume correlated with fewer adverse out-

TABLE 5.—Potentially Avoidable Deaths and Adverse Outcomes Per Year

Treated at Low Volume Hospitals, n/Total (%)	Unruptured Aneurysms		Ruptured Aneurysms	
	716/1792 (40)		2093/3645 (57)	
	Adverse Outcome	In-Hospital Deaths	Adverse Outcome	In-Hospital Deaths
Observed poor outcomes	64	7	348	85
Estimated poor outcomes with selective referral to high-volume hospitals	51 (47-56)	6 (6-7)	306 (274-343)	76 (70-82)
Potential Improvement in aggregate outcome	13 (8-17)	1 (CI 0-1)	41 (5-74)	9 (4-15)
Improvement, %	20	11	12	11

Note: Data are n (95% confidence interval). Table shows theoretically avoidable adverse outcomes and in-hospital deaths resulting from selective transfer of all patients with cerebral aneurysms to high-volume hospitals for curative treatment. Because of rounding, estimated poor outcome and potential improvement do not always sum to observed poor outcome.

(Courtesy of Berman MF, Solomon RA, Mayer SA, et al: Impact of hospital-related factors on outcome after treatment of cerebral aneurysms. *Stroke* 34:2200-2207, 2003. Reproduced with permission of *Stroke*. Copyright 2003 American Heart Association.)

comes and lower in-hospital mortality among patients with UCA or SAH. The use of endovascular treatment correlated with fewer adverse outcomes after treatment of unruptured aneurysms (Table 2). The effect of hospital volume on outcome was more pronounced after aneurysm clipping than after endovascular therapy (Table 3).

Conclusion.—Both hospital volume and the use of endovascular therapy are associated independently with better outcomes in patients with UCA and SAH (Table 5). A program of regionalization and selective referral for cerebral aneurysm treatment may improve outcomes in this patient population.

▶ These authors present compelling data regarding regionalization of health care for patients with intracranial aneurysms. They have reviewed 6 years of discharge data from all hospitals in New York State and their findings are consistent. Both for ruptured and unruptured aneurysms, adverse outcome and in-hospital mortality are decreased with increasing volume of patients treated either surgically or with endovascular techniques. Small increases in volume—in increments of 10 cases per year—are associated with statistically significant improvement in outcomes. This is more dramatic in treatment of unruptured aneurysms as compared to ruptured aneurysms.

The authors predict a decrease in adverse outcome of 20% and in-hospital mortality of 11% if all patients with unruptured aneurysms were treated in high-volume centers. For ruptured aneurysms, the decrease in adverse outcomes (12%) is more modest, with a similar decrease in hospital mortality. Many clinical trials of new therapies have failed to show such a dramatic improvement.

The authors point out that regionalization is difficult for many reasons and could potentially have an adverse impact by overwhelming the resources in the high-volume centers. However, it is an option to improve patient outcome that must be seriously considered. One would expect that even if the resources of high-volume centers were originally taxed with regionalization, it would result in further expansion of those resources and potentially further improvements in care.

S. Black, MD

Educational Levels of Hospital Nurses and Surgical Patient Mortality
Aiken LH, Clarke SP, Cheung RB, et al (Univ of Pennsylvania, Philadelphia; Children's Hosp of Philadelphia)
JAMA 290:1617-1623, 2003   1–10

Background.—Both the United States public and physicians cite nurse understaffing as one of the most significant threats to patient safety in hospitals. Education in nursing is obtained in 3-year diploma programs in hospitals, associate degree nursing programs in community colleges, and baccalaureate nursing programs in colleges and universities. By 2001, 36% of nurses came from the baccalaureate programs, 61% from associate degree programs, and only 3% from hospital diploma programs. The relation between the educational composition of a hospital's registered nurse (RN) staff and patient outcomes was examined, along with any predictive function education holds for patient mortality rates.

Methods.—To determine if the proportion of hospital RNs educated at the baccalaureate level or higher influences the risk-adjusted mortality and failure to rescue (death occurring in surgical patients with serious complications) rates, cross-sectional analyses of outcomes data were performed. Included were 232,342 patients who had general, orthopedic, or vascular surgery and were discharged from 168 nonfederal adult general Pennsylvania hospitals. The data from these cases were linked to administrative and survey information on educational composition, staffing, and other aspects of the hospitals. The 30-day risk-adjusted patient mortality and failure to rescue data were correlated with the educational levels of nursing staff.

Results.—A strong association was found between the educational composition of hospitals and other hospital characteristics, such as nurse workloads. Hospitals with higher percentages of nurses with baccalaureate or master's degrees were generally larger and had postgraduate medical training programs and high-technology facilities. In addition, these hospitals tended to have slightly less experienced nurses and significantly lower mean workloads. A statistically significant association was found between the proportion of nurses in a hospital who had bachelor's and master's degrees and the risks of death and failure to rescue before and after controlling for hospital and patient factors. A 10% increase in the proportion of nurses with higher degrees resulted in a diminished risk of death and failure to rescue by a factor of 0.95, or 5%. As a result, the odds of death and failure to rescue within 30 days of admission would be 19% lower in hospitals where 60% of the nurses held baccalaureate or higher degrees than in hospitals where this was true for only 20% of the nurses. Years of experience in nursing did not significantly predict death or failure to rescue.

Conclusions.—Patient outcomes are improved in hospitals where the majority of nurses have baccalaureate or higher degrees in nursing. Surgical patients, including those with significant complications, cared for in such hospitals have a substantial survival advantage over those receiving care in hospitals where fewer nurses have these more advanced degrees.

▶ Hospital inpatient mortality rate is very important to both individual physicians, patients, and hospital administrators in not only making personal decisions about choosing a hospital, but also for insurance companies in negotiating managed care contracts with hospital administrators. The data in this manuscript may not be surprising but have very important implications for critical care policies in the future.

M. Wood, MD, FRCA

Alpha-2 Adrenergic Agonists to Prevent Perioperative Cardiovascular Complications: A Meta-Analysis
Wijeysundera DN, Naik JS, Beattie S (Univ of Toronto; Univ Health Network, Toronto)
Am J Med 114:742-752, 2003   1–11

Background.—The surgical stress response is important in the pathogenesis of cardiovascular complications after cardiac and noncardiac surgery. The $\alpha_2$adrenergic agonists currently used, such as clonidine, dexmedetomidine, and mivazerol, attenuate this stress response, which may decrease cardiovascular complications. The effects of $\alpha_2$adrenergic agonists on perioperative mortality rate and cardiovascular complications were studied in a meta-analysis.

Methods.—The literature search included MEDLINE, EMBASE, the Cochrane Clinical Trials Register, the Science Citation Index, and the bibliographies of articles selected. There was no language restriction. The 23 trials included were randomized, controlled studies of preoperative, intraoperative, or postoperative administration of clonidine, dexmedetomidine, or mivazerol that reported death, myocardial infarction, ischemia, or supraventicular tachyarrhythmia. A total of 3395 patients were enrolled. The fixed-effects model was used to determine treatment effects.

Findings.—Overall, the use of $\alpha_2$adrenergic agonists significantly decreased mortality rate and ischemia. During vascular surgery, mortality rate and myocardial infarction were reduced. The use of $\alpha_2$adrenergic agonists during cardiac surgery decreased ischemia and correlated with a trend toward lower mortality rate and risk of myocardial infarction.

Conclusions.—This meta-analysis suggests that the use of $\alpha_2$adrenergic agonists decreases mortality rate and myocardial infarction after vascular surgery. These agents appear to decrease ischemia during cardiac surgery and may also affect mortality rate and myocardial infarction.

▶ Beta-adrenergic blocking drug administration during the perioperative period reduces morbidity but is infrequently used. This meta-analysis shows that α_2-adrenergic agonists may also prevent cardiovascular complications. The meta-analysis used here suffers from many problems, including publication bias whereby positive studies are much more likely to be published than negative studies. Although meta-analysis certainly provides useful information on which to base future studies and raise novel hypotheses, it should not be regarded as a substitute for correctly powered randomized trials.

M. Wood, MD, FRCA

Correlation of Thrombophilia and Hypofibrinolysis With Pulmonary Embolism Following Total Hip Arthroplasty: An Analysis of Genetic Factors
Westrich GH, Weksler BB, Glueck CJ, et al (Hosp for Special Surgery, New York; New York Presbyterian Hosp; Molecular Diagnostics Lab, Cincinnati, Ohio)
J Bone Joint Surg Am 84-A:2161-2167, 2002   1–12

Introduction.—The increased thromboembolic risk linked with total hip arthroplasty (THA) is multifactorial. Advances in both surgical and anesthetic methods, along with improved understanding of the pathogenesis and prevention of thromboembolic disease, have markedly decreased the prevalence of pulmonary embolism (PE) after THA.

Several inherited deficiencies or dysfunctional mutations in proteins of the clotting cascade have recently been determined to increase thrombolic risk. Combinations of these genetic factors with one another or with traditional risk factors multiply, not add to, the net risk of thromboembolism. The prevalence of abnormalities identified by new molecular and functional screening tests for thrombophilia and hypofibrinolysis was assessed to ascertain whether it was higher patients in whom a PE had developed after THA without thromboembolic complications.

TABLE 1.—Frequency of Thrombophilic Abnormalities in the Pulmonary Embolism and Control Groups

| | Group | | |
| | Pulmonary | | *P* |
Thrombophilic Abnormality	Embolism	Control	Value*
Prothrombin G20210A mutation (heterozygous and homozygous)†	4/14	0/14	0.05
Mean no. of thrombophilic genes	1.71	1.07	0.05
Subject had ≥2 of the following†	10/14	5/14	0.06
Plasminogen activator inhibitor-1 4G/4G mutation (homozygous)			
Prothrombin G20210A mutation (heterozygous and homozygous)			
Platelet glycoprotein IIb/IIIa A1/A2 or A2/A2 mutation			
Methylenetetrahydrofolate reductase C677T mutation (homozygous)			
Antithrombin-III level <70% of normal			
Homocysteine level ≥13.5 µmol/L			
Fibrinogen level >400 mg/dL (>11.76 µmol/L)			
Protein-C level <65% of normal			
Subject had ≥1 of the following†	7/14	0/14	<0.01
Antithrombin-III <70% of normal			
Prothrombin G20210A mutation (heterozygous and homozygous)			

*As determined with the 1-sided Fisher test. In contrast to the significant factors listed in the table, there was no significant difference between groups with regard to the prevalence of subjects with a protein-S level of less than 60% of normal, protein-C level of less than 65% of normal, and antithrombin-III level of less than 70% of normal, abnormal dilute Russel viper venom time, factor-V Leiden (heterozygous or homozygous), activated protein-C resistance, platelet glycoprotein IIb/IIIa A1/A2 or A2/A2 mutation, plasminogen activator inhibitor-1 4G/4G mutation, methylenetetrahydrofolate reductase CG77T mutation (homozygous), a homocysteine level of 13/5 µmol/L or greater, or a fibrinogen level of more than 400 mg/dL (more than 11.76 µmol/L) (P < .05).

†The values are give as the number of subjects with the factor/the number of subjects tested in the group.

(Republished with permission of the Journal of Bone and Joint Surgery, Inc. Westrich GH, Weksler BB, Glueck CJ, et al: Correlation of thrombophilia and hypofibrinolysis with pulmonary embolism following total hip arthroplasty: An analysis of genetic factors. *J Bone Joint Surg Am* 84-A:2161-2167, 2002. Reproduced by permission of the publisher via Copyright Clearance Center, Inc.)

Methods.—Fourteen patients with documented PE after THA and 14 matched control subjects who had undergone THA without any clinical indications of thromboembolism were assessed for risks of thrombophilia and hypofibrinolysis. Functional tests of hemostasis were performed that included testing of prothrombin time; activated partial thromboplastin time; levels of fibrinogen, serum homocysteine, protein-C, protein-S, and antithrombin-III; activated protein-C resistance; and dilute Russel viper venom time. Molecular genetic testing was conducted for factor-V Leiden, prothrombin promoter G20210A, methylenetetrahydrofolate reductase C677T, plasminogen activator inhibitor-1 4G/4G, and platelet glycoprotein IIb/IIIa A1/A2 or A2/A2 mutations.

Results.—The total number of genetic thrombophilic abnormalities was higher in the PE group (24 abnormalities) than in the control subjects (15 abnormalities; $P = .05$). Only patients with PE had heterozygosity or homozygosity for the prothrombin G20210A mutation (4/14 patients; $P = .05$) and a reduced antithrombin-III level (3/14 patients; $P = .10$) versus control subjects. Patients with PE were more likely than control subjects to have a minimum of 1 thrombophilic abnormality (7/14 patients with PE had a low antithrombin-III level or the prothrombin G20210A gene mutation versus 0/14 in control subjects; $P < .01$) (Table 1). The presence of the prothrombin G20210A gene mutation was significantly associated with PE ($r = 0.41$; $P = .03$), as was the presence of at least 1 abnormality (a low antithrombin-

TABLE 2.—Simple Correlations Between Risk Factors and Development of Pulmonary Embolism

Risk Factor	No. of Subjects Tested	Correlation*	P Value†
Antithrombin-III level <70% of normal	27	0.37	0.06
Prothrombin G20210A mutation (heterozygous and homozygous)	28	0.41	0.03
Antithrombin-III level <70% of normal and/or prothrombin G20210A mutation (heterozygous and homozygous)	28	0.58	<0.01
Prothrombin G20210A mutation and/or plasminogen activator inhibitor-1 4G/4G mutation (homozygous)	28	0.45	0.02
Antithrombin-III level <70% of normal and/or prothrombin G20210A mutation and/or plasminogen activator inhibitor-1 4G/4G mutation (homozygous)	28	0.53	<0.01

*Pulmonary embolus = 1, no pulmonary embolus = 0, abnormal = 1, and normal = 0.
†In contrast to the significant correlations listed in the table, there was no significant correlation between the development of pulmonary embolism and the presence of plasminogen activator inhibitor-1, 4G/4G mutation, platelet glycoprotein IIb/IIIa (A2/A2) mutation, methylenetetrahydrofolate reductase C677T mutation (homozygous), a homocysteine level of 13.5 μmol/L or greater, a body-mass index of 30 kg/m^2 or greater, activated protein-C resistance, a fibrinogen level of more than 400 mg/dL (more than 11.76 μmol/L), a protein-C level of less than 65% of normal, a protein-S level of less than 60% of normal, or an antithrombin-III level of less than 70% of normal, and/or the presence of plasminogen activator inhibitor-1 4G/4G mutation ($P > .05$).

(Republished with permission of the Journal of Bone and Joint Surgery, Inc. Westrich GH, Weksler BB, Glueck CJ, et al: Correlation of thrombophilia and hypofibrinolysis with pulmonary embolism following total hip arthroplasty: An analysis of genetic factors. *J Bone Joint Surg Am* 84-A:2161-2167, 2002. Reproduced by permission of the publisher via Copyright Clearance Center, Inc.)

III level or the presence of the prothrombin G20210A gene mutation) ($r =$ 0.58; $P = .001$) (Table 2).

Conclusion.—Genetic thrombophilia and hypofibrinolysis were more common in patients who had PE after THA than in those who did not have these abnormalities. The presence of multiple genetic thrombophilic polymorphisms, especially prothrombin G20210A and antithrombin-III rather than any single genetic prothrombotic abnormality, seems to signal an increased thromboembolic risk in patients undergoing THA.

▶ Polymorphisms are frequently being recognized as affecting clinical outcome, eg, β-receptor polymorphism and mortality in cardiac failure. This report demonstrates that genetic factors may affect surgical outcome. If simple blood tests can be used as predictors of outcome in surgery, not only mortality but also morbidity, more aggressive perioperative management may be instituted in certain patients.

M. Wood, MD, FRCA

Urgent Adenotonsillectomy. An Analysis of Risk Factors Associated With Postoperative Respiratory Morbidity
Brown KA, Morin I, Hickey C, et al (McGill Univ, Montreal)
Anesthesiology 99:586-595, 2003   1–13

Background.—In 1999, overnight oximetry performed at home or in the hospital was used to screen children suspected of having obstructive sleep apnea syndrome (OSAS). As a result, more children had urgent adenotonsillectomy performed during the hospital stay. Diagnosing OSAS raised the risk for postoperative respiratory morbidity from about 1% to 20%, and respiratory complications were excessive. The frequency and type of respiratory complications after urgent adenotonsillectomy were compared with those of children having a sleep study and adenotonsillectomy for OSAS. Risk factors predicting respiratory complications were noted.

Methods.—The study group included 43 boys and 11 girls; the mean age was 4.0 years and the mean weight 22.4 kg. Laboratory criteria for OSAS were met by 51 children; 31 had severe OSAS defined by an arterial oxygen saturation (SaO_2) nadir under 80%. Tests to establish OSAS included polysomnography in the sleep laboratory, cardiorespiratory sleep studies at home, overnight oximetry in the home or the hospital, and/or awake capillary carbon dioxide tension.

Retrospective chart review provided data on preoperative status (including evaluation for OSAS), anesthetic management, and postoperative respiratory interventions. Routinely, children are extubated awake in the operating room and transported to the postoperative unit in lateral decubitus position. Oxygen is given by face mask attached to a Jackson Rees circuit close to the child's face immediately after surgery. Morphine is given until the patient can tolerate oral codeine, and oximetry is performed the first night postoperatively.

Respiratory complications noted were desaturation and airway obstruction. Children were divided into those requiring postoperative medical interventions for respiratory complications and those not requiring it. Minor interventions included oxygen therapy beyond the usual period and/or repositioning. Major interventions required physician assessment, included giving racemic epinephrine, Ventolin, or Lasix; airway instrumentation with an oropharyngeal or nasopharyngeal airway or endotracheal tube; and ventilation. Both types were documented.

Results.—There was a median of 2 days between sleep study and surgery for the study group. All fasted before surgery and none received rapid-sequence induction. Sevoflurane was used for 21 patients and halothane for 2; 93% received propofol during induction and 27 had a muscle relaxant. Isoflurane was used for maintenance in all cases, and 98% received an opioid. Intraoperative dexamethasone was used for 13 children. Eight were admitted to the pediatric ICU and 47 to the postanesthesia care unit. Medical intervention was needed by 26 children who had postoperative opioids.

The 75 control children had positive sleep study findings and were hospitalized the night after surgery. The control group's preoperative SaO_2 nadir was 86.0%; 7 had a nadir under 80%. Children with a nadir under 80% had surgery a median of 4 days after the sleep study, but the median for control subjects was 60 days. Sevoflurane was used for 35 children, halothane for 2, and an unknown for 12. Propofol was given to 93% of control subjects, 22% had muscle relaxants, and all were given intraoperative opioids.

More study group children had co-morbid conditions (45.5% vs 13.6%) and had more severe disease compared with the control group. Sixty percent of the study group required medical interventions, with 49% performed in the first hour postoperatively; one third had multiple desaturation episodes. Five children developed pneumonia. Radiographs showed evidence of bilateral infiltrates consistent with pulmonary aspiration in one patient. Twenty-two children needed minor medical interventions; all had postoperative oxygen desaturation within 5.8 hours of postoperative unit admission. Eleven needed major medical interventions, with 7 receiving racemic epinephrine and 6 receiving tracheal reintubation. Major medical interventions were made for all children with preoperative hypercarbia.

Three control group children needed medical intervention during emergence from anesthesia and 16 needed such intervention postoperatively; 13 interventions were minor and 3 major. Risk factors for postadenotonsillectomy respiratory morbidity included associated medical conditions, an SaO_2 nadir of less than 80%, and the requirement for intraoperative dexamethasone.

Conclusion.—Major respiratory events occurred after urgent adenotonsillectomy in 20.3% of the study group and 6.1% of the control subjects. The difference in OSAS severity between the groups does not allow direct comparison, but the impression that the complication rate in the study group was excessive was confirmed. Postoperative reintubation was required in 11.1% of the children and postoperative pneumonia developed in 9.3%. Some respiratory complications did not occur until over 8 hours postoperatively. Those requiring minor interventions tended to have episodic, repeated desaturation, while those requiring major interventions showed worsening airway obstruction from their admission to the postoperative unit. When a co-morbid condition was present, the odds ratio for a medical intervention was 8.15%.

Most children who had major complications had no co-morbidity or asthma. Severity of OSAS was an independent risk factor. The 2-day interval between the sleep test and surgery may have been insufficient for optimal preoperative preparation. Aggressive preoperative preparation (administration of antibiotics, bronchodilators, and oral or nasal steroids) might decrease postsurgical respiratory morbidity.

▶ In a retrospective review of pediatric patients undergoing adenotonsillectomies, the authors have identified a group at high risk for postoperative respiratory complications requiring significant interventions. This group consists of patients being evaluated for OSAS felt to need urgent adenotonsillectomy. Often the indication for urgent tonsillectomy was severe nocturnal hypoxemia (<80% Sao$_2$).

The patients undergoing urgent tonsillectomy had a respiratory complication requiring intervention 60% of the time. Twenty percent of the patients required a major intervention such as intubation or racemic epinephrine administration and 40% more minor interventions. The patients undergoing elective adenotonsillectomy for OSAS had a respiratory complication rate of 36%, with only 7% requiring major intervention. Some of this difference is likely due to the greater percentage of patients requiring urgent surgery with severe OSAS as compared to those having elective surgery. However, as the authors suggested, the lack of time for optimal preoperative preparation may also play a role.

These patients—both children with OSAS undergoing adenotonsillectomy and those requiring urgent surgery—have relatively high rates of respiratory complications, only half or less occurring in the early postoperative period. These patients clearly require hospital admission postoperatively and careful monitoring throughout the day and evening of surgery.

S. Black, MD

Pulmonary Hypertension as a Risk Factor for Death in Patients With Sickle Cell Disease

Gladwin MT, Sachdev V, Jison ML, et al (NIH, Bethesda, Md; Howard Univ, Washington, DC)
N Engl J Med 350:886-895, 2004   1–14

Background.—Pulmonary hypertension is a sequela of most forms of hereditary and chronic hemolytic anemia, including sickle cell disease, and retrospective studies have suggested a prevalence of pulmonary hypertension of 20% to 40% in patients with sickle cell disease. There may be a relation between frequent reports of sudden death in adults with sickle cell disease in the absence of coronary artery disease and the high risk of sudden death in patients with sickle cell disease and pulmonary hypertension. However, the prevalence of pulmonary hypertension in adults with sickle cell disease, the mechanism of development, and the possible prognostic significance of this association are unknown. Pulmonary hypertension as a risk factor for death in patients with sickle cell disease was characterized.

Methods.—Doppler echocardiographic assessments of pulmonary-artery systolic pressure were performed in 195 consecutive patients, including 82 men and 113 women with a mean age of 26 ± 12 years. Pulmonary hypertension was prospectively defined as a tricuspid regurgitant jet velocity of at least 2.5 m/s. The mean duration of follow-up was 18 months, and data were censored at the time of death or if a patient was lost to follow-up.

Results.—Doppler-defined pulmonary hypertension was identified in 32% of patients. With multiple logistic regression analysis with a tricuspid regurgitant jet velocity of less than 2.5 m/s or 2.5 m/s or more as a dichotomous variable, it was found that a self-reported history of cardiovascular or renal complications, increased systolic blood pressure, high lactate dehydrogenase levels, high levels of alkaline phosphatase, and low transferrin levels were significant independent correlates of pulmonary hypertension. Fetal hemoglobin level, white cell count, and platelet count and the use of hydroxyurea therapy were found to be unrelated to pulmonary hypertension. There was a strong association between an increased risk of death and a tricuspid regurgitant jet velocity of at least 2.5 m/s compared with a velocity of less than 2.5 m/s. This association persisted on a proportional hazards regression model after adjustment for other possible risk factors.

Conclusions.—Pulmonary hypertension identified by Doppler echocardiography is a common finding in adult patients with sickle cell disease. Pulmonary hypertension in these patients would appear to be a complication of chronic hemolysis that is resistant to hydroxyurea therapy and is associated with a high risk of death. These findings support the need for therapeutic trials focusing on this population.

▶ Pulmonary hypertension, which was prospectively defined as a tricuspid regurgitant jet velocity of at least 2.5 m/s as measured during transthoracic echocardiography, occurred in 32% of patients. These numbers were confirmed in about half of the study patients with right heart catheterization. Based on multiple logistic regression analysis, independent correlates of pulmonary hypertension were a self-reported history of cardiovascular or renal complications, increased systolic blood pressure, high lactate dehydrogenase levels (a marker of hemolysis), high levels of alkaline phosphatase, and low transferrin levels. Fetal hemoglobin level, white blood cell count, platelet count, and the use of hydroxyurea therapy were not significant predictors of pulmonary hypertension.

Compared with a tricuspid regurgitant jet velocity of less than 2.5 m/s, a tricuspid regurgitant jet velocity of at least 2.5 m/s was associated with an increased risk of death. Adjustment for other possible risk factors in a proportional hazards regression model did not affect this association.

Pulmonary hypertension appears to be common in adults with sickle cell disease and is associated with a poor outcome. Therapeutic trials of oxygen, warfarin, transfusion, and pulmonary vasodilator and remodeling medications are urgently required to evaluate their potential to decrease the substantial morbidity and mortality rates associated with pulmonary hypertension in this population. We as anesthesiologists need to factor in this additional potential risk when providing anesthesia for these patients. This does not mean that all patients with sickle cell disease need a preoperative echocardiogram, but the preoperative plan must factor in the potential presence of what appears to be a common problem for these patients. Even more disturbing is how poorly the sickle cell patients with pulmonary hypertension do over time. This suggests that increased vigilance is necessary during the perioperative period with these patients.

M. F. Trankina, MD

Quality of Reporting of Randomised Controlled Trials in the Intensive Care Literature: A Systematic Analysis of Papers Published in *Intensive Care Medicine* Over 26 Years

Latronico N, Botteri M, Minelli C, et al (Univ of Brescia, Italy; Centro per lo Studio dello Malattie Rare Alda e Cele Dacco, Villa Camozzi, Italy)
Intensive Care Med 28:1316-1323, 2002   1–15

Background.—Evidence-based medicine may be defined as the systematic collection, analysis, synthesis, and application of the best clinical evidence for the integration of individual clinical expertise. One of the highest levels of evidence for evaluation of the efficacy of health care interventions is the randomized, controlled trial (RCT). RCTs are usually used by clinicians as a guide to daily practice. However, these trials are of value only if they are rigorously designed and performed and completely reported. Unclear or incomplete reporting of data makes it difficult to interpret RCTs and may jeopardize an otherwise well planned and conducted trial. The number and quality of the reporting of RCTs published in *Intensive Care Medicine* was assessed.

Methods.—Systematic analysis was used to evaluate RCTs published in *Intensive Care Medicine* from its inception to December 2000 as identified by a search of the MEDLINE database and the authors' research. The Jadad scale and individual assessment of key methodologic components—specifically the randomization process, blinding, and reporting and handling of loss to follow-up—were used to evaluate the quality of reporting. Included in the analysis were data regarding the design characteristics of and analytical approach to the study.

Results.—A total of 173 RCTs, of which 63% were derived from European countries, were included in the analysis. Of these, 44 (25.4%) RCTs were adequately reported, according to a Jadad scale score of more than 2. Analysis of individual methodologic components showed a variable percentage of adequate reporting, ranging from 3.5% for randomization to 10.4% for blinding and to 49.1% for loss to follow-up. The sample sizes were small, with a median of 30 patients, and rationale for its estimation was reported in 7.5%. However, 81.5% of RCTs reported statistically significant results, a finding that suggests that the treatment effects were strong or that a publication bias existed or that the uncertainty principle was not fulfilled.

Conclusion.—Randomized, controlled trials represent the best evidence for the efficacy of medical interventions, but only when high standards of transparent reporting are used. Rigorous attention to the methodologic quality of reporting and adherence to recently published guidelines (CONSORT II) may facilitate transparent reporting in randomized controlled trials.

▶ This is a very thorough assessment of the RCTs published in *Intensive Care Medicine*, a solid journal that is sponsored by the European Society of Intensive Care Medicine. It is based on the CONSORT statement[1]—a system developed by scientists and editors to improve the quality of reporting of RCTs— that more attention should be paid to study design and reporting. Fascinating was that out of 173 RCTs published since the journals inception, only 13 had the patient and physician blinded. The good news is that the frequency of RCTs is on the rise. With respect to the clinical evidence, one must give credit to specialties, such as *Cardiology*, as they have been leaders in areas conducting RCTs and outcome measures.

J. D. Lang, Jr, MD

Reference

1. Altman DG, et al: The revised CONSORT statement for reporting randomized trials: Explanation and elaboration. *Ann Int Med* 134:663-694, 2001.

One-Year Outcomes in Survivors of the Acute Respiratory Distress Syndrome
Herridge MS, for the Canadian Critical Care Trials Group (University Health Network, Toronto; et al)
N Engl J Med 348:683-693, 2003   1–16

Background.—The acute respiratory distress syndrome (ARDS) is characterized by bilateral pulmonary infiltrates on frontal chest radiography, a ratio of arterial oxygen tension to the fraction of inspired oxygen of 200 or less, and the absence of clinical evidence of left atrial hypertension. Improved survival rates among patients with ARDS have heightened the need for an understanding of the long-term effects of this condition and its treatment. Long-term pulmonary and extrapulmonary function were characterized in a prospectively identified cohort of patients who survived ARDS.

Methods.—A total of 109 survivors of ARDS were evaluated at 3, 6, and 12 months after discharge from the ICU. The patients were interviewed at each visit and underwent a physical examination, pulmonary function testing, a 6-minute walk test, and a quality of life evaluation.

Results.—Survivors of ARDS were young (median age, 45 years) and severely ill (median Acute Physiology, Age, and Chronic Health Evaluation score, 23) and had a long stay in the ICU (median, 25 days). The patients had lost 18% of baseline body weight by discharge from the ICU and stated that muscle weakness and fatigue were the source of their functional limitation. Lung volume and spirometric measurement results were normal by 6 months, but carbon dioxide diffusion capacity was low throughout the 12 months of follow-up.

None of the patients required supplemental oxygen at 12 months, but 6% had arterial oxygen saturation values below 88% during exercise. There was an increase in the median score for the physical role domain of the Medical Outcomes Study 36-Item Short-Form General Health Survey from 0 at 3 months to 25 at 12 months (compared to a score of 84 in the normal population). Distance traveled on the 6-minute walk test increased from a median of 281 meters at 3 months to 422 meters at 12 months. Factors associated with a better functional status during the 1-year follow-up were the absence of systemic corticosteroid treatment, the absence of illness acquired during the ICU stay, and rapid resolution of lung injury and multiorgan dysfunction.

Conclusion.—This study found persistent functional disability among survivors of ARDS at 1 year after discharge. In addition, most patients were found to have extrapulmonary conditions, the most prominent of which were muscle wasting and weakness.

▶ A revealing study that gives the intensivist some perspective on what occurs in these acutely ill patients once they leave the ICU. It also allows the intensivist and other physicians involved in longitudinal care to council the patient and family about expectations. Also, more aggressive physical therapy may be warranted as a result of this study. It also makes you wonder what role steroids administered for nonresolving lung injury and relative adrenal insufficiency may have played (in fact, the absence of corticosteroid treatment during the ICU stay had the strongest association with a longer walk distance over the 6-minute testing interval). Surprisingly, pulmonary function was not significantly impaired at 3, 6, or 12 months post ICU discharge.

J. D. Lang, Jr, MD

Use of *Ephedra*-Containing Products and Risk for Hemorrhagic Stroke
Morgenstern LB, Viscoli CM, Kernan WN, et al (Univ of Texas at Houston; Univ of Michigan, Ann Arbor; Yale Univ, New Haven, Conn; et al)
Neurology 60:132-135, 2003   1–17

Background.—Products containing ephedra are commonly marketed for weight loss and energy enhancement. A recent survey of 14,000 adults in the United States found that 1% of respondents had used an over-the-counter product containing ephedra in the previous 2 years. Use of ephedra has been associated with hemorrhagic stroke in 2 published case series. In a recent report from Health Canada, most of the cases of hemorrhagic stroke among the 60 patients in the series involved doses that exceeded currently recommended limits or were combined with other stimulants. Together, these studies have provided uncontrolled evidence that the use of ephedra may increase the risk for hemorrhagic stroke. The purpose of this study was to provide more reliable evidence of this potential association.

Methods.—The Hemorrhagic Stroke Project was a case-control study investigating the association of phenylpropanolamine with the risk for hemorrhagic stroke. The case subjects were aged 18 to 49 years and were capable of completing an interview within 30 days of their event. Control subjects were identified by random telephone dialing and matched 2:1 with cases on the basis of telephone exchange, sex, race, and age. The control subjects were interviewed within 7 days of the focal time, which was defined by the onset of symptoms that caused the patient to seek medical attention. The focal times for the control subjects corresponded to the patients' focal times. Patients and controls were asked to report all medications taken within 2 weeks of the focal time and about specific classes of drugs, including diet remedies.

Results.—A total of 702 patients and 1376 control subjects were included in the study. There were 19 exposures to ephedra among patients and control subjects, with most involving products containing multiple botanical ingredients. Sixteen (84%) involved products that contained guarana or other sources of caffeine. For use of ephedra at any dose in the 3 days prior to the stroke, the adjusted odds ratio (OR) was 1.00 (95% confidence interval [CI], 0.32-3.11). For daily doses of ephedra less than or equal to 32 mg/d, the OR was 0.13 (95% CI, 0.01-1.54), and for daily doses larger than 32 mg/d the OR was 3.59 (95% CI, 0.70-18.35).

Conclusion.—It appears that the use of ephedra is not associated with an increased risk for hemorrhagic stroke, except perhaps when used at higher doses.

▶ This is a case-control study so it is subject to all of the retrospect bias of case-control studies. However, all of us know the risks of high doses of ephedra or ephedrine when given acutely in the operating room. This study found that 32 mg a day increased the risk of hemorrhagic stroke 3-fold. Usually, one starts to put a lot of credence in this type of epidemiologic data when risk ratios go over 2.4 or under 0.7. This study found a risk ratio of over 3; thus, maybe a daily dose of more than 32 mg of ephedra increases the risk of stroke.

What's the dose in the common diet formulation that is given over the counter? It is supposed to be under 14 mg per dose, but, in fact, some preparations that the FDA has surveyed have well over 20 mg. This dose issue may be important. Before you think this study doesn't pertain to you or your family or your patients, these are patients that are 18 to 49 years old. This wasn't just older people with strokes. And ephedra weight loss products are taken by up to 30 million people a year.

M. F. Roizen, MD

2 Preoperative Evaluation

The Effect of Alterations in a Preoperative Assessment Clinic on Reducing the Number and Improving the Yield of Cardiology Consultants
Tsen LC, Segal S, Pothier M, et al (Harvard Med School, Boston)
Anesth Analg 95:1563-1568, 2002   2–1

Background.—For patients with known or suspected cardiac disease who are scheduled for noncardiac surgery, it is wise to conduct an evaluation with a cardiologist before surgery is undertaken. Preoperative consultations can be ordered by attending anesthesiologists who are on the staff of a preoperative assessment testing clinic (PATC) and performed by a senior attending cardiologist. Because few consultations led to a diagnosis of new or unstable cardiac disease or required more cardiologist-ordered tests before surgery, procedural, educational, and staffing alterations in the PATC were made. The effect of these changes on cardiology consultation, resulting interventions, and patient outcomes was assessed.

Methods.—The changes in PATC procedures, which included the use of more stringent consultation algorithms, a cardiac assessment and electrocardiogram interpretation educational program, and altered staffing of anesthesiologists and ancillary personnel, were made in 1996. The 1196 PATC anesthesiologist–requested cardiology consultations for patients having elective surgery between 1993 and 1999 were retrospectively reviewed, comparing those 3 years before (917 consultations, PRE group) and 3 years after (279 consultations, POST group) the changes were implemented. All consultations were performed by a single senior cardiologist. The data collected included age, sex, reason for consultation, cancellations, surgical procedure, and outcomes.

Results.—The number of consultations performed fell significantly and accounted for 1.46% of the PRE total noncardiovascular surgeries and 0.49% of the POST surgeries. At both time periods, patients undergoing thoracic and orthopedic procedures accounted for the majority of cases. The 3 most common reasons for the consultations were ECG abnormalities, changes in known cardiac disease, and symptoms of cardiac disease. The POST group requested consultations for ECG changes alone significantly less often than the PRE group. Compared with the PRE group, the POST group was composed of more men, more older patients, and more patients who were scheduled for hospital admission rather than day surgery. Most consultants at both times found minimal or stable known cardiac disease, yet significantly more interventions were performed in the POST group than the PRE group. These interventions included exercise stress testing, echocardiograms, or both. Cancellations were equivalent in the 2 groups, as were the number and type of postoperative complications that occurred.

Conclusions.—The changes instituted in PATC consultation algorithms, education, and staffing led to a significant decline in the use of preoperative cardiology consultations. Among the consultations performed after the alterations, significantly more required further testing to evaluate the patient's cardiac status than in those performed before the changes were made.

▶ PATCs can be useful in reducing patient cancellations on the day of surgery, hence improving cost-efficiency, but are very expensive. These authors showed that by changing the process in the clinic, they could decrease the use and improve the benefit of preoperative cardiac consultations.

M. Wood, MD, FRCA

Should Same Anaesthetist Do Preoperative Anaesthetic Visit and Give Subsequent Anaesthetic? Questionnaire Survey of Anaesthetists
Simini B for the GiViT1 Group (Ospedale Generale Provinciale, Lucca, Italy; et al)
BMJ 327:79-80, 2003   2–2

Background.—The purposes of the preoperative anesthetic visit are to assess the fitness of the patient for surgery, discuss with the patient the most appropriate anesthetic technique, reassure the patient, obtain informed consent, and prescribe premedicant drugs. In the past patients were visited by the same physician who later anesthetized them, but today the preoperative visit and the subsequent anesthetic are usually not performed by the same anesthetists. It has been determined that patients would prefer to be anesthetized by the physician who conducted the preoperative anesthetic interview, but the opinion of anesthetists regarding this question have not been explored. The opinions of anesthetists were solicited in regard to whether the preoperative anesthetic visit and the anesthesia delivery should be performed by the same anesthetist.

Methods.—A questionnaire was sent in 2002 to a group of Italian anesthetists. Two scenarios were presented. In the first scenario, patients were anesthetized by the anesthetist who visited them; in the second scenario, patients were visited by one anesthetist and the anesthesia was delivered by another anesthetist. The anesthetists were asked which scenario was used in their institution, which scenario they preferred, and to select at least 1 reason for their choice from a list included with the questionnaire.

Results.—The response rate was 76%. The majority of respondents (81.3%) preferred the first scenario, in which one anesthetist conducts the visit and administers the anesthesia. However, the majority of anesthesia departments (89.9%) used the second scenario, in which one anesthetist visited the patient and another administered the anesthesia. The most common reasons for preferring the "one patient, one anesthetist" scenario involved litigation concerns and the view that the preoperative tests and drugs are best ordered by the anesthetist delivering the anesthetic. The most common reasons given for preferring the "1 patient, 2 anesthetists" approach involved ease of organization and the necessity for uniform preoperative criteria.

Conclusions.—The policy of "1 patient, 2 anesthetists" is used by most anesthesia department in Italy but is at odds with professional standards and with the opinion of a majority of anesthetists and patients.

▶ A provocative questionnaire! The authors ask, why is clinical practice so far from ideal? Would there be a difference in real measured outcomes data if the same anesthesiologist performed the preoperative visit and the anesthetic? We do not know, but food for thought.

M. Wood, MD, FRCA

Guideline Chaos: Conflicting Recommendations for Preoperative Cardiac Assessment
Gordon AJ, Macpherson DS (VA Pittsburgh Healthcare System, Pa; Univ of Pittsburgh, Pa)
Am J Cardiol 91:1299-1303, 2003   2–3

Introduction.—The American College of Cardiology/American Heart Association (ACC/AHA) and the American College of Physicians (ACP) have published guidelines for evaluating preoperative cardiac risks in patients undergoing noncardiac surgery. The ACC/AHA and ACP guidelines were reviewed to determine if they differ in preoperative recommendations for a group of patients and whether they differ from actual provider recommendations.

Methods.—Patient characteristics and physician recommendations were abstracted in a retrospective cohort investigation by using electronic medical records of consecutive patients attending a Medical Preoperative Evaluation Clinic (MPEC) of the Veteran Affairs Pittsburgh Healthcare System between January 1 and April 1, 1998. Physicians in the MPEC were instructed to dictate relevant items from the patient examination, including description of planned surgery type, relevant medical history, history or lack thereof of significant cardiac or pulmonary disease, focused physical examination findings, and evaluation of cardiac risk and recommendations, including the need for invasive or noninvasive preoperative testing. Patient characteristics were used to ascertain which preoperative cardiac testing should have been ordered if each guideline was followed.

Results.—Most of the 138 patients identified underwent moderate-risk surgeries. The recommendations for preoperative testing were discordant between guidelines in 17% of the cohort ($\kappa = 0.38$). Guidelines did not agree on the need for noninvasive stress testing (NST) in any patient. Extreme differences in recommendations were observed in 9 patients (7%). Physicians ordered NST more frequently than either guideline (27 patients). In this subgroup of patients in whom physicians ordered a NST, the 2 guidelines differed significantly ($\kappa = 0.26$).

Conclusion.—When applied to actual patients being evaluated for surgery, the ACC/AHA and ACP guidelines significantly differed in recommendations for preoperative cardiac testing.

▶ This small study retrospectively applies ACC/AHA and ACP guidelines for preoperative cardiac evaluation of patients to existing preoperative evaluations. There are problems with this approach, in particular that there were no forms used to guide data collection and recording. As a result, data critical to application of the ACC/AHA guidelines, functional capacity, were not routinely available. As this is one critical factor in guiding recommendations, its absence would negatively affect retrospective application of ACC/AHA guidelines. The finding that the 2 guidelines differ is not surprising, given that ACP guidelines recommend testing only for patients undergoing vascular surgery. These guidelines would also be expected to be less helpful for the vast majority of patients at risk for cardiac disease for nonvascular surgery. Nonetheless, the study is important as it reminds us of the need to further study guidelines and their impact.

M. F. Trankina, MD

Obesity in General Elective Surgery
Dindo D, Muller MK, Weber M, et al (Univ Hosp Zurich, Switzerland)
Lancet 361:2032-2035, 2003   2–4

Introduction.—Obesity increases the risk for minor wound infections in numerous types of surgical procedures. The effect of obesity on other types of postoperative complications is speculative due to the use of different definitions and classifications for obesity and the lack of a uniform approach to reporting surgical complications. How obesity effects surgical outcome in elective general surgery was examined in 6336 patients followed up prospectively in a single institution for more than 10 years.

Methods.—Excluded were patients undergoing emergency, vascular, thoracic, and bariatric surgeries; transplantation procedures; patients under immunosuppression; and surgeries performed with the patient under local anesthesia. Postoperative mortality was examined for nonobese and obese patients (body mass index less than 30 kg/m^2 vs 30 kg/m^2 or greater). Obesity was additionally stratified into mild obesity (30.0-34.9 kg/m^2) and severe obesity (35 kg/m^2 or greater) (Table 1). Risk factors were assessed by univariate and multivariate models.

Results.—A total of 808 of 6336 (13%) patients were obese; 569 (9%) were mildly obese and 239 (4%) were severely obese. The morbidity rates in patients who were obese versus those who were not obese were similar (122

TABLE 1.—Patient Characteristics

Variable	Non-Obese* (n=5528)	Overall† (n=808)	P‡	Obese Grade I§ (n=569)	Grade II/III¶ (n=239)
Patient factors					
Age (years)	52 (17·1)	52·6 (14·4)	0·49	55·2 (14·0)	48·8 (13·2)
Female sex	2554 (46%)	494 (61%)	<0·0001	292 (51%)	173 (72%)
BMI (kg/m²)	24·0 (2·8)	34·9 (6·0)	<0·0001	31·3 (1·3)	41·7 (6·8)
Medical history					
Diabetes mellitus	321 (6%)	110 (14%)	<0·0001	58 (10%)	39 (16%)
Hypertension	918 (17%)	249 (31%)	<0·0001	154 (27%)	89 (37%)
Malignant disease	1454 (26%)	184 (23%)	0·21	154 (27%)	54 (23%)
Pathological cardiac history	1078 (20%)	288 (36%)	<0·0001	166 (29%)	111 (47%)
Pathological respiratory history	1365 (25%)	212 (26%)	0·2	153 (27%)	65 (27%)
Regular tobacco use	2637 (48%)	365 (45%)	0·31	250 (44%)	117 (49%)
ASA classification			<0·0001‖		
I	2615 (47%)	247 (31%)		188 (33%)	61 (26%)
II	1896 (34%)	402 (50%)		259 (46%)	147 (62%)
III	896 (16%)	102 (13%)		73 (13%)	29 (12%)
IV	122 (2%)	5 (1%)		3 (1%)	2 (1%)
Operative data					
Type A	2725 (49%)	340 (42%)	<0·0001‖	274 (48%)	66 (28%)
Type B	2278 (41%)	437 (54%)		271 (48%)	165 (69%)
Type C	525 (10%)	32 (4%)		23 (4%)	8 (3%)
Minimally invasive surgery	1973 (36%)	377 (47%)	<0·0001	198 (35%)	146 (61%)

Note: Values are mean (standard deviation) or number of patients (percentage).
*Body mass index (*BMI*) less than 30 kg/m².
†BMI 30 kg/m² or greater.
‡ Comparisons between patients with BMI less than 30 kg/m² and 30 kg/m² or greater.
§BMI 30·0–34·9 kg/m².
‖*P* for trend < ,0001.
¶BMI 35 kg/m² or greater.
Abbreviation: ASA, American Society of Anesthesiologists.
(Courtesy of Dindo D, Muller MK, Weber M, et al: Obesity in general elective surgery. *Lancet* 361:2032-2035, 2003. Reprinted with permission from Elsevier Science.)

TABLE 2.—Overall Morbidity and Complication Grades

Variable	Non-Obese* (n=5528)	Obese			
		Overall† (n=808)	P‡	Grade I§ (n=569)	Grade II/III¶ (n=239)
Complication					
Overall‖	896 (16%)	122 (15%)	0·26	84 (15%)	38 (16%)
Grade I	415 (8%)	53 (7%)	0·17	37 (7%)	16 (7%)
Grade II	238 (4%)	26 (3%)	0·06	18 (3%)	8 (3%)
Grade III	260 (5%)	44 (6%)	0·25	23 (4%)	12 (5%)
Grade IV	122 (2%)	20 (3%)	0·36	13 (2%)	7 (3%)
Grade V	72 (1%)	6 (1%)	0·12	6 (1%)	0

Note: Values are number of patients (percentage).
*Body mass index (*BMI*) <30 kg/m^2.
†BMI 30 kg/m^2 or greater.
‡Comparisons between patients with BMI < 30 kg/m^2 and 30 kg/m^2 or greater.
§BMI 30.0-34.9 kg/m^2.
‖One or more complications.
¶BMI 35 kg/m^2 or greater.
(Courtesy of Dindo D, Muller MK, Weber M, et al: Obesity in general elective surgery. *Lancet* 361:2032-2035, 2003. Reprinted with permission from Elsevier Science.)

[15.1%] of 808 vs 901 of 5528 [16.3%] who were not obese; P = .26), with the exception of a higher rate of wound infections after open surgery in patients who were obese (17 [4%] of 431 vs 92 [3%] of 3555; P = .03).

The rate of complications did not vary between patients who were mildly obese (91 [16.0%] of 569), severely obese (36 [15.1%] of 239), or nonobese (901 [16.3% of 5528; P = .19) (Table 2). Multivariate regression analyses showed that obesity was not a risk factor for the development of postoperative complications. The additional medical resource use as estimated by a new classification of complications revealed no differences between patients who were and were not obese.

Conclusion.—Obesity by itself is not a risk factor for postoperative complications. Forcing obese patients to lose weight before surgery or to exclude them from elective general surgery is not supported by these findings.

▶ This article is fascinating in that it shows that obesity alone is not a risk factor for postoperative complications. However, obese patients had more comorbidities, such as diabetes and hypertension. Bias might occur in that very obese patients with severe illness might not be selected for surgery. Obese patients underwent more laparoscopic procedures than nonobese patients. So there are details that indicate that this is not a perfect study. It is not possible to conclude that there is absolutely not an increased risk for obese patients, but rather that these types of data should be taken into account before excluding obese patients from elective surgery.

M. Wood, MD, FRCA

Improving the Process of Informed Consent in the Critically Ill
Davis N, Pohlman A, Gehlbach B, et al (Univ of Chicago)
JAMA 289:1963-1968, 2003   2–5

Background.—Patients in the ICU are often not able or even not asked to provide informed consent for invasive procedures. A universal consent form covering the 8 invasive procedures most commonly performed in the ICU was developed, and its effect on obtaining informed consent was assessed.

Methods.—The study included 270 patients who were admitted consecutively to the ICU during a baseline period (n = 125) and an intervention period (n = 145). During the 2-month baseline period, the number of invasive procedures performed in the ICU for which informed consent was obtained was recorded. During the next 3 months, a universal informed consent form was developed that covered the 8 invasive procedures most commonly performed in the ICU (lumbar puncture; thoracentesis; paracentesis; intubation/mechanical ventilation; and placement of an arterial catheter, central venous catheter, pulmonary artery catheter, or peripherally inserted central catheter). Handouts describing each of these procedures were attached to the form, and were also available in the ICU waiting area. Physicians and nurses were introduced to the universal consent form during ICU orientation. Then, during the next 2 months, the number of invasive procedures performed for which informed consent had been obtained was again recorded. During both the baseline and the intervention periods, patients or their proxies completed a questionnaire to assess their understanding of the procedures.

Results.—At baseline, only 155 (53%) of the 292 invasive procedures were performed after informed consent had been obtained. This number increased significantly to 308 (90%) of 340 procedures after the universal consent form was available (absolute difference, 37.4%). During the intervention period, the universal consent form was provided to 83 patients, and all but 1 signed it. Most (91%) of these 82 patients underwent at least 1 of the procedures covered by the form. In both the baseline and the intervetion periods, most of the consents were provided by proxies (71.6% and 65.6%, respectively; between-group difference not significant). According to the questionnaire, the proportions of patients or proxies who said they understood the indications for and risks of the procedures were also similar in the 2 periods.

Conclusion.—A universal consent form covering the 8 invasive procedures most commonly performed in the ICU dramatically improved the frequency with which informed consent was obtained. Patient or proxy comprehension of the procedures was not adversely affected by the process.

▶ Much can be learned from this study. All parties (physicians, patients and proxies) are well served by the authors' universal consent form and handouts, educating the proxies about the various procedures they are being asked to allow to be performed. This study has impacted our ICU, and we are now in the process of adapting the methodology followed by the authors. Patient autonomy is very important, and progressive ways to ensure that freedom of choice to some degree should always be strived for in the dynamic environment of the ICU.

J. D. Lang, Jr, MD

3 Anesthesia-Related Pharmacology and Toxicology

Gender Differences in Drug Effects: Implications for Anesthesiologists
Pleym H, Spigset O, Kharasch ED, et al (St Olav's Univ Hosp, Trondheim, Norway; Norwegian Univ of Science and Technology, Trondheim, Norway; Univ of Washington, Seattle)
Acta Anaesthesiol Scand 47:241-259, 2003   3–1

Background.—Differences are found in the pharmacokinetics and pharmacodynamics of drugs related to the practice of anesthesia between the sexes. An overview was compiled on these differences and their clinical relevance.

Methods.—MEDLINE searches were used to obtain the data for review. Key words used were "human," "gender," "sex," and the specific names of various drugs.

Results.—The compositions of male and female bodies differ, so the same dose per kilogram of body weight results in different plasma concentrations depending on whether the drug is lipophilic or water soluble. Lipophilic drugs have a volume of distribution per kilogram of body weight in women that is higher than in men, with the reverse true for water-soluble drugs. Thus, for opioids and benzodiazepines (lipophilic drugs), women have a higher volume of distribution than men, and for muscle relaxants (water-soluble drugs), men have a higher volume of distribution. These gender differences can influence the optimal dosage of drugs given in one or a few single doses but not that of steady-state drug concentrations. Women have a reduced total liver blood flow compared to men, so their liver clearance of a drug is generally lower. Gender differences in drugs metabolized by the hepatic cytochrome P-450 (CYP) system can be important with respect to anesthesia. Anesthetic drug properties are not influenced by contraceptive pills, pregnancy, the menstrual cycle, or menopause, although age does play a role. Gender-sensitive dosing is recommended with the use of vecuronium, pancuronium, and rocuronium when a rapid onset or short duration of action is needed. Female subjects have a 20% to 30% greater sensitivity to the muscle relaxant effects of these agents than male subjects. For propofol, male subjects show greater sensitivity than female subjects, so the dose may need to be diminished by 30% to 40% to achieve similar recovery times in men. Opioid receptor agonists, morphine, and several kappa receptor agonists are handled with greater sensitivity by female bodies than by men, who require 30% to 40% higher doses to achieve pain relief equivalent to that obtained in women. If female subjects receive the same doses as men, respiratory depression and other adverse effects are more likely to occur.

Conclusions.—Because of the significant differences in how male and female patients handle drugs relevant to anesthesia, sex should be considered in dosage calculations. Further study is required to optimize drug treatment between the sexes.

▶ I selected this article because it is an extremely useful review on drug pharmacokinetics/pharmacodynamics and gender. Knowledge such as this might result in a more logical administration of anesthetic drugs to female patients.

M. Wood, MD, FRCA

Pharmacodynamics and Pharmacokinetics of Propofol in a Medium-Chain Triglyceride Emulsion
Ward DS, Norton JR, Guivarc'h P-H, et al (Univ of Rochester, NY; RTP Pharma Inc, Montreal; Univ of Pennsylvania, Philadelphia)
Anesthesiology 97:1401-1408, 2002   3–2

Introduction.—Current formulations of propofol use soybean oil emulsion rather than water since propofol is insoluble. These soybean emulsions can produce elevated plasma triglycerides and support bacterial growth. An alternative formulation of propofol is a 2% emulsion in a medium-chain triglyceride solution (IDD-D Propofol; RTP Pharma Inc, Verdum, PQ, Canada) with Diprivan was evaluated in a double-blind, crossover, phase 1 investigation.

Methods.—Two consecutive protocols for propofol with Diprivan were used in 24 patients (12 in each group). Patients in protocol 1 received a single bolus of 2.5 mg/kg; those in protocol 2 received the same induction dose followed by a 30-minute infusion at 0.2 mg/kg/min. Venous samples were obtained for propofol concentration and biochemical measurements. Induction and emergence times were ascertained by termination of voluntary counting and responding to command, respectively.

Results.—Plasma concentrations were not significantly different between the 2 formulations. Induction time was 14% longer with IDD-D Propofol than with Diprivan (24 patients, protocols 1 and 2 combined; mean, 53.3 seconds and 46.9 seconds, respectively; $P = .002$). Emergence time was not significantly different for protocol 1 (Fig 1) and was marginally longer ($P = .04$) for IDD-D Propofol in protocol 2 (1197 seconds for 11 patients and 1254 seconds for 12 patients, respectively). As expected, due to the inherent

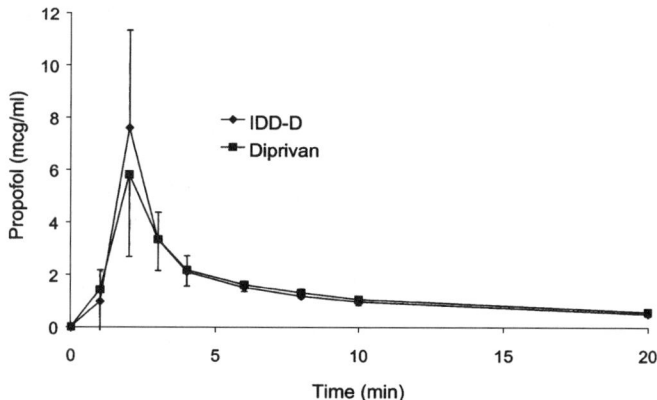

FIGURE 1.—Average (±standard deviation) plasma propofol concentrations for protocol 1. There was no significant difference between the plasma concentrations of the 2 drugs at any of the times shown, before correcting for multiple comparisons. Most data points are the average of samples from each of the 12 subjects. There were some samples that were not obtained because of technical difficulties, but the number of patients was 9 or more for all points. (Courtesy of Ward DS, Norton JR, Guivarc'h P-H, et al: Pharmacodynamics and pharmacokinetics of propofol in a medium-chain triglyceride emulsion. *Anesthesiology* 97:1401-1408, 2002. Copyright American Society of Anesthesiologists, Inc. Used with permission of Lippincott Williams & Wilkins Publishers.)

characteristics of the formulations, plasma triglycerides were elevated with Diprivan and not with IDD-D Propofol; octanoate, a metabolite of medium-chain triglycerides, was elevated only with IDD-D Propofol. Octanoate was elevated to concentrations less than those regarded as toxic.

Plasma concentrations of other biochemical markers of medium-chain triglyceride metabolism (eg, ketones) demonstrated no significant changes. Of interest, there were significant differences between male and female research subjects in the propofol plasma concentrations and time to awakening with both drugs.

Conclusion.—Differences between the 2 propofol formulations were slight and not clinically important. Similar gender differences were observed for both formulations in plasma concentrations and awakening times.

▶ This study highlights the pharmacokinetics and pharmacodynamics of 2 propofol formulations. The authors found no important clinical differences.

M. Wood, MD, FRCA

Modeling of the Sedative and Airway Obstruction Effects of Propofol in Patients With Parkinson Disease Undergoing Stereotactic Surgery
Fábregas N, Rapado J, Gambús PL, et al (Univ of Barcelona; Univ of Navarra, Spain)
Anesthesiology 97:1378-1386, 2002   3–3

Background.—Patients with Parkinson's disease (PD) have an anatomic alteration of the neurons of the extrapyramidal system that manifests as rigidity and tremor along with respiratory dysfunction. When pharmacologic management is unsuccessful and the patient reaches an advanced stage of PD, stereotactic pallidotomy and the implantation of electrodes to stimulate specific subthalamic regions may improve symptoms. Patients require sedation for the procedure yet must be able to awaken rapidly for electrocorticography or neuropsychiatric testing. Propofol offers this anesthetic profile, but the relation between drug kinetics and depth of sedation in PD patients has not been assessed. An assessment was carried out to determine the optimal plasma propofol concentration that produces sedation with minimal risk of respiratory obstruction for patients with advanced PD having functional stereotactic pallidotomy.

Methods.—Functional stereotactic pallidotomy was performed in 21 patients with advanced PD. All were administered propofol by target-controlled infusion to produce an initial steady state concentration of 1 µg/mL. The Ramsay Sedation Scale was used to measure the degree of sedation, and a 4-category score was obtained to determine airway obstruction. Propofol levels were determined from blood samples.

Results.—The propofol concentrations that the target-controlled infusion device predicted were significantly greater than the measured plasma propofol concentrations. The steady-state plasma concentration associated with 50% probability (C_{50}) was estimated to be 0.1 µg/mL for a Ramsay score of 3, 1.02 µg for a Ramsay score of 4, and 2.28 µg/mL for a Ramsay score of 5. The C_{50} estimates for airway obstruction scores of 2 and 3 were 0.32 and 2.98 µg/mL, respectively. The profiles that were obtained suggest that for a typical steady-state propofol plasma concentration of 0.35 µg/mL, the likelihood of obtaining an adequate level of sedation is greatest while the risk of severe airway obstruction is least.

Conclusions.—With a steady-state propofol concentration of 0.35 µg/mL, a sedation score of 3 and minimal or no airway obstruction can be achieved in patients with PD undergoing stereotactic and electrode implantation surgery.

▶ The anesthetic management of PD is anecdotal, and carefully conducted clinical studies are lacking. This study shows that a low concentration of propofol (0.35 µg/mL) is required to produce sedation and minimal airway obstruction in patients undergoing stereotactic surgery.

M. Wood, MD, FRCA

Side Effects of Opioids During Short-Term Administration: Effect of Age, Gender, and Race
Cepeda MS, Farrar JT, Baumgarten M, et al (Javeriana Univ, Bogota, Colombia; Univ of Pennsylvania, Philadelphia; Univ of Maryland, Baltimore)
Clin Pharmacol Ther 74:102-112, 2003   3–4

Background.—Opioids are used extensively in pain management, yet the factors that increase the risk of developing side effects and the incidence of side effects with specific opioids remain largely unexplored. Within the framework of short-term opioid use, the type of opioid and the age, sex, and race of the patient were evaluated for their effect on the incidence of the side effects of nausea and vomiting and respiratory depression.

Methods.—A cohort of 8855 subjects drawn from 35 community-based and tertiary hospitals had been evaluated retrospectively and were secondarily analyzed for drug side effects. All subjects were at least aged 16 years and had received meperidine (69.0%), morphine (27.0%), or fentanyl (6.0%) in treatment, usually for acute pain. Whether these patients had nausea and vomiting or respiratory depression was assessed.

Results.—Nausea and vomiting developed in 26% of the patients. Respiratory depression was noted in 1.5% of cases, with 53% of these considered life-threatening; 22 patients died. Route of administration was the only factor that changed the odds ratio for the risk factors evaluated. The odds for fentanyl and morphine to produce nausea and vomiting were similar, but meperidine produced less nausea and vomiting than either of the other agents. The odds of developing nausea and vomiting were increased when the IV drug route was used and when the dose increased. The odds declined when the patients were older than 80 years, male, and black. The odds ratio for any of the risk factors for developing respiratory depression was changed by more than 15% only by the route of administration. Meperidine had a lower risk of respiratory depression than morphine. Age increased the risk of developing respiratory depression substantially, but sex, race, and higher doses had no significant impact.

Conclusions.—For short-term use, meperidine offered a better side effect profile than either morphine or fentanyl. Patients in the meperidine group had a lower incidence of nausea and vomiting and respiratory depression than patients receiving the other agents. Increased age was a significant predictor of the development of respiratory depression. In addition, women were found to have nausea and vomiting more often than men. Race requires further investigation to determine its effects.

▶ Meperidine is not used as often as morphine in the postoperative recovery area but may, under certain circumstances, be a useful and even safer drug than morphine. One caveat: meperidine is metabolized to normeperidine, a long-acting metabolite that produces adverse effects in the central nervous system with seizures.

M. Wood, MD, FRCA

Food and Drug Administration Black Box Warning on the Perioperative Use of Droperidol: A Review of the Cases
Habib AS, Gan TJ (Duke Univ, Durham, NC)
Anesth Analg 96:1377-1379, 2003   3–5

Introduction.—A recent editorial indicated that the use of small-dose droperidol has been a highly cost-effective antiemetic for over 30 years. The drug at IV doses of 0.625 to 1.25 mg has been widely accepted as a first-line treatment for management of postoperative nausea and vomiting. The decision by the Food and Drug Administration (FDA) to issue a "black box" warning concerning the use of droperidol for the treatment and prevention of postoperative nausea and vomiting has been challenged by several anesthesiologists. A database search was performed.

Findings.—The Freedom of Information Act was accessed, and information was requested concerning the cases upon which the FDA warning was based. In response, data were received that was contained in the adverse event reporting system—a computerized database that contained a summary of all adverse events reported to the FDA. There were 273 cases reported to the FDA between November 1, 1997, and January 2, 2002. Copies were requested of the individual case reports (MedWatch forms) in which cardiac adverse events were reported after use of droperidol at doses of 1.25 mg or below.

The forms had information voluntarily submitted to the FDA or to the drug manufacturer by consumers or health care professionals. The reporting person ascertained whether droperidol was the primary or secondary suspect. Of the 10 cases in the FDA database in which serious cardiovascular events were possibly associated with the administration of droperidol at doses of 1.25 mg or less, there were several confounding factors that made it impossible to establish the exact cause of the adverse cardiac event. Possible cardiac events and torsade or prolonged QT were observed in 74 and 17 cases, respectively. It is estimated that over 11 million ampules of droperidol were sold in the United States in 2001. This would make the incidence of cardiac events and torsade/prolonged QT 74 in 11 million and 17 in 11 million, respectively.

Conclusion.—Of the 10 cases in which arrhythmias occurred after administration of small doses of droperidol, there was no evidence of a cause-and-effect relationship.

▶ Droperidol and other related antiemetic 5 HT 3 receptor antagonist drugs can cause torsade and/or prolonged QT interval leading to arrhythmias and even death. The authors provide commentary on the FDA "black box" warning, which has markedly reduced the use of droperidol in the United States.

M. Wood, MD, FRCA

The P-Glycoprotein Inhibitor Quinidine Decreases the Threshold for Bupivacaine-Induced, but not Lidocaine-Induced, Convulsions in Rats

Funao T, Oda Y, Tanaka K, et al (Osaka City Univ, Japan)
Can J Anesth 50:805-811, 2003   3–6

Background.—Bupivacaine is a long-acting local anesthetic with high lipid solubility and more than 90% protein binding. When local anesthetics are accidentally injected IV in a toxic dose, CNS effects are seen first, then cardiovascular collapse. CNS side effects are only seen if the local anesthetic diffuses into the brain across the blood-brain barrier. The ability of bupivacaine to do so has not been determined. P-glycoprotein (P-gp) is an important component of the blood-brain barrier that can actively pump drugs out of the CNS. The CNS toxicity of local anesthetics can be affected by various drugs; the specific effects of P-gp inducers or inhibitors on CNS toxicity produced by local anesthetics have not been studied previously. Local anesthetics are usually used along with P-gp inhibitors such as verapamil, quinidine, and cyclosporine. The effect of quinidine on lidocaine- and bupivacaine-induced convulsions was explored in a rat model.

Methods.—Male Sprague-Dawley rats were randomly assigned to 4 groups of 10 animals each. The groups received 15 mg/kg of quinidine or saline solution, then were given either 4 mg/kg per minute infusion of lidocaine or 1 mg/kg per minute infusion of bupivacaine until they convulsions occurred. The groups were thus labeled quinidine plus lidocaine (QL), quinidine plus bupivacaine (QB), saline plus lidocaine (L), and saline plus bupivacaine (B). High-performance liquid chromatography was used to measure the concentrations of lidocaine and its primary metabolite (monoethylglycinexylidide [MEGX]) and bupivacaine in plasma and in the brain at the onset of convulsions.

Results.—The L and QL groups showed no differences in the cumulative doses of lidocaine that produced convulsions, no differences in the total and unbound lidocaine in plasma or total lidocaine in the brain, and no differences in the concentration of total or unbound MEGX in the plasma or total MEGX in the brain. The B and QB groups showed no differences in the cumulative doses of bupivacaine required to induce convulsions and no differences in the brain concentration of total bupivacaine. However, there were significantly lower plasma concentrations of total and unbound bupivacaine in the QB group and significantly higher brain/plasma concentration ratios of total bupivacaine in the B group.

Conclusions.—Quinidine reduced the plasma concentration and increased the brain/plasma concentration ratio of bupivacaine at the point when convulsions developed. Quinidine inhibits P-gp activity at plasma concentrations less than were used in this assessment. Thus, bupivacaine may be a substrate of P-gp. The inhibition of P-gp by quinidine resulted in a greater concentration of bupivacaine in the brain and reduced the concentration in the plasma that was needed to produce convulsions. Lidocaine-induced convulsions were not affected by quinidine. Therefore, the administration of bupivacaine along with a P-gp inhibitor requires careful monitoring to avoid CNS toxicity.

▶ This study shows a drug interaction between the P-gp inhibitor quinidine and bupivacaine in a rat model.

M. Wood, MD, FRCA

A Pharmacogenetic Study of Uridine Diphosphate–Glucuronosyltransferase 2B7 in Patients Receiving Morphine

Sawyer MB, Innocenti F, Das S, et al (Univ of Chicago; St Jude Children's Research Hosp, Memphis, Tenn)

Clin Pharmacol Ther 73:566-574, 2003   3–7

Introduction.—Glucouronidation is an important metabolic pathway for endogenous compounds and xenobiotics. It is catalyzed by uridine diphosphate-glucuronosyltransferase (UGT) enzymes. The UGTs have a crucial role in drug biotransformation since glucuronidated substrates are more readily eradicated through the biliary system and kidney. Among the human UGTs, UGT2B7 has a wide substrate specificity and is responsible for the glucuronidation of steroids, retinoids, zidovudine, morphine, and the anticancer drug epirubicin. Functional mutations in the *UGT2B7* gene may have important clinical consequences. The variation in the *UGT2B7* gene was examined in patients receiving patient-controlled analgesia with morphine.

Methods.—Blood samples were obtained from 12 patients at 24 and 26 hours after the start of patient-controlled analgesia. Concentrations of morphine and its glucuronides were determined in patient plasma. The *UGT2B7* gene was sequenced in phenotypic extremes of the distribution of morphine-6-glucuronide/morphine plasma ratios.

Results.—A new 161C/T promoter variant was in complete linkage disequilibrium with the 802C/T variant and was more common in low glucuronidators ($P = .039$). Both variants were genotyped in all 86 patients. Complete linkage disequilibrium was verified. Trend analysis revealed decreased morphine-6-glucuronide/morphine ratios in patients with T/T, C/T, and C/C genotypes (T/T>C/T>C/C) ($P = .031$). Morphine levels were lower in T/T patients (median, 18 ng/mL; range, 18-1490 ng/mL) versus C/T and C/C patients combined (median, 66 ng/mL; range, 18-3995 ng/mL) ($P = .04$). Morphine-6-glucuronide and morphine-3-glucuronide concentrations were significantly lower among C/C patients (median, 18 ng/mL; range, 0-66 ng/mL; and median, 152 ng/mL; range, 30-434 ng/mL, respectively) versus C/T and T/T ng/mL, respectively ($P = .45$ and $P = .004$, respectively) (Fig 2).

Conclusion.—Inter-individual variations in morphine glucuronidation may be due to the genetic variation in *UGT2B7*.

▶ Glucuronidation of morphine to morphine-3-glucuronide and morphine-6-glucuronide is an important pathway. The authors report here a pharmacogenetic study in patients receiving morphine during the postoperative period by patient-controlled analgesia. Blood samples were taken to measure morphine and its glucuronides, and also gene sequencing was done to show that inter-

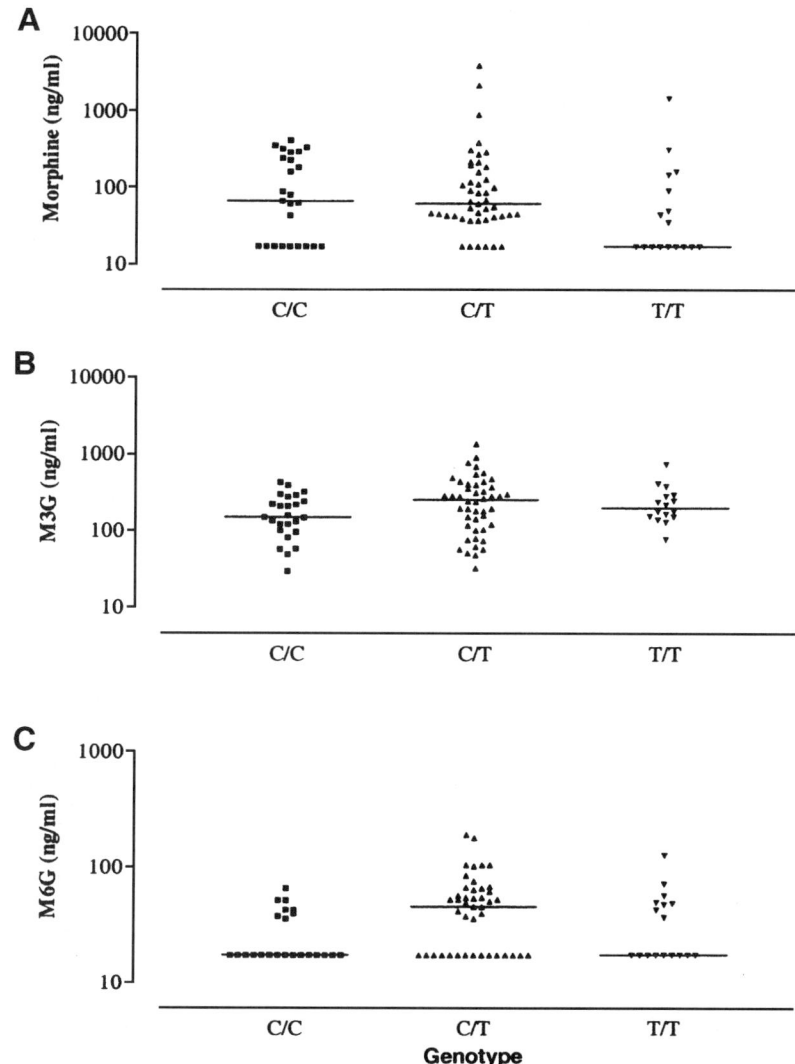

FIGURE 2.—Morphine (**A**), morphine-3-glucuronide (*M3G*) (**B**), and morphine-6-glucuronide (*M6G*) (**C**) plasma concentrations (log scale) stratified by genotype. M6G levels were undetectable (value set at 0) in 2 C/C and 2 C/T patients and are not included in the graph. For samples with either morphine or M6G levels below the limit of quantification, the value was set to 18 ng/mL for both compounds (half of the limit of quantification). *Bars* represent medians. (Courtesy of Sawyer MB, Innocenti F, Das S, et al: A pharmacogenetic study of uridine diphosphate—Glucuronosyltransferase 2B7 in patients receiving morphine. *Clin Pharmacol Ther* 73:566-574, 2003.)

individual differences in morphine glucuronidation may be due to genetic variation of UGT2B7—an enzyme responsible for the glucuronidation of morphine. Subtle differences (and not so subtle) in patient response to patient-controlled analgesia may be due to genetic polymorphism.

M. Wood, MD, FRCA

Polymorphisms in Human *MDR1* (P-glycoprotein): Recent Advances and Clinical Relevance

Marzolini C, Paus E, Buclin T, et al (Vanderbilt Univ, Nashville; Univ Dept of Adult Psychiatry, Prilly-Lausanne, Switzerland; Univ Hosp of Lausanne, Switzerland)
Clin Pharmacol Ther 75:13-33, 2004   3–8

Background.—Drug transporters play a vital role in drug disposition and response. P-glycoprotein (P-gp) is the encoded product of the multidrug resistance (*MDR1*) gene and was first studied to determine its role in mediating the multiple drug resistance phenotype found in certain cancers. It has broad substrate specificity. The current data on its role in drug disposition were outlined, with special focus on how genetic variations in the transporter alter drug pharmacokinetics and disease outcomes. The inconsistencies of effect observed in *MDR1* polymorphisms were also noted.

P-gp Facts.—P-gp moves drugs from the intracellular to the extracellular domain and may also interact with drug molecules limited to the cell membrane lipid bilayer. Its mechanisms of action have been compared to a vacuum cleaner. The function and anatomic position of P-gp suggest that it forms a protective barrier to keep toxins out of the body and excrete compounds into the bile, urine, and intestinal lumen. Thus, these compounds do not accumulate in critical organs such as the brain, gonads, and bone marrow or in the fetus. A broad range of substrates, inhibitors, or inducers of this transporter exist. Many drug substrates of P-pg are also substrates of drug-metabolizing enzymes, particularly cytochrome P450 (CYP) 3A4. Animal models confirm that the colocalization of P-gp and CYP3A4 in the small intestine and liver means P-gp is a significant contributor to the oral bioavailability, distribution, and excretion of drugs. When P-gp is inhibited, many drug-drug interactions result.

MDR1 Polymorphisms.—In animals, naturally occurring polymorphisms are linked to a complete loss of transporter function, and similar genetic defects in humans appear possible. Twenty-nine single-nucleotide polymorphisms (SNPs) have been identified in the *MDR1* gene thus far. SNPs at exon 21 and 1b may be associated with altered transporter function or expression. Linkage disequilibrium has been found between SNPs at exon 26 and at exon 21, so differences in P-gp function may result from nonsynonymous polymorphism in exon 21. Three common haplotype combinations are found in all ethnic groups. More than 70% of the subjects in most studies have these, which confirms the presence of a strong linkage disequilibrium between exon 26 and 21. Marked differences in the allele frequency of exon 26 and 21 SNP were found between various ethnic groups, which may explain why some have selective advantages against certain disorders. This influences disease risk, as has been seen in renal cell carcinoma, parkinsonism, and HIV infection. Conflicting results may result from confounding factors, which require further study. Among these factors are the lack of clarification about the molecular basis of the *MDR1* exon 26 C3435T effect and contributions from linkage disequilibrium, diet, and environmental chemicals. In addition, tissues may express P-gp at various levels, and the selection of P-gp probe drugs has not been standardized.

Conclusions.—In evaluating P-gp with respect to drug disposition and response, careful attention to haplotypes, environmental factors, and sample size is required. Demographic data must be standardized so that the P-gp expression of individuals with a disease is not compared with its expression in a population without the disease. Further study of substrate specificity, regulation, and species-related differences in the structure and function of P-gp is also needed, as are standardized assay methods.

▶ I selected this review article to highlight the importance of transporters in drug delivery, for example, to the central nervous system. Many drugs are substrates for P-gp, and the potential for drug interactions is great.

M. Wood, MD, FRCA

Selective Depression by General Anesthetics of Glutamate Versus GABA Release From Isolated Cortical Nerve Terminals
Westphalen RI, Hemmings HC (Cornell Univ, New York)
J Pharmacol Exp Ther 304:1188-1196, 2003   3–9

Background.—General anesthetics exhibit both presynaptic and postsynaptic mechanisms, with prolongation of synaptic inhibition serving an important role in the depressant effects of volatile anesthetics and several IV anesthetics. Essential to understanding the neurophysiologic outcomes of presynaptic anesthetic actions is a grasp of the effects general anesthetics have on the release of the major excitatory transmitter glutamate and the major inhibitory transmitter γ-aminobutyric acid (GABA). A dual-isotope method was used to simultaneously compare the effects of isoflurane (a volatile agent) and propofol (an IV agent) on the release of glutamate and GABA from rat synaptosomes.

Methods.—The isolated rat cerebrocortical nerve terminals, or synaptosomes, were labeled with L-[^{3}H]glutamate and [^{14}C]GABA. Release was measured by superfusion with pulses of 30 mmol/L potassium ion channel blockers or 1 mmol/L 4-aminopyridine (4AP) with or without 1.9 mmol/L of free calcium.

Results.—The release of glutamate and GABA by 4AP was significantly inhibited by both isoflurane and propofol. The 4AP-evoked glutamate release was preferentially inhibited by isoflurane over GABA release at various clinical concentrations. Selective inhibition of 4AP-evoked release of glutamate over GABA was exhibited by tetrodotoxin and riluzole, which are sodium ion channel blockers. This may indicate that isoflurane selectively inhibits glutamate release by sodium channel blockade. The release of glutamate and GABA induced by elevated potassium was not influenced by either isoflurane or propofol.

Conclusions.—Isoflurane and propofol were both able to inhibit the release of glutamate and GABA by 4AP. Isoflurane preferentially inhibited glutamate release, which was most likely by sodium channel blockade. Thus, the inhibition of excitatory amino acid transmitter release forms an important part of the mechanisms of neuronal depression produced by volatile anesthetics in clinical concentrations. Propofol's presynaptic effects are weaker in relation to its clinically relevant concentrations. Isoflurane selectively depresses glutamate release, stimulates spontaneous GABA release, and potentiates postsynaptic GABA receptors, yielding complementary actions that produce depressed excitatory and augmented inhibitory CNS transmissions.

▶ Isoflurane and propofol have different effects on glutamate and GABA release in nerve terminals. As new mechanisms of producing anesthesia are defined, the potential exists for the development of more specific target-limited intravenous and inhalational anesthetics.

M. Wood, MD, FRCA

4 Anesthesia Techniques and Monitors

Ultrasound-Guided Supraclavicular Brachial Plexus Block
Chan VW, Perlas A, Rawson R, et al (Univ of Toronto; Toronto Western Hosp)
Anesth Analg 97:1514-1517, 2003   4–1

Background.—The use of US guidance in brachial plexus blocks may enhance success and lower complication rates. US imaging may help localize the brachial plexus accurately, enabling needle advancement to the target nerves. State-of-the-art US technology for supraclavicular brachial plexus blocks was evaluated.

Methods.—Forty outpatients were included in the study. Clinicians used US imaging to identify the brachial plexus before the block, guide the block needle to the target nerves, and visualize the pattern of spread of the local anesthetic. Nerve stimulation before injection was also performed to confirm needle position. The block technique used aligned the needle path and US beam.

Findings.—In 95% of the patients, the block was successful after 1 attempt. One failure was attributed to subcutaneous injection, and 1 was attributed to partial intravascular injection. There were no instances of pneumothorax.

Conclusions.—A high-resolution US probe appears to identify reliably the brachial plexus and surrounding structures in the supraclavicular region. Nerves can be localized quickly through real-time guidance during needle advancement. Identifying distinct patterns of local anesthetic spread on US can further verify that needle location is accurate.

Ultrasound Guidance Speeds Execution and Improves the Quality of Supraclavicular Block
Williams SR, Chouinard P, Arcand G, et al (Université de Montréal)
Anesth Analg 97:1518-1523, 2003   4–2

Background.—The use of ultrasonic guidance in supraclavicular blocks may increase the percentage of successful procedures, reduce execution time, and decrease the incidence of complications. The quality, safety, and execution time of supraclavicular block of the brachial plexus were investigated by using ultrasonic guidance and neurostimulation compared with a supraclavicular method of anatomic landmarks and neurostimulation.

Methods.—Eighty patients were enrolled in the randomized trial. The 40 patients in group US received supraclavicular block guided in real time by a 2-dimensional ultrasonic image, with neurostimulator confirmation of correct needle placement. The 40 patients with group NS underwent supraclavicular block by using the subclavian perivascular approach, also with neurostimulator confirmation. Bupivacaine 0.5% and lidocaine 2% were used, with epinephrine 1:200,000 as the anesthetic mixture. Patients were assessed over a 30-minute period for onset of motor and sensory block for the musculocutaneous, median, radial, and ulnar nerves.

Findings.—At 30 minutes, 95% of group US and 85% of group NS had partial or complete sensory block of all nerve territories. Also, 55% of group US and 65% of group NS had a complete block of all nerve territories. In 85% of group US and 78% of group NS, surgical anesthesia without supplementation was obtained. None of the group US patients, compared with 8% of group NS patients, needed general anesthesia. In group NS but not group US, the quality of ulnar block was significantly inferior to the quality of block in other nerve territories. The quality of ulnar block did not differ significantly between groups NS and US. Block was achieved in a mean 9.8 minutes in group NS and 5 minutes in group US. Neither group had major complications.

Conclusions.—US-guided neurostimulator-confirmed supraclavicular block provides a more complete block than supraclavicular block with anatomic landmarks and neurostimulator confirmation. The former method also can be performed more rapidly than the latter.

▶ State-of-the-art US technology is increasingly being used to enhance successful peripheral nerve blockade, as these 2 studies illustrate (Abstracts 4–1 and 4–2)

M. Wood, MD, FRCA

Preventing Complication of Central Venous Catheterization
McGee DC, Gould MK (Stanford Univ, Calif; Veterans Affairs Palo Alto Health Care System, Calif)
N Engl J Med 348:1123-1133, 2003   4–3

Background.—Although central venous catheters permit the monitoring of hemodynamic variables that cannot be accurately measured otherwise and allow medications and nutritional support to be administered safely, their use is accompanied by adverse events that can be life threatening as well as costly.

Types of Catheters and Sites of Insertion.—Antimicrobial-impregnated catheters lower the rate of catheter-related bloodstream infections and thus decrease direct medical costs. Resistant organisms present an important concern with the use of these catheters. No difference in complication rates was noted between single- and multiple-lumen catheters, so the type chosen should reflect the need, either delivering medications or providing nutritional support. Central venous catheterization can be achieved via the internal jugular, subclavian, or femoral venous access routes.

Complications.—Mechanical complications include arterial puncture, hematoma, and pneumothorax—with similar risks for these whether internal jugular or subclavian venous catheterization is used—and greater risks for the femoral venous route. However, the rate of serious mechanical complications is similar between subclavian and femoral insertion. Infectious complications may arise because of infection at the exit site that leads to migration of the pathogen along the external catheter surface, contamination of the catheter hub, or hematogenous seeding of the catheter. The lowest rate of infectious complications occurs with subclavian venous catheterization.

Thrombotic complications are a significant risk, with venous thrombosis found in 33% of patients in medical ICUs; 15% of these are related to catheters. The lowest risk for thrombotic complications is seen with subclavian venous catheterization. Factors that influence the risk of complications associated with insertion include the physician's experience with catheterization, the use of US guidance, the prompt identification of arterial puncture, the prevention of air embolism, and the use of prophylactic antibiotics, although the last has the potential to increase the emergence of antibiotic-resistant organisms.

Antibiotic ointments have been used to maintain the insertion site but carry the risk of colonization by fungi, promote the emergence of antibiotic-resistant organisms, and do not lower the rate of catheter-related bloodstream infections; therefore, their use is discouraged. While catheter hubs can be a source of contamination, 2 types of antiseptic-containing hubs decrease the risk of infection; needleless access devices have been associated with increased infection rates.

The probability that a patient will acquire a catheter-related infection increases the longer the catheter is left in place; however, scheduled routine exchanges of catheters over a guide wire have been linked to an increased rate of catheter-related infections, along with a higher risk of having a mechanical complication. Therefore, the scheduled replacement of central venous catheters is not recommended. Even with all preventive efforts in place, some patients develop catheter-related infections. Care for these includes prompt identification, empirical antibiotic therapy if sepsis or septic shock is present, and removal of the catheter.

Conclusion.—Catheter-related complications are seen in a significant number of patients each year. In this report, the principal problems are outlined, and methods for reducing the frequency of complications in adult patients are noted.

▶ A superb review article of central venous catheter techniques and the complications that accompany their use. It really drives home the message that frequent (scheduled) catheter changes can increase the risk of mechanical and infectious complications, a habit hard to break around my workplace.

J. D. Lang, Jr, MD

Ultrasound Imaging of the Axillary Vein—Anatomical Basis for Central Venous Access
Galloway S, Bodenham A (Leeds Gen Infirmary, England)
Br J Anaesth 90:589-595, 2003   4–4

Background.—When central venous access is desired, usually the jugular, subclavian, femoral, or brachial veins are cannulated. If the surface landmark techniques are inadequate to achieve subclavian catheterization, US may be used to place a catheter in the infraclavicular axillary vein. The anatomical relationships between the axillary vessels were evaluated to determine how best to safely approach the axillary vein for cannulation.

Methods.—US was used in 50 subjects (mean age, 64.3 years; range, 30 to 90 years) to examine the infraclavicular regions from under the mid clavicular point and at 2 cm and at 4 cm farther laterally. The arms were held at 0°, 45°, and 90° of abduction. Measurements were obtained at each point, with the artery and vein seen in cross-section. Included were measures of the depth from the skin, the diameters of the vessels, and the distance between the vessels. A scale of 0 to 3 was applied to the degree of overlap present, from no overlap to complete overlap. When visible, the distance between the rib cage and axillary vein was documented. The vein was also imaged longitudinally; the angle of ascent in relation to skin, the length of the vein, and the vein's depth were noted.

Results.—The clavicular length ranged from 12 to 19 cm (mean, 15 cm) in the 50 patients. Forty-one scans were complete with respect to visualizing both vessels. The body mass index for patients whose scans were incomplete was 27.2, while that for patients with complete scans was 25.2. Various relationships were noted between the various subclavian vein tributaries; generally the cephalic vein was smaller than the axillary vein and joined it laterally. In about 12% of the scans, the cephalic vein arose more medially.

Fourteen percent of the subjects had abnormalities, generally unusual combinations of tributaries but also incompressible vessels with no obvious thrombus. Twelve percent of patients had thrombus, with half idiopathic in origin. The brachial plexus could not be visualized reliably. The mean venous diameter was 1.3 cm with a 10° head-down tilt; the mean arterial diameter in this position was 0.8 cm. A median arteriovenous overlap of two thirds was noted with the subject in a 10° head-down tilt.

In 388 of the 900 slices, the rib cage was seen, with 72% in the 0-cm slice, 26% in the 2-cm slice, and 2% in the 4-cm slice. On longitudinal scans, the mean depth of the deepest part of the vein was 2.7 cm and the mean angle between skin and vein was 13.3°, with a range of 1° to 29°.

Conclusion.—The axillary vein and artery are farther apart and farther from the rib cage the more laterally one moves. Thus, the axillary vein would be a good site for central venous access placement. The diameter of the vein, however, decreases with lateral positioning. US is appropriate for locating the vein, given its depth and lack of surface landmarks that reliably mark its position.

▶ An insightful study and legitimate alternative site for vascular access, especially for those chronic patients in the ICU with thrombosis of other traditional sites. This study takes advantage of technology that is now cost effective and that should be commonly available and in use in the settings such as the ICU and operating room.

J. D. Lang, Jr, MD

Performance of Noninvasive Partial CO_2 Rebreathing Cardiac Output and Continuous Thermodilution Cardiac Output in Patients Undergoing Aortic Reconstruction Surgery
Kotake Y, Moriyama K, Innami Y (Keio Univ, Tokyo)
Anesthesiology 99:283-288, 2003   4–5

Background.—Maintaining optimal cardiac output is an important goal of intraoperative hemodynamic management. Noninvasive cardiac output monitoring (NICO) by the partial CO_2 rebreathing method has many advantages but has not been fully validated. NICO and continuous thermodilution (CCO) were compared with standard bolus thermodilution (BCO) in 28 patients undergoing aortic reconstruction surgery.

Study Design.—The study group consisted of 28 patients undergoing elective aortic reconstruction for infrarenal abdominal aortic aneurysm. Anesthetic management was standardized. After tracheal intubation, cardiac output was continuously monitored by both NICO and CCO. BCO was assessed after anesthetic induction (postinduction), during aortic cross-clamping (XC), at reperfusion of the unilateral iliac artery (declamp), and during peritoneal closure (endop). NICO monitoring was ended postoperatively, but CCO could be maintained at the physician's discretion. Correlations between NICO or CCO and BCO data were analyzed by linear regression. A Bland-Altman plot was used to compare the bias and precision of the different methods.

Findings.—The bias and precision from all the measurements between NICO and BCO was − 0.58 ± 0.9 L/min, and for CCO and BCO it was 0.38 ± 1.17 L/min. The bias between NICO and BCO was small after anesthetic induction and during cross-clamp, but increased after reperfusion. The bias between CCO and BCO was small until reperfusion but increased significantly during peritoneal closure.

Conclusions.—Cardiac output monitoring by NICO is accurate after anesthetic induction but underestimates cardiac output after aortic cross-clamping and declamping. Cardiac output monitoring by CCO has less bias but overestimates cardiac output at the end of surgery. NICO appears to be a useful method for noninvasive monitoring of cardiac output during elective aortic reconstructive surgery.

▶ This is an excellently done article and will prove to be a classic in its field on cardiac output monitoring and comparison of techniques. If you are interested in the field, this is an excellent article to learn from.

M. F. Roizen, MD

The EmulSiv™ Filter Removes Microbial Contamination From Propofol But Is Not a Substitute for Aseptic Technique
Hall WCE, Jolly DT, Hrazdil J, et al (Univ of Alberta, Edmonton, Canada)
Can J Anesth 50:541-546, 2003   4–6

Introduction.—The incidence of patient-acquired infections from anesthetic practices has been considered insignificant, but this presumption was challenged after the introduction of propofol. Failure in aseptic anesthetic technique became apparent when postoperative infections and sepsis acquired from the use of propofol during anesthesia were documented. The EmulSiv filter (EF; Pall Biomedical Products Co, East Hill, NY) was specifically created for use with lipid emulsion drugs like propofol. The ability of the EF to remove extrinsic microbial contaminants from propofol was examined with 10 microbes.

Methods.—The microbial agents used in the study were *Staphylococcus aureus, Escherichia coli, Moraxella osloensis, Klebsiella pneumoniae, Enterobacter agglomerans, Candida albicans, Serratia marcescens, Moraxella catarrhalis, Haemophilus influenzae,* and *Campylobacter jejuni.* The first 7 in the list had been documented in outbreaks of propofol contamination; the 3 remaining microbial agents were assessed because of their unusual structure or small size. Study solutions consisted of 10-mL and 20-mL samples of inoculated propofol filtered through the EF. These volumes were selected to represent common adult and pediatric doses. Unfiltered inoculated propofol solutions served as controls.

Results.—The EF was effective in removing *E coli, S aureus, K pneumoniae, M catarrhalis,* and *C albicans* from contaminated propofol. A small number of *H influenzae* colony-forming units (CFU), however, evaded filtration in both 10-mL and 20-mL samples. In the 10-mL sample only, *C jejuni* CFU evaded filtration. Filter efficacy was 100% in both sample sizes for *M osloensis, E agglomerans,* and *S marcescens.*

Conclusion.—Bacteria such as *E coli* were too large to pass through the EF, but organisms such as *H influenzae,* which are pleomorphic and variable in size, and *C jejuni,* which is a coiled spiral, may be able to "squeeze" through. Even the use of an effective filter such as the EF is no substitute for meticulous aseptic technique in the handling and administration of propofol.

▶ While the use of this filter decreases bacterial counts in a laboratory set-ting, as is demonstrated in this study, it is not clear how the filter would per-form in clinical practice where there are extra steps during which contamina-tion could occur when using this device. It is a low enough contamination rate with propofol that it is unclear what the result would be. I hope the authors will do that clinical (real life) study.

M. F. Roizen, MD

Using Amsorb to Detect Dehydration of CO_2 Absorbents Containing Strong Base

Knolle E, Linert W, Gilly H (Univ of Vienna; Technical Univ of Vienna; L Boltzmann Inst for Experimental Anesthesiology and Research in Intensive Care, Vienna)
Anesthesiology 97:454-459, 2002   4–7

Background.—In clinical practice, the drying out of carbon dioxide absorbents from exposure to fresh gas flow in an anesthesia machine can re-sult in pathologically increased concentrations of carboxyhemoglobin in the patient. It cannot be determined in a clinical setting when this desiccation is occurring. However, Amsorb (Armstrong, Coleraine, Northern Ireland)—a recently developed absorbent that contains no strong bases and produces no carbon monoxide, even when completely dry—has been observed to change color from white to violet when dried. Whether Amsorb in combination with different strong base-containing carbon dioxide absorbents signals de-hydration of these absorbents was investigated.

Methods.—This study involved 5 different carbon dioxide absorbents, each of which was topped with 70g of Amsorb. The absorbents were dried in an anesthesia machine with oxygen. When a color change was detected in the Amsorb, the samples were tested for change in weight and formation of carbon monoxide from 7.5% desflurane or 4% isoflurane. In a second ex-periment, Amsorb was layered at the drying gas outflow site. In still other experiments, Amsorb was tested for color change from drying and rehydrat-ing and from drying with nitrogen. In the final experiment, a mixture of Amsorb and 1% NaOH was dried and examined for color change.

Results.—In the experiments in which Amsorb was layered at the inflow, the Amsorb changed color when the water content of the samples was mar-ginally reduced (to a mean of 13.6%) with no formation of carbon monox-ide. In the experiment in which Amsorb was layered at the outflow, it changed color when the mean water content was reduced to 8.8%, and vary-ing degrees of carbon monoxide formation were detected. The change in color was independent of the drying gas and could be reversed by rehydra-tion. In the final experiment, the addition of NaOH to Amsorb prevented the color change.

Conclusion.—The addition of Amsorb as a top layer at the fresh gas in-flow provides a reliable indication of dehydration in strong base-containing absorbents. It is assumed that the mechanism of this color change is the absence of strong base in Amsorb.

▶ This study attempts to find ways of avoiding the Monday morning syndrome of carbon monoxide production when desflurane, enflurane, and isoflurane are first exposed to dry absorbents. That the use of this substance needs to be machine specific and probably tested under different humidity conditions in each operating room means to me that the solution they have proposed is not readily generalizable. It would be nice if they had, in fact, tested this in a more generalizable solution to see if it depends on atmosphere humidity over the weekend, etc. Like good studies, this one raises more questions than answers.

M. F. Roizen, MD

5 Cardiothoracic and Vascular Anesthesia

Selective COX-2 Inhibition Improves Endothelial Function in Coronary Artery Disease
Chenevard R, Hürlimann D, Béchir M, et al (Univ Hosp Zürich, Switzerland; Kantonsspital St Gallen, Switzerland)
Circulation 107:405-409, 2003   5-1

Background.—The gastrointestinal toxicity of conventional nonsteroidal anti-inflammatory drugs (NSAIDs) and aspirin stems from the inhibition of COX-1, which synthesizes gastroprotective prostaglandins. The selective COX-2 inhibitors (such as celecoxib, rofecoxib, and valdecoxib) were developed in response to the finding that the anti-inflammatory and pain-relieving effects of NSAIDs and aspirin are derived mainly from the inhibition of inducible COX-2–dependent inflammatory pathways.

Clinical trials have demonstrated the efficacy of coxibs compared with NSAIDs in the treatment of patients with arthritis, with a lower incidence of gastrointestinal side effects, However, there is an ongoing debate as to whether the gastrointestinal safety of these COX-2 inhibitors is obtained at the cost of increased cardiovascular side effects. The effects of selective COX-2 inhibitors on clinically useful surrogates for cardiovascular disease, particularly endothelial function, were investigated.

Methods.—A total of 14 male patients with a mean age of 66 ± 3 years and with severe coronary artery disease who were undergoing stable background therapy with aspirin and statins were included in this double-blind, placebo-controlled, crossover study. The patients were treated with celecoxib, 200 mg twice a day, or placebo for 2 weeks. Flow-mediated dilation of the brachial artery, high-sensitivity C-reactive protein, oxidized LDL, and prostaglandins were measured after each treatment period.

Results.—Endothelium-dependent vasodilation was significantly improved with celecoxib compared with placebo, while endothelium-independent vasodilation, as assessed by nitroglycerin, was unchanged. High-sensitivity C-reactive protein and oxidized LDL were significantly lower after celecoxib than after placebo, while prostaglandins were unchanged.

Conclusion.—These findings are the first to demonstrate that selective COX-2 inhibition results in improved endothelium-dependent vasodilation and reduced low-grade chronic inflammation and oxidative stress in patients with coronary artery disease. It would appear from these findings that the use of selective COX-2 inhibition may improve outcomes in patients with cardiovascular disease.

▶ One of disappointments of COX-2 inhibitor therapy is that the epidemiologic data have not shown it to be as beneficial as aspirin for decreasing aging of our arteries. This study seems to indicate that the epidemiologic data may not prove true in randomized intervention studies; that is, COX-2 inhibitors may be as good as aspirin in the intervention studies. Such studies have not been published yet, but this study shows that—at least from a point of vasodilation, stress testing, and anti-inflammatory effect the COX-2 inhibitors appear much better than placebos. Are they as good as aspirin? We don't know. That is one of the deficits of this study. It did not compare COX-2 with aspirin; it only compared COX-2 with placebo.

M. F. Roizen, MD

Increased Serum Homocysteine and Sudden Death Resulting From Coronary Atherosclerosis With Fibrosis Plaques

Burke AP, Fonseca V, Kolodgie F, et al (Armed Forces Inst of Pathology, Washington, DC; Veteran's Affairs Med Ctr, Little Rock, Ark; Louisiana State Univ, New Orleans)
Arterioscler Thromb Vasc Biol 22:1936-1941, 2002   5–2

Background.—Elevation of serum homocysteine is associated with coronary artery disease. This study compared homocysteine levels in men who died suddenly of coronary artery disease to a control group of men who died of noncoronary causes.

Study Design.—Postmortem serum homocysteine was determined in 87 men with coronary thrombus, 35 men with severe coronary disease without thrombus, and 46 controls who died of other causes. The average age of death was 50 years for all 3 groups. Atherosclerotic plaques were classified.

Findings.—Median serum homocysteine was 10.4 µmol/L in men with acute thrombus, 12.1 µmol/L in men with organized thrombus, 12.5 µmol/L in men without thrombus, and 9.8 µmol/L in control subjects. Median serum homocysteine was 12.1 µmol/L in men with healed infarcts. The number of fibrous plaques was associated with log-normalized homocysteine independent of other risk factors such as age, albumin, smoking, hypertension, and serum cholesterol. Homocysteine levels in the upper tertile (>15 µmol/L) were associated with sudden death without acute or organized thrombus, independent of other risk factors. Diabetes mellitus increased the association.

Conclusion.—Elevated serum homocysteine was associated with sudden death in men in the absence of acute coronary thrombosis, especially when diabetes was also present. Elevated serum homocysteine levels were associated with fibrous plaques and were not associated with thin-cap atheromas, suggesting that their association with atherosclerosis differs from that of hypercholesterolemia.

▶ This is 1 in a series of now about 15 articles showing that homocysteine level correlates with aging of the arteries and with development of fibrous plaques. The mechanism for this harm from homocysteine is not known, but we start seeing reports of tests in preoperative evaluation clinics of homocysteine level. But you don't have to really worry about this yourself. Just take 800 μg of folate a day, plus appropriate RDA or daily values of B6, B12 (requirement of B12 increases dramatically with age as we start malabsorbing it over the age of about 60), and you'll have a low homocysteine level.

The message here is you want a homocysteine level less than 9, and it is easy to obtain it by taking folate, B6, and B12. By the way, an elevated homocysteine level of 20 was the equivalent (as far as increasing the risk of arterial aging events including sudden death) of having type II diabetes or low-density lipoprotein cholesterol of over 200.

M. F. Roizen, MD

Use of Continuous Quality Improvement to Increase Use of Process Measures in Patients Undergoing Coronary Artery Bypass Graft Surgery: A Randomized Controlled Trial
Ferguson TB Jr, for the Society of Thoracic Surgeons and the National Cardiac Database (Louisiana State Univ, New Orleans; et al)
JAMA 290:49-56, 2003   5–3

Introduction.—Randomized trials assessing the effectiveness of continuous quality improvement (CQI) as an approach to quality improvement in medicine have generated mixed results. A randomized trial of CQI in medicine was performed on a national scale to determine whether low-intensity CQI intervention can be used to speed the national adoption of 2 coronary artery bypass graft (CABG) surgery process-of-care measures: preoperative β-blockade therapy and internal mammary artery (IMA) grafting in patients 75 years of age or older.

Methods.—Three hundred fifty-nine academic and nonacademic hospitals that performed CABG surgery in 267,917 patients and were participating in the Society of Thoracic Surgeons National Cardiac Database between January 2000 and July 2002 were randomly assigned to either a control arm or 1 of 2 groups that used CQI interventions created to increase the use of process-of-care measures. Each intervention group received measure-specific information, including a call to action to a physician leader; educational products; and periodic longitudinal, nationally benchmarked, site-specific feedback. The primary outcome measure was differential incorporation of the targeted care processes into practice at the intervention sites versus control sites. Preintervention (January-December 2000)/postintervention (January 2001-July 2002) site differences were measured; a hierarchical patient-level analysis was used.

Results.—Between January 2000 and July 2002, the use of both process measures increased nationally (β blockade, 60.0%-65.6%; IMA grafting, 76.2%-82.8%). The use of β-blockade was significantly greater at β-blockade intervention sites (7.3%) compared with control sites (3.6%) in the preintervention/postintervention ($P = .04$) and hierarchical analyses ($P < .001$). The use of IMA grafting tended to increase at IMA intervention sites, compared with control sites (8.7% vs 5.4%; $P = .20$ and $P = .11$ for preintervention/postintervention and hierarchical analyses, respectively). Both interventions tended to have more influence at lower volume CABG sites (for interaction; $P = .04$ for β-blockade; $P = .02$ for IMA grafting).

Conclusion.—A multifaceted, physician-guided, low-intensity CQI effort can enhance the adoption of care processes into national practice within the context of a medical specialty society infrastructure.

▶ This is an unusual study—a randomized trial of quality improvement with 2 interventions, viz, β-adrenergic blockade and IMA grafting for elderly patients in the setting of cardiac surgery performed on a national scale. The point is that national practice changed. Could this mechanism be used to achieve an intervention on a national level in anesthesiology? Should anesthesiology societies develop infrastructure and clinical databases such as seen for the Society of Thoracic Surgeons and the National Cardiac Database?

M. Wood, MD, FRCA

Efficacy and Safety of the Cyclooxygenase 2 Inhibitors Parecoxib and Valdecoxib in Patients Undergoing Coronary Artery Bypass Surgery

Ott E, for the Multicenter Study of Perioperative Ischemia (McSPI) Research Group and the Ischemia Research and Education Foundation (IREF) Investigators (Ischemia Research and Education Found, San Francisco, Calif; et al)
J Thorac Cardiovasc Surg 125:1481-1492, 2003   5–4

Introduction.—High-risk populations have not been specifically evaluated in earlier selective cyclooxygenase 2 (COX-2) inhibitor analgesia clinical trials. Thus, experience is limited concerning the efficacy and safety in these patients. Patients undergoing coronary artery bypass grafting (CABG) surgery were evaluated by a new parenteral combined with oral COX-2 selective inhibitor.

Methods.—A total of 462 patients with New York Heart Association classes I to III younger than 77 years from 58 institutions in the United States, Canada, Germany, and the United Kingdom were evaluated in a multicenter, phase III, placebo-controlled, double-blind, randomized, parallel-group investigation. Patients were allocated in a 2:1 ratio to either parecoxib/valdecoxib or standard care (control subjects). IV study drugs were given within 30 minutes after extubation and every 12 hours for a minimum of 3 days. Oral treatment at a dose of 40 mg was subsequently administered every 12 hours for a total of 14 days. Patient-controlled analgesia was administered as needed. Evaluation of the analgesic efficacy of parecoxib/valdecoxib was primarily based on morphine and morphine equivalent use. Additional efficacy assessments included daily pain intensity, physician global assessment of study medication, and pain effect on quality of life. Clinical adverse events were investigated at each site from time of initial dose through the 30-day postdosing period.

Results.—Patients in the parecoxib/valdecoxib group required significantly less morphine or morphine equivalent compared with control subjects during the 0- to 24-hour (P = .009), 24- to 48-h (P = .017), 72- to 96-hour (P = .002), 96- to 120-hour (P = .004), and 120- to 144-hour (P = .037) periods. Patients (P < .001) and physicians (P < .001) rated the study medication as significantly better than control therapy. The modified Brief Pain Inventory questionnaire used during the oral dosing period identified significant improvements in the parecoxib/valdecoxib treatment group in 6 of 8 domains evaluated. There were no significant between-group differences in overall adverse events; serious adverse events were observed twice as often in the study medication versus control group (19.0% vs 9.9%; P = .015); the rate of sternal wound infection was higher in the parecoxib/valdecoxib group than the control group (3.2% vs 0%; P = .035).

Conclusion.—In patients undergoing CABG surgery, parecoxib/valdecoxib provided effective postoperative analgesia. The 14-day treatment regimen was linked with an increased incidence of sternal wound infections. Further investigation is needed before these COX-2 inhibitors can be recommended for use in patients undergoing CABG surgery.

▶ This is a large and well-conducted prospective randomized trial of COX-2 inhibitors after CABG. Patients were started on IV COX-2 inhibitors within 24 hours of surgery and then continued with oral agents up to day 14 postoperatively. There are 2 very important findings. First, these agents were effective analgesic agents, decreasing opioid use and decreasing pain compared with placebo at all times studied. Second, serious adverse events were significantly more likely to occur in the patients receiving COX-2 inhibitors. Total serious adverse events, defined as potentially life threatening or requiring readmission, and sternal wound infections were more common. This raises serious concerns that these drugs, while effective, might be unacceptably dangerous in this patient population. While the authors suggest that these patients reflect only about 30% of total CABG patients, looking at the inclusion and exclusion criteria they reflect the healthiest subgroup. While different dosing regimens—either lower doses, or shorter duration of treatment—might be acceptable, until such dosing regimens are studied and demonstrated to be both safe and effective, anesthesiologist should be cautious when considering use of COX-2 inhibitors in cardiac surgery patients.

M. F. Trankina, MD

Assessment of Neurocognitive Impairment After Off-Pump and On-Pump Techniques for Coronary Artery Bypass Graft Surgery: Prospective Randomised Controlled Trial

Zamvar V, Williams D, Hall J, et al (Univ Hosp of Wales, Cardiff; Providence Health System, Portland, Ore; UK Natl External Quality Assurance Scheme, Sheffield, England)

BMJ 325:1268-1271, 2002   5–5

Introduction.—Neurologic injury is an important complication after coronary artery bypass graft (CABG) surgery and consists of 2 types. Type 1 injuries include stroke, transient ischemic attack and coma (incidence, 3%-6%); type 2 injury is more subtle and includes impairment of cognitive function. The impact of on-pump and off-pump techniques on neurocognitive impairment was examined in patients undergoing CABG surgery for triple vessel disease in a randomized controlled investigation.

Methods.—Sixty patients undergoing CABG surgery for triple vessel disease were prospectively randomly assigned to either an off-pump or an on-pump technique. The primary outcome measures were a change in scores in 9 standard neuropsychometric tests administered preoperatively and at 1 and 10 weeks postoperatively.

Results.—The on-pump group demonstrated a significantly greater deterioration in scores for 2 and 3 tests at 1 and 10 weeks postoperatively, respectively, compared with the off-pump group. The on-pump group had a significantly higher rate of major deterioration in 1 of the tests both at 1 and 10 weeks postoperatively (Table 1). The rate of neurocognitive impairment at 1 week postoperatively was 27% (8/30) in the off-pump group and 63% (19/30) in the on-pump group ($P = .004$); at 10 weeks postoperatively, it was 10% (3/30) in the off-pump group and 40% (12/30) in the on-pump group ($P = .017$).

Conclusion.—Off-pump CABG surgery is associated with less neurocognitive impairment than the on-pump technique.

▶ This is an important study describing CNS cognitive defects "off pump" and "on pump"—important because it is a prospective randomized trial. As expected from previous studies, "off pump" CABG results in less neurocognitive impairment than "on pump" techniques. Only 60 patients were studied, so it is not a large multicenter trial. Nonetheless, as an accompanying editorial[1] notes, the results were striking.

M. Wood, MD, FRCA

Reference

1. Taggart D: Off-pump coronary artery bypass may be associated with lesser postoperative neurocognitive impairment (editorial). *BMJ* 325:1255-1256, 2002.

TABLE.—Percentage of Patients in Each Group Who Had Deterioration of 1 Standard Deviation or Greater in Individual Tests at 1 Week and 10 Weeks Postoperatively

Test	1 Week Postoperatively				10 Weeks Postoperatively			
	Off-Pump (n=30)	On-Pump (n=29)	Difference %	95% CI	Off-Pump (n=30)	On-Pump (n=30)	Difference %	95% CI
Rey auditory verbal learning test	13.3	34.5	21.2	(−0.7 to 41.0)	10.0	23.3	13.3	(−6.1 to 32.1)
Part A of trail making test	26.7	44.8	18.2	(−6.0 to 39.8)	6.7	16.7	10.0	(−7.4 to 27.6)
Part B of trail making test	23.3	44.8	21.5	(−2.6 to 42.6)	10.0	30.0	20.0	(−0.5 to 39.0)
Grooved pegboard test using dominant hand	13.3	31.0	17.7	(−3.7 to 37.6)	0	20.0	20.0	(4.5 to 37.3)*
Grooved pegboard test using non-dominant hand	6.7	48.3	41.6	(19.3 to 59.6)*	3.3	16.7	13.3	(−2.9 to 30.5)
Digit symbol substitution test	6.7	24.1	17.5	(−1.4 to 36.1)	3.3	13.3	10.0	(−5.6 to 26.6)
Digit span forward test	10.0	27.6	17.6	(−2.7 to 36.9)	0	10.0	10.0	(−3.1 to 25.6)
Digit span backward test	6.7	20.7	14.0	(−4.2 to 32.4)	0	0	0	(−11.4 to 11.4)
Controlled oral word association test	6.7	27.6	20.9	(1.4 to 39.7)*	3.3	10.0	6.7	(−8.2 to 22.5)

*Excludes 0.

Abbreviation: CI, Confidence interval.

(Courtesy of Zamvar V, Williams D, Hall J, et al: Assessment of neurocognitive impairment after off-pump and on-pump techniques for coronary artery bypass graft surgery: Prospective randomized controlled trial. *BMJ* 325:1268-1271, 2002. Reprinted with permission from the BMJ Publishing Group.)

A Comparison of On-pump and Off-pump Coronary Bypass Surgery in Low-risk Patients

Nathoe HM, for the Study Group (Univ Med Ctr, Utrecht, The Netherlands; et al)

N Engl J Med 348:394-402, 2003   5–6

Background.—Coronary artery bypass grafting is an important component in the management of ischemic heart disease. Bypass with cardiac arrest, or "on-pump," provides a blood-free and motion-free surgical field, which facilitates the safe construction of the anastomoses. However, it is believed that the use of cardiopulmonary bypass is a major determinant of perioperative morbidity, hospital stay, and costs. As a result, "off-pump" coronary bypass surgery has been reintroduced into clinical practice. It is thought that the off-pump procedure may reduce perioperative morbidity and costs, but it is unclear whether outcomes for off-pump and on-pump surgery are similar. The cardiac outcome and cost effectiveness of on-pump coronary bypass surgery were compared with those of the off-pump bypass surgery.

Methods.—In this multicenter, randomized trial, 139 patients with predominantly single- or double-vessel coronary disease were assigned to on-pump surgery, and 142 similar patients were assigned to off-pump surgery. The main outcome measures were cardiac outcome and cost effectiveness 1 year after surgery. Bootstrapping was used to address the uncertainty regarding the cost-effectiveness ratio.

Results.—At 1-year follow-up, the rate of freedom from death, stroke, myocardial infarction, and coronary intervention was 90.6% after on-pump surgery and 88% after off-pump surgery. In a subgroup of patients selected randomly, graft patency was 93% after on-pump surgery and 91% after off-pump surgery. On-pump surgery cost per patient was $14,908 compared with $13,069 cost per patient for off-pump surgery, a difference per patient of $1839 or 14.1%. On-pump surgery resulted in an increase in quality-adjusted years of life of 0.83 compared with 0.82 for off-pump surgery. In 95% of bootstrap estimates, off-pump surgery was more cost effective than on-pump surgery.

Conclusions.—Coronary bypass surgery in low-risk patients resulted in no difference in cardiac outcome at 1 year between patients who underwent on-pump procedures and those who underwent off-pump procedures. However, off-pump surgery was found to be more cost effective.

▶ The performance of coronary artery bypass grafting without the use cardiopulmonary bypass has become popular in recent years. The complexity of anesthetic management is greater than that for routine on-pump surgery, but despite the lack of randomized clinical trials, perioperative morbidity (eg, stroke) was believed to be less. This article shows the value of randomized controlled trials, in that there was no significant difference in cardiac outcome between these 2 techniques. However, the lack of significant difference between the 2 groups suggests that off-pump surgery is a viable alternative. In addition, off-pump surgery was more cost-effective.

M. Wood, MD, FRCA

Platelet Function After Coronary Artery Bypass Grafting: Is There a Procoagulant Activity After Off-Pump Compared With On-pump Surgery?
Møller CH, Steinbrüchel DA (Univ of Copenhagen)
Scand Cardiovasc J 37:149-153, 2003   5–7

Introduction.—The extracorporeal circulation of the blood initiates a diffuse systemic inflammatory response, which produces a greater risk of respiratory, renal, and neurologic complications and interferes with hemostasis. The cause of this disorder is multifactorial; transient platelet dysfunction is considered one of the most important components, which is attributed to coating of platelet surfaces by fibrin degradation products, loss of surface receptors, and α-degranulation. By avoiding extracorporeal circulation and full heparinization, respiratory, renal, and neurologic complications are not avoided but may be diminished. This may preserve hemostasis, which may result in procoagulant activity with a higher risk of venous thrombosis and a potential danger to the patency of coronary anastomoses. Thirty patients were prospectively evaluated to determine whether this possibly better preserved hemostasis produces procoagulant activity of the platelets.

Methods.—Of 30 patients evaluated, 15 underwent on-pump coronary artery bypass (CABG) and 15 underwent off-pump coronary artery bypass (OPCAB). Platelet function was assessed 4 times within the first 24 hours: preoperatively, immediately postoperatively, and 4 hours and 1 day postoperatively by a bedside whole blood clotting test.

Results.—A significant increase in platelet activating factor–induced platelet aggregation was seen postoperatively after OPCAB (*P* < .01). Two patients did not achieve preoperative values within 1 day postoperatively and 2 patients had a more than 2-fold increase. Platelet aggregation immediately after on-pump CABG was diminished to nearly half of postoperative values; within 1 day postoperatively, normal platelet aggregation was regained in half the cohort.

Conclusion.—After OPCAB, platelets were more easily activated during the early postoperative period. A temporary platelet dysfunction was observed after CABG with cardiopulmonary bypass that appeared to be overcome within the first postoperative day.

▶ This small prospective study evaluated one aspect of platelet function after cardiac surgery, comparing cardiopulmonary bypass procedures with off-pump procedures. The results suggest that after OPCAB platelets are more easily activated immediately and for at least the first 24 hours postoperatively compared with preoperatively. In contrast, after CABG platelets are initially less easily activated, with return to baseline function by 24 hours. Because this study did not follow platelet activation past 24 hours, and it was not designed to investigate complications related either to bleeding or to a procoagulant state, clinical implications can only be speculated on. The lack of platelet inhibition after OPCAB may be beneficial by preventing early bleeding complications but may predispose to thromboembolic complications. Only larger studies looking at platelet function for longer periods and at complications will answer this important question.

M. F. Trankina, MD

The Effects of Magnesium Prime Solution on Magnesium Levels and Potassium Loss in Open Heart Surgery
Jian W, Su L, Yiwu L, et al (Hebei Med Univ, Shijiazhuang, People's Republic of China)
Anesth Analg 96:1617-1620, 2003   5–8

Introduction.—Magnesium deficiency can impair cardiac conduction, increase the risk for arrhythmias, predispose to coronary artery spasm, and encourage neurologic irritability. Few measures have been taken to prevent hypomagnesemia and its effects during the perioperative period in pediatric patients undergoing cardiopulmonary bypass (CPB). The effects of magnesium supplementation in the CPB prime solution on magnesium levels and potassium loss with open heart surgery were examined in pediatric patients.

Methods.—Forty pediatric patients with normal heart, liver, and kidney function undergoing open heart surgery with CPB for repair of ventricular septal defect were randomly assigned to treatment with either magnesium sulfate (0.25 mmol/kg) or saline placebo supplementation to the prime solution. Ionized magnesium (IMg) and urinary magnesium and potassium, along with arterial blood, were obtained at defined time points during and after CPB. After the procedure, calcium and potassium were supplemented to normal levels.

Results.—Patients in the magnesium group had a large IMg blood concentration during CPB and normal levels postoperatively. The IMg levels were significantly lower for patients in the placebo group. Creatinine, potassium, and calcium levels were within the reference range for patients in both groups at all evaluation points. There were no between-group differences in requirement for calcium, potassium, or furosemide. After aortic cross-clamp removal, 5 (25%) patients in the placebo group and 2 (10%) in the magnesium group had ventricular fibrillation (P = not significant).

Conclusion.—Adding magnesium to the prime solution can prevent hypomagnesemia during and after CPB and can reduce the urinary potassium loss after CPB. Routine supplementation of magnesium sulfate may be beneficial in pediatric patients undergoing cardiac surgery with CPB.

▶ The authors in a homogenous group of patients undergoing a single cardiac surgical procedure (ventricular septal defect repair) demonstrated that adding IMg to the cardiopulmonary bypass prime solution prevented hypomagnesemia during and after CPB. The patients without IMg added to the prime solution had only transient hypomagnesemia. Given that there were no complications from the IMg administration and the known contribution of hypomagnesemia to postbypass dysrhythmias and cardiac dysfunction, this seems a reasonable intervention to consider.

M. F. Trankina, MD

Volume Expansion With Albumin Decreases Mortality After Coronary Artery Bypass Graft Surgery
Sedrakyan A, Gondek K, Paltiel D, et al (Yale Univ, New Haven, Conn; Bayer Corp, West Haven, Conn)
Chest 123:1853-1857, 2003   5–9

Introduction.—Albumin and nonprotein colloids are often used as blood volume expanders perioperatively in patients undergoing coronary artery bypass graft (CABG) surgery. Cost concerns motivate a trend to replace albumin with low-cost nonprotein colloids during cardiac surgery. Earlier reports have demonstrated that nonprotein colloid volume expanders are linked with excessive postoperative bleeding. A large administrative dataset that specifically reported information on colloid use was used to ascertain whether albumin use is associated with decreased risk of death.

Methods.—Discharge data obtained for the Solucient Clinical Pathways Database from 19,578 patients undergoing CABG surgery was used from 182 United States hospitals in 1997 and 116 U.S. hospitals in 1998. Excluded were patients simultaneously undergoing cardiac aneurysm excision surgery and those who received both albumin and a nonprotein colloid expander. Those who underwent simultaneous cardiac valve repair or replacement were included. Comorbidity profiles were created. Demographic, institutional, and procedure-related variables were included. Mortality was considered to be in-hospital and all-cause deaths. A multivariable model was created.

Results.—Albumin was administered in 8084 cases (41.3%). The use of albumin and nonprotein colloids was not associated with patient characteristics. The mortality rate was lower in the albumin versus nonprotein colloid group (2.47% vs 3.03%; $P = .02$). After adjusting for the effect of 16 covariates, multivariable logistic regression analysis revealed that albumin use was linked with 25% lower odds of death versus nonprotein colloid use (odds ratio, 0.80; 95% confidence interval, 0.67-0.96). When albumin versus nonprotein colloids were used, approximately 5 to 6 lives were saved for every 1000 patients who underwent CABG. Patients with simultaneous CABG and valve procedures benefited more from albumin administration than those with isolated CABG procedures (odds ratio, 0.61 vs 0.86).

Conclusion.—Colloid administration in CABG is not associated with patient characteristics and is more likely to be linked to institutional preferences. It appears that the use of albumin versus colloid is associated with a lower rate of mortality after CABG surgery.

▶ While this study has all the limitations of a retrospective look at an administrative, rather than clinical, dataset, it reports an interesting observation. The authors report a decreased risk of mortality associated with the use of albumin as opposed to nonprotein colloid solutions even by multivariate analysis, including many variables known to be associated with alteration of mortality rates after cardiac surgery. Of concern in interpreting these data is the failure to include myocardial infarction, congestive heart failure, and atrial fibrillation in the analysis. The rationale given is understandable. Still, these conditions are well known to increase mortality rate in CABG patients, and their exclusion from the multivariate analysis should be considered. The incidence of these conditions was similar in the 2 groups and may well not have affected the results. In addition to the reduction in morality rate with use of albumin, a number of other treatment options were associated with decreased mortality— notably the use of mammary grafts and, as in other major procedures, performance of the procedure in high-volume centers.

M. F. Trunkina, MD

Intraoperative Transesophageal Echocardiography in Pediatric Congenital Cardiac Surgery: A Two-Center Observational Study
Bettex DA, Schmidlin D, Bernath M-A, et al (Univ Hosp of Zurich, Switzerland; Univ Hosp of Lausanne, Switzerland)
Anesth Analg 97:1275-1282, 2003   5–10

Introduction.—Practice guidelines for perioperative transesophageal echocardiography (TEE) established for the American Society of Cardiovascular Anesthesiologists and the American Society of Anesthesiologists state that there is strong evidence for the usefulness of TEE in surgery for congenital heart disease because it significantly improves clinical outcome in these patients. Although anesthesiologists are primarily responsible for the interpretation of intraoperative TEE during adult cardiac surgery, their role in TEE during congenital cardiac surgery is under debate. Reports were reviewed from 865 routine TEE examinations performed between January 1994 and March 2002 in patients younger than 7 years who were undergoing surgery for congenital heart disease.

Methods.—Median patient age was 36 months (range, 1 day to 16 years). All patients weighing less than 3.5 kg underwent routine TEE examination in the absence of formal contraindications. In those who weighed less than 3.5 kg, the insertion of a 9.1 mm × 8.8 mm was attempted only for any complex defect or after surgical indications. Surgical procedures were categorized as either low, moderate, or high risk. The primary end point was incidence of surgical and medical management decisions from TEE findings, and secondary end points were diagnostic impact (diagnostic exclusions and new diagnoses) and surgical outcome. Anesthesiologists with an advanced level of education in TEE performed 50% of the procedures. All examiners had performed 500 or more TEE examinations.

Results.—Supervision by an anesthesiologist with an advanced level of education was sought in 36.7% of cases; supervision by a cardiologist was sought in 3.8% of cases. Surgical modifications of management were reported in 12.7% of cases, including the need for a repeat bypass run in 7.3% and medical modifications in management in 19.4% of cases. Diagnostic impact of TEE was seen in 18.5% of cases, along with a suboptimal yet acceptable outcome in 27.6%. The TEE findings predicted preoperative difficulties in 4.0% of cases.

Conclusion.—Routine TEE was useful in the repair of congenital heart defects, which was competently performed by a regular team of cardiac anesthesiologists appropriately educated in TEE.

▶ This study systematically reviewed the impact of intraoperative TEE on the operative course in children undergoing repair of congenital cardiac anomalies. There are several interesting points. First, in the vast majority of cases the exams were done by anesthesiologists with experience in TEE, with cardiology consultation required in fewer than 4% of the cases. It is important to note that in these 2 centers, the anesthesiologist performing the exam was not responsible for the anesthetic management during the period of the exams. A second anesthesiologist was present at that time. Second, there was a very high incidence of interventions made based solely or in part on the TEE exam. It is not possible to know how many, if any, of these interventions were unnecessary. These would represent false-positive findings on TEE. At least with regards to the patients requiring repeat bypass (7%), there would appear to be no false-positives. All patients in whom a need for repeat bypass was suggested by the TEE exam had that confirmed by additional examinations. The false-negative rate would also appear to be low, with 1.8% of patients requiring reoperation—nonemergently—for abnormalities that might have been detected with intraoperative TEE. This study would suggest that anesthesiologists with experience in intraoperative TEE can offer a clinically important service in patients with congenital cardiac disease.

M. F. Trankina, MD

Payer Status Is Related to Differences in Access and Outcomes of Abdominal Aortic Aneurysm Repair in the United States
Boxer LK, Dimick JB, Wainess RM, et al (Univ of Michigan, Ann Arbor)
Surgery 134:142-145, 2003   5–11

Introduction.—Lower socioeconomic status and delayed access to health care are associated with increased mortality rates from cardiovascular disease. Because timely access is particularly important with repair of an abdominal aortic aneurysm (AAA), it was hypothesized that outcomes would differ among patients with private insurance, patients with Medicaid, and the uninsured.

Methods.—Patient and provider information was obtained from the National Inpatient Sample database for the period 1995-2000. Eligible patients were younger than 65 years and had a primary diagnosis code for intact or ruptured AAA. Data gathered on the study population of 5363 patients included age, sex, race, payer status, income based on zip code, in-hospital mortality rates, and comorbid conditions.

Results.—The mean age of the study patients was 59; 86% were men and 72% were white. Rupture of the AAA was present in 13.6% of cases and was more common in patients with no insurance (36%) or Medicaid (18%) than in those with private insurance (13%). In multivariate analysis, the variables with a statistically significant association with rupture were age, payer status, and emergent admission. Mild liver failure was the only comorbidity examined that increased the risk of rupture. Operative mortality rates were higher for patients with no insurance or with Medicaid than for patients with private insurance, particularly when rupture (45.3% and 33.1% vs 26.2%, respectively) had occurred. Age, female gender, payer status, type of admission, and mild liver failure were significant indicators of in-hospital mortality rate on multivariate analysis.

Conclusion.—Compared with patients who have private insurance, uninsured patients and patients with Medicaid are seen more often for emergent treatment of ruptured AAAs than for elective repair. Mortality rates after both intact and ruptured AAA repairs are higher for patients with Medicaid or no insurance. Payer status thus appears to affect both timely access to and outcomes of AAA repair.

▶ Several important points to make in understanding this study. First, it was limited to patients who are younger than 65, and thus a peer group that, in fact, should have had optimal care and optimal mortality rates because of their younger age (mortality rate for AAA surgery increases as the natural logarithm of their age changes). This difference is reflected in patients' 30-day mortality rates, not 6 months later mortality rates, so that care outside the hospital after discharge was not different.

But the authors did not specify, except of course for patients with ruptured aneurysm, whether the health status and prior health care were different between the insured and the uninsured. They could have done that easily by looking at, for example, the incidence of gingivitis and periodontitis in the population as a surrogate for the other marker. That would have been a wonderful addition to the study and hopefully in the future will be done. Nevertheless, I believe the authors have made an important contribution, but the rationale—that is, blaming the lack of insurance and the lack of access for the increased mortality rate—may be misguided and inappropriate.

M. F. Roizen, MD

Endovascular Repair With Bifurcated Stent-Grafts Under Local Anaesthesia to Improve Outcome of Ruptured Aortoiliac Aneurysms
Lachat ML, Pfammatter Th, Witzke HJ, et al (Zurich Univ, Switzerland)
Eur J Vasc Endovasc Surg 23:528-536, 2002   5–12

Background.—The mortality and morbidity rates of ruptured aortoiliac aneurysms (rAIAs) treated by conventional open surgery continue to range from 30% to 70%, despite significant improvements in anesthetic and surgical techniques. Promising results have been obtained with the less invasive endovascular technique, but studies thus far have evaluated stent-grafting performed with the patient under general anesthesia. The hemodynamic instability that can occur during induction of general anesthesia is an important concern. The use of local anesthesia for endovascular aneurysm repair (EVAR) of rAISs was evaluated. It was hypothesized that the use of local anesthesia would provide more hemodynamic stability during this procedure.

Methods.—A total of 21 consecutive patients with rAIA were enrolled in this study. All but 1 patient underwent EVAR under local anesthesia and the remaining patient was treated under general anesthesia. Hemodynamics were stabilized during assessment of EVAR feasibility by CT scan and during the procedure by controlled hypertension (MAP, 50-60 mm Hg) and moderate fluid resuscitation.

Results.—The median duration of the procedure was 120 minutes. Hemodynamic status remained stable in all but 3 patients who required transfemoral balloon occlusion of the supra-renal aorta. Perioperative intubation was necessary in 5 patients because of respiratory distress (2 patients) or retroperitoneal access (3 patients). Temporary deterioration of renal function occurred in 6 patients of whom 2 required hemofiltration. Sealing of the rAIA was confirmed by CT scan in all patients at discharge. The 30-day mortality rate was 9.5% (2 deaths). At a median follow-up of 19 months, there were no deaths; however, 3 endovascular reinterventions, 1 crossover femorofemoral bypass, and 1 open surgical graft repair were performed.

Conclusion.—This series is the first to demonstrate that EVAR of rAIAs can be safely performed under regional anesthesia, which allows the use of commercially available stent-grafts and improves outcomes.

▶ While the rationale for this study is a peculiar one, the loss of abdominal muscle tone during induction of general anesthesia in patients with ruptured aneurysms may worsen outcome. It is clear that you may want to use this technique with monitored anesthesia care as the usual technique for EVAR, as we have started to do. It should be noted however that 25 of these patients required emergency intubations because of respiratory distress, and that another 25% or so required additional vascular surgery procedures.

M. F. Roizen, MD

Use of Mortality Rate After Aortic Surgery as a Performance Indicator

Michaels JA (Sheffield Teaching Hosps, England)
Br J Surg 90:827-831, 2003   5-13

Introduction.—In November 2002, a newspaper report indicated that mortality after aneurysm repair varied widely among hospitals. This finding raised considerable concerns, but factors such as case mix and population differences may have produced distortions in the data. Hospital episode statistics were analyzed to examine the variation in mortality rate between hospitals after aortic surgery.

Methods.—Hospital episode statistics were obtained for all acute hospitals in England and Wales for the period from April 1996 to March 2001. Five subgroups of aortic surgery were considered: complex (with inclusion of suprarenal or visceral artery surgery), elective, emergency, and urgent aortic surgery, and unoperated aortic aneurysm. The number of patients in each category and the number of deaths were recorded for each hospital. In-hospital mortality was calculated for all patients older than 40 years who underwent abdominal aortic procedures or died in the hospital with a primary diagnosis of aortic aneurysm.

Results.—A total of 38,319 episodes occurred during the study period: 8.9% complex, 46.8% elective, and 44.4% emergency. The elective mortality rate was 6.4% overall, whereas mortality after emergency procedures was 35.0%. The exclusion of urgent procedures increased the mortality rate after emergency operation to 41.6%; inclusion of unoperated cases increased the rate to 63.1%. Procedures classified as complex had a mortality rate of 22.1%. A median of 68 elective procedures were carried out by individual hospitals. Overall elective mortality rates were 5.8% for hospitals undertaking the largest number of procedures and 7.3% for hospitals with the least activity. Hospitals varied widely in the proportion of elderly patients, tertiary referrals, and the proportion of emergency admissions that had surgery.

Conclusion.—A comparison of mortality rates after aortic surgery may yield misleading findings because of the differences between hospitals in case mix and selection. Some hospitals will always end up as outliers, and the handling of such outcome data remains a major challenge.

▶ The authors should be congratulated for such an outstanding analysis, but it would be even more helpful if they developed a risk assessment process that could be easily applied and account for the large differences in mortality rate. Otherwise use of crude mortality statistics may favor case selection and economic status of hospitals rather than surgical and perioperative skill.

M. F. Roizen, MD

Effects on Coagulation of Intravenous Crystalloid or Colloid in Patients Undergoing Peripheral Vascular Surgery

Ruttmann TG, James MFM, Finlayson J (Univ of Cape Town, South Africa)
Br J Anaesth 89:226-230, 2002   5–14

Background.—Previous studies have shown that hemodilution with 0.9% saline and other crystalloid solutions causes enhanced coagulation. The colloids are highly effective volume expanders, but there are lingering questions as to the effects of the colloids on coagulation. Many studies of the effects of colloids on coagulation have used a crystalloid control or have not allowed for any crystalloid the patient may have received in addition to the colloid. It has not yet been demonstrated that hemodilution-related coagulation enhancement is relevant in a clinical setting or whether this effect occurs on the basis of a stress response or the hemodilution-induced enhancement of coagulation. This study investigated whether hemodilution-enhanced coagulation can be demonstrated under regional anesthesia, whether this effect occurs before surgery, and whether the effect is influenced by the type of fluid used.

Methods.—Patients scheduled for peripheral vascular surgery on the lower limb who were candidates for regional anesthesia were randomly assigned to received either crystalloid (20 patients) or colloid IV fluid (20 patients). Epidural analgesia was administered. Samples of venous blood were obtained before fluid administration, after completion of the epidural and initial fluid load, during surgery before heparin, and after 24 hours. The main outcome measures were thromboelastograph analysis and measures of full blood count, international normalized ratio, activated partial thromboplastin time, D-dimers, and thrombin-antithrombin complex.

Results.—In patients who received crystalloid, coagulation was enhanced compared with baseline after initial fluid load and before heparin administration. There was no enhancement of coagulation in the colloid group, and there were no changes from baseline after 24 hours.

Conclusion.—The results of this study provide confirmation that the enhanced perioperative coagulation mechanism is related to dilution rather than to surgery and is initiated by rapid hemodilution of crystalloid. The use of colloid rather than crystalloid for rapid fluid loading should be considered in vasculopathic patients undergoing surgery.

▶ This is a fascinating article, one that made me say "I didn't know that. I didn't even know that it was remotely possible that crystalloid administered prior to surgery can trigger a clotting response." I always thought it was the stress of surgery that increased coagulation postoperatively, but maybe it has something to do with the foreign substance in the crystalloid or as these authors postulate, a response to the volume infusion of the crystalloid leading to a pro-coagulant state. I suppose it should be logical that anything given prior to surgery could trigger some response, but it still is surprising to me that I was totally unaware of this phenomenon. Is this real or is it a figment of the thromboelastograph? I do not know the answer to that question, but I expect that further study will tell us if, when we start to give crystalloid, we also have to give heparin or something similar with the crystalloid. I think this is a very important study and one which I look forward to reports of further studies.

M. F. Roizen, MD

Absence of Adverse Outcomes in Hyperkalemic Patients Undergoing Vascular Access Surgery
Olson RP, Schow AJ, McCann R, et al (Duke Univ, Durham, NC)
Can J Anesth 50:553-557, 2003   5–15

Introduction.—Significant hyperkalemia is considered a contraindication to anesthesia, but delaying vascular access surgery if the patient is hyperkalemic may be counterproductive. Eight cases in which vascular access procedures for hemodialysis proceeded despite uncorrected hyperkalemia were retrospectively reviewed for patient characteristics and outcomes.

Methods.—A list of all vascular access procedures for hemodialysis performed by a single surgeon from 1995 to 2000 were matched with preoperative potassium (K) results recorded in the hospital laboratory database. Charts of cases in which the preoperative K was greater than 6.0 mmol·L^{-1} were reviewed.

Results.—Of the 1472 cases recorded during the study period, 1350 had a preoperative K concentration recorded; 45 (3.3%) of these were greater than 6.0 mmol·L^{-1}. Complete data were available on 8 patients who proceeded to surgery with high K concentrations (mean, 7.0 mmol·L^{-1}). The mean age of the 8 patients was 53 years; 5 had diabetes. Techniques of anesthesia included general anesthesia (n = 1), monitored anesthesia care with local anesthetic infiltration of the surgical site (n = 5), local anesthetic (n = 1), and regional anesthetic (n = 1). Hyperglycemia, present in 2 cases, was treated with IV insulin. No adverse events occurred perioperatively, and ECG tracings performed within 2 hours of surgery showed no changes suggestive of hyperkalemia.

Conclusion.—Hyperkalemia is the most frequent perioperative complication in patients with renal failure. However, none of these 8 patients who underwent vascular access surgery with a high K concentration exhibited adverse effects or clinical or ECG signs of hyperkalemia. Thus, asymptomatic hyperkalemia may not be an absolute contraindication to vascular access procedures.

▶ This is a significant problem in patients undergoing access since the access is clearly for dialysis, and many such patients have hyperkalemia. It is interesting that such patients did not suffer adverse effects. Perhaps it is knowing about the hyperkalemia and making sure these patients don't hypoventilate that was so important. In any case, this is an important contribution to the anesthesia literature and one that I will probably quote multiple times. The authors should be commended for such an excellent article.

M. F. Roizen, MD

6 Pediatric Anesthesia

Massage Therapy by Mothers Enhances the Adjustment of Circadian Rhythms to the Nocturnal Period in Full-Term Infants
Ferber SG, Laudon M, Kuint J, et al (Tel Aviv Univ, Israel; Neurim Pharmaceuticals Ltd, Tel Aviv, Israel; Bar Ilan Univ, Ramat Gan, Israel)
J Dev Behav Pediatr 23:410-415, 2002   6–1

Background.—The ontogeny of the circadian rhythm in infants is initiated before birth, and it is believed that this rhythm is essentially intrinsic. The fetal biological clock is an endogenous system that has the capacity to generate circadian rhythms and to respond to maternal entraining signals. Fetal diurnal rhythms are entrainable by maternal cues to the day-night rhythms by the third trimester of pregnancy. Social cues become important in the first weeks of life, while light becomes the dominant environmental cue only at a later stage. Findings from a number of studies have indicated that most infants would be entrained to their mothers' ordinary daily schedule without expression of the overt free-running rhythm of the biological clock.

In the first weeks of life, neonates are more active at night than are older infants. As a result, there is considerable maternal distress associated with the disruption of nightly sleep. Several studies have suggested that massage therapy is beneficial for mother-infant interaction, particularly in depressed mothers. This study investigated the effect of massage therapy on phase adjustment of rest-activity and melatonin secretion rhythms to the nocturnal period in full-term infants.

Methods.—The rest-activity cycles of 21 infants were measured by actigraphy before and after 14 days of massage therapy beginning at age 10 ± 4 days (treatment group, 13 infants) and at 6 and 8 weeks of age (treatment group and 8 control infants). Excretion of 6-sulphatoxymelatonin was assessed in urine samples at 6, 8, and 12 weeks of age in both groups.

Results.—At 8 weeks of age, the control infants showed 1 peak of activity at about midnight (11 PM to 3 AM) and another one at about noon (11 AM to 3 PM). In contrast, the treated group showed a major peak of activity early in the morning (3 AM to 7 AM) and a secondary peak in the late afternoon (3 PM to 7 PM). At 12 weeks, the nocturnal 6-sulfphatoxymelatonin excretions were significantly higher in the treated infants than in the control infants (1346.38 ± 209.40 (g/night vs 823.25 ± 121.25 µg/night).

Conclusion.—Massage therapy by mothers in the perinatal period acts as a powerful time cue and enhances coordination of the developing circadian system with environmental cues.

▶ This is a fascinating study in our journal for anesthesiologists: *The Journal of Developmental and Behavorial Pediatrics.* What this study said may be important: that mother and child both slept better when the child received 2 weeks of backrubs given in a specific fashion. The massage therapy was given between 10 and 14 days after birth for 2 weeks, for 30 minutes, including lightly stroking the infants back in a circular motion with 1 hand. This study shows that, in fact, both mother and child could sleep better for the next 6 months after this either bonding or goal-setting behavior that occurred between 8:00 PM and 9:00 PM. For those of us involved in trying to get sleep when we have new children or for those involved in caring for pediatric patients, I think this is a valuable study and maybe there are lessons for us as adults as well.

M. F. Roizen, MD

EMLA® Cream Versus Dorsal Penile Nerve Block for Postcircumcision Analgesia in Children

Choi WY, Irwin MG, Hui TWC, et al (Pamela Youde Nethersole Eastern Hosp, Chai Wan, Hong Kong; Queen Mary Hosp, Hong Kong)
Anesth Analg 96:396-399, 2003   6–2

Background.—Circumcision, a common pediatric operation, can be painful, with pain relief most often provided by caudal epidural block or dorsal penile nerve block (DPB). However, DPB has a failure rate of 4% to 8% and may cause bleeding or hematoma at the site of injection. Caudal blocks can produce prolonged time to micturition, lower limb motor block, and heightened potential for local anesthetic toxicity. For alleviating pain during circumcision, the topical eutectic mixture of local anesthetic (EMLA) cream has greater efficacy than placebo but less than DPB. The use of EMLA cream preoperatively in children over age 2 years has not been assessed, but it was hypothesized that the analgesic efficacy and complication rate would be the same as with DPB.

Methods.—The evaluation followed a double-blind, randomized design and lasted 6 months. Elective inpatient circumcision was scheduled for 63 boys with American Society of Anesthesiologists physical status I or II, age 2 to 12 years. None of the patients had an allergy to amide type local anesthetics or EMLA cream, had recently ingested sulfonamides or nitrites, had congenital or idiopathic methemoglobinemia, or had atopic dermatitis. Group D underwent DPB, while group E was administered 2 to 4 g of EMLA cream with the use of a syringe on the distal half of the penile skin (excluding the mucosal surface), which was covered with a clear plastic occlusive dressing 1 hour or more before the procedure.

Anesthetic induction was accomplished by IV injection of 3 to 4 mg/kg of propofol and maintained with spontaneous breathing of 66% nitrous oxide in oxygen and isoflurane via a face mask; the end-tidal isoflurane concentration was 0.6% to 0.9%. Inadequate analgesia was defined as having the respiratory rate or heart rate increase over 25% from baseline during surgery, for which an IV bolus dose of fentanyl 0.5 µg/kg was given every 5 minutes to a maximum dose of 2 µg/kg. Failed analgesia was declared when this intervention did not reduce the sympathetic activity. These patients were excluded from the rest of the study.

Results.—Operation duration, time to postoperative self-recognition, number of patients who required fentanyl during surgery, and total dose of fentanyl required were similar for the 2 groups. Those having analgesia with DPB had a median duration of analgesia (from the first dose of paracetamol) twice that of those having EMLA cream. However, only 33.3% of patients with EMLA cream required paracetamol while 50% of the DPB group required it. Most patients having EMLA cream required either no paracetamol or just 1 dose after surgery.

Conclusion.—The preoperative application of topical EMLA cream was both safe and effective in providing postcircumcision analgesia. EMLA cream offers the advantages of technical simplicity and avoidance of the serious complications of DPB that occur on rare occasions. DPB had a longer period of analgesia than EMLA cream because bupivacaine has a greater duration of action, making it a good drug for this purpose. Fewer patients who had EMLA cream applied required paracetamol compared with patients who had DPB, but the total dose of paracetamol did not differ between the 2 groups.

▶ This comparison of preoperative application of EMLA cream to DPB for postcircumcision pain demonstrated similar quality of analgesia with both techniques, with a shorter duration of action (195 minutes compared to 100 minutes) with EMLA application. Patients with both forms of analgesia required only short-duration postoperative nonnarcotic pain medication. The techniques appear to have similar analgesic efficacy intraoperatively as the intraoperative narcotic requirements were not different. Each technique has potential advantages and disadvantages in the outpatient setting. While EMLA application is technically simpler, it does require an hour application compared with the essentially immediate onset with the nerve block. Which technique would be superior likely depends on the nature of the practice rather than any clear advantage, disadvantage, or risk to either technique.

S. Black, MD

Traditional Versus New Needle Retractable IV Catheters in Children: Are They Really Safer, and Whom Are They Protecting?

Coté CJ, Roth AG, Wheeler M, et al (Northwestern Univ, Chicago)
Anesth Analg 96:387-391, 2003   6–3

Background.—To reduce the incidence of accidental needle-stick injury, the government has mandated that retractable needle systems for IV catheters be available, but some experience with these new systems has revealed that successful venipuncture may be more difficult to recognize and to achieve. Use of the "traditional" IV catheters (JELCO, Johnson & Johnson) was compared with use of the "new" ones (Angiocath Autoguard, BD Medical Systems Inc).

Methods.—Outcome measures for the prospective study were difficulty of IV access, number of catheters used, and splatters or spills of blood on skin, linen, floor, clothing, and operating room table. Catheter type was assigned by week in the operating room, and completion of a questionnaire was requested after catheter placement to determine the number of catheters used, patient age and weight, operative procedure, spilling or splattering of blood, and time from initial skin puncture to successful running of IV fluid.

Results.—Over 20 operative days, 473 catheter insertions were attempted in 330 patients, with 328 by anesthesia trainees and 145 by anesthesia attendings. Trainees achieved 219 successful insertions and attendings achieved 95. No significant differences were noted between the trainees and attendings in number of patients needing more than 1 catheter attempt. A larger proportion of children aged 3 years and under required more than 1 catheter for establishing access when compared with older children. More patients over age 3 years needed more than 1 new catheter for successful IV placement compared with those receiving a traditional catheter, but in children aged 3 years or younger, there was no difference.

During attempted IV placement for 42 patients, 77 spatters or spills of blood occurred, with a larger absolute number of blood splatters or spills occurring with the new compared with the traditional catheters and with attendings more than with trainees. Poor flashback influenced 18 new catheter insertions but no traditional insertions. No significant difference in insertion time was noted.

Conclusion.—Some institutions have interpreted the new regulations as meaning that needleless systems, safety needles, and retractable IV catheter needle systems are the only choices allowed, but the legislation states that the final decision as to which needle or system to use is left to the health provider. The goal is reducing needlestick injury, the injury most often associated with transmission of HIV infection, but HIV can be acquired by non-needlestick injuries, so changing catheter systems may not always be the answer.

A clinically relevant finding was that the use of this brand of retractable IV catheter compared with traditional catheters was linked to a statistically significant increase nearly 4-fold in blood spattering and spilling. The difference in contamination rate between the new and traditional catheters was largely related to attending physicians and not trainees, despite 5 months of previous experience with these devices by the attendings. Possible explanations for the difference include the longer experience of trainees with the "new" catheters compared with attendings; the potential for reporting bias based on the starting hypotheses; or the possibility that younger physicians are more willing to adapt to and adopt new technology and devices with greater safety precautions compared with older physicians, who may be more experienced with traditional technology, find it difficult to change, or see the new device as less easy to use. Whether the potential for needlestick injury with the retractable needle system is offset by the potential for transmission of pathogens through increased cutaneous blood exposure was not determined. Both the traditional and the new systems should be available for the practitioner to choose.

▶ The authors compared traditional IV catheters and retractable needle IV catheters. They found "more difficulty" with use of the retractable needle catheters in the form of more patients requiring multiple catheters for successful cannulation. They also noted more splatters and spills with the new catheters. While it is correct that exposure other than needle sticks is important to consider, the results might well be due to the idea suggested by the authors, namely, that the clinicians with more experience with traditional catheters were resistant to the use of newer catheters. The authors' conclusion and recommendations seem reasonable, that both forms of catheters should be available. It would be interesting to review the issue in several more years as the "safe catheters" are more widely used.

S. Black, MD

Caudal Anesthesia in Children: Effect of Volume Versus Concentration of Bupivacaine on Blocking Spermatic Cord Traction Response During Orchidopexy
Verghese ST, Hannallah RS, Rice LJ, et al (Children's Natl Med Ctr, Washington, DC; George Washington Univ, Washington, DC)
Anesth Analg 95:1219-1223, 2002   6–4

Background.—Testicular innervation derives from the aortic and renal plexuses and sympathetic fibers connected to the T10 and T11 segments of the spinal cord through the thoracic splanchnic nerves. Therefore, analgesia for testicular surgery is achieved by using a T10-level block. Children having orchidopexy surgery require blockade at a higher level, up to T4, to block the peritoneal stimulation accompanying traction on the spermatic cord. The rostral spread of caudal analgesia depends on the volume of local anesthetic injected, but the dose, volume, and concentration of the injected drug influence the quality and level of the blockade.

Higher-level blocks are produced by using larger volumes of local anesthetic solution. The effect of 2 volumes and concentrations of bupivacaine on the level and intensity of caudal blockade when the dose of bupivacaine was held constant at 2 mg/kg was investigated.

Methods.—The 50 children having unilateral orchiopexy (age range, 1-6 years) were divided into 2 groups. Caudal block was achieved using a fixed 2 mg/kg dose of bupivacaine immediately after induction. The 23 children in group 1 received 0.8 mL/kg of 0.25% bupivacaine (low volume/high concentration), and the 27 children in group 2 received 1.0 mL/kg of 0.2% bupivacaine, prepared by diluting 0.8 mL/kg of the 0.25% solution into a 1 mL/kg solution using saline solution free of preservatives (high volume/low concentration). In addition, epinephrine 1:400,000 and 0.1 mL of sodium bicarbonate per 10 mL of local anesthetic solution were used.

All patients had mask anesthesia maintained by using 6 L of fresh gas flow in a circle system; the ratio of N_2O to oxygen was 2:1. Children received 2% halothane during the first 10 minutes, the incision was made, and the inspired concentration of halothane was adjusted based on the patient's response to the surgical stimulus. The intensity and level of rostral spread of the caudal blockade were evaluated when the surgeon placed digital traction on the spermatic cord during orchidopexy. Expired halothane concentration was measured throughout; a patient response of tachycardia, hypertension, hyperventilation, or phonation prompted an increased concentration to reverse the response.

An Objective Pain Scale score was obtained, with rescue fentanyl 1 µg/kg given for a score of 6 or more. Acetaminophen suppository was given for pain in the short-stay recovery unit.

Results.—The anesthetic time, discharge time, halothane minimum alveolar anesthetic concentration, and postoperative analgesic therapy were similar in the 2 groups. Heart rate, blood pressure, or respiratory rate increased 15% to 20% from baseline in 65.2% of the group 1 children and 29.6% of the group 2 children. Group 1 children also had an incidence of phonation requiring acute increase in the halothane concentration; group 2 children required less frequent increases. Rescue therapy using fentanyl or acetaminophen was given at equal rates, and the ability to ambulate and length of stay related to motor weakness were similar.

Conclusion.—These children had excellent intraoperative and postoperative analgesia with bupivacaine 0.25% plus light general anesthesia. Clinical experience that a caudal injection volume of 0.75 mL/kg of 0.25% bupivacaine cannot block peritoneal stimulation during spermatic cord traction was supported by the patients' phonation, hyperventilation, and increased blood pressure and heart rate with this volume. Performing a caudal block with more dilute bupivacaine is more effective than using less of a more concentrated solution, which can prolong motor blockade of the lower extremities.

▶ In this study, a simple change in technique (diluting the local anesthetic concentration for a bupivacaine caudal) in patients undergoing orchidopexy improved the quality of the intraoperative anesthetic. By diluting the local anesthetic, they were able to give a larger volume and the same dose of the bupivacaine as using a smaller volume of the standard concentration, thus giving more rostral spread of the anesthetic without increasing risk of toxicity. This more rostral spread improved the intraoperative course by more effectively blunting the response to spermatic cord traction. Since the risk for toxicity is unchanged and the postoperative pain relief unchanged, this improved operative course comes without any disadvantages.

S. Black, MD

Use of Discharge Abstract Databases to Differentiate Among Pediatric Hospitals Based on Operative Procedures: Surgery in Infants and Young Children in the State of Iowa
Dexter F, Wachtel RE, Yue JC (Univ of Iowa, Iowa City; Natl Chengchi Univ, Taipei, Taiwan)
Anesthesiology 99:480-487, 2003   6–5

Introduction.—A pediatric hospital may seek to differentiate its clinical services from those of other facilities, but little is known about the demographics of pediatric surgery and the types of procedures performed in pediatric versus nonpediatric hospitals. Furthermore, criteria do not exist for quantifying differences among facilities in the types of procedures performed. Discharge abstracts from the state of Iowa were used to study inpatient and outpatient operative procedures in young children (0-2 years).

Methods.—The period of interest extended from January 1, 2001 to June 30, 2001. Cases examined were those performed in the 117 hospitals and 2 hospital-affiliated freestanding outpatient surgery centers statewide. Only 2 hospitals were considered pediatric hospitals by virtue of sponsoring an accredited pediatric residency or having major participation in an accredited pediatric residency. A total of 5671 operative procedures (requiring an incision) had been performed during 462 inpatient admissions and 3143 outpatient visits. Facilities were compared for number of procedures, number of different types of procedures, physiologic complexity of procedures, and several other factors.

Results.—Of the 93 facilities performing at least 1 procedure in young children, the 90 that performed 15 or fewer types of procedures provided surgical care for 80% of procedures. Less than 0.15% of procedures performed at these 90 facilities were considered physiologically complex. Such procedures, however, accounted for 26% of procedures at the larger pediatric hospital and 7% at the smaller pediatric hospital, and the larger hospital had performed 64% of all physiologically complex procedures during the study period. The larger pediatric hospital reported 181 different types and the smaller pediatric hospital 73 different types of procedures.

Conclusion.—Discharge abstract data showed that the 2 pediatric hospitals in Iowa provided more diverse, comprehensive, and physiologically complex procedures than nonpediatric hospitals. When pediatric hospitals want to show how they differ from nonpediatric hospitals, diversity of procedures performed should be stressed over volume issues.

▶ This is a wonderfully innovative and important article that uses physiologic complexity to differentiate or to be able to differentiate pediatric from nonpediatric hospitals. The conclusion of this article is wonderfully written and says a lot: "Hospitals frequently aim to help government agencies, charitable organizations, and philanthropic individuals appreciate their services. In this article, we describe how inpatient and outpatient discharge abstract databases can be used to quantify pediatric operative procedures."

This article provides a wonderful rationale for allowing children's hospitals to develop and differentiate themselves.

M. F. Roizen, MD

Adverse Effect of Nitrous Oxide in a Child With 5,10-Methylenetetrahydrofolate Reductase Deficiency

Selzer RR, Rosenblatt DS, Laxova R, et al (Univ of Wisconsin, Madison; McGill Univ, Montreal)
N Engl J Med 349:45-50, 2003   6–6

Introduction.—Nitrous oxide irreversibly oxidizes the cobalt atom of vitamin B$_{12}$, thus inhibiting the activity of the cobalamin-dependent enzyme methionine synthase (or 5-methyltetrahydrofolate-homocysteine S-methyltransferase; Enzyme Commission code EC 2.1.1.13). It has been shown that methionine synthase catalyzes the remethylation of 5-methyltetrahydrofolate and homocysteine to tetrahydrofolate and methionine. Reported is the neurologic deterioration and death of a child anesthetized twice with nitrous oxide before being diagnosed with 5,10-methylenetetrahydrofolate reductase (MTHFR; EC 1.5.1.20) deficiency (Online Mendelian Inheritance in Man number 236250) was established.

> *Case Report.*—Boy, 3 months, appeared normal until a mass in the left leg was detected. Before surgery, it was not known that the patient's father and one of his uncles had serum levels of total homocysteine above 20.0 μmol/L and above 30.0 μmol/L, respectively. The proband's sibling was receiving lifelong therapy with high-dose vitamin B supplements and had a homocysteine level of 4.3 μmol/L. The father and his sibling had never received nitrous oxide.
>
> The patient was premedicated with atropine and anesthesia was induced with sodium thiopental and succinylcholine. After intubation, anesthesia was maintained with 0.75% halothane and 60% nitrous oxide in oxygen for 45 minutes. The surgical biopsy specimen showed an infantile fibrosarcoma. Resection of the mass was performed on day 4 after biopsy. The patient underwent induction of anesthesia with halothane and was anesthetized for 270 minutes with 0.75% halothane and 60% nitrous oxide. He was discharged on postoperative day 7 in apparently good health.
>
> Seventeen days later (25 days post resection), the patient was admitted for seizures and episodes of apnea. He was severely hypotonic, without reflexes and with ataxic ventilation. Cranial CT revealed generalized atrophy of the brain, with enlarged prepontine

and medullary cisterns. The patient's urine was positive for homo-cysteine (1.30 µmol/mg of creatinine) and negative for organic acids and methylmalonic acid. Plasma homocysteine was elevated (0.6 mg/dL) and the methionine level was low at 0.06 mg/dL). The vita-min B_{12} level, serum folate level, and level of folate in the CSF were normal.

The infant died at 130 days of age (46 days after surgery) after a respiratory arrest. Autopsy revealed asymmetric cerebral atrophy and severe demyelination, with astrogliosis and oligodendroglial cell depletion in the midbrain, medulla, and cerebellum. The values for MTHFR activity in cultured fibroblasts were 1.22 and 0.8 nmol of formaldehyde produced/mg of protein/h (normal mean value, 5.04 ± 1.36) with and without flavinadenine dinucleotide, respectively.

The patient was heterozygous for a novel mutation, 1755G→A in exon 10. This causes a substitution of isoleucine for methionine at residue 581 (M581I) (GenBank accession number, NM−005957). Restriction-enzyme analysis verified the presence of the 1755G→A mutation in the heterozygous father, his father, his brother, 1 uncle, and 1 aunt. This was not seen in 100 control chromosomes. The in-fant was also heterozygous for a 677C→T mutation in exon 4 (re-sulting in a substitution of valine for alanine at residue 222) and a 1298A→C mutation in exon 7 (resulting in a substitution of alanine for glutamic acid at residue 429).

The father was homozygous (TT) for the 677C→T mutation and homozygous (AA) at 1298A. The infant's mother was heterozygous for both common polymorphisms and homozygous (wild type) at 1755G. The patient had a sibling whose haplotype was identical in all coding regions. Genomic analysis of the genes encoding methio-nine synthase, methionine synthase reductase, and cystathionine β-synthase was performed to determine genotypes at these loci for all members of the pedigree.

Conclusion.—About 45 million persons in North America undergo anes-thesia every year. Nitrous oxide is a major component in about half of these procedures. Due to the growing use of nitrous oxide, patients with known mutations related to mild or severe abnormalities in folate-cycle enzymes are increasingly likely to receive nitrous oxide. Based on the findings in this pa-tient, it is recommended that patients with a diagnosis of severe MTHFR de-ficiency do not receive nitrous oxide as an anesthetic.

▶ Nitrous oxide was first prepared by Priestley in 1772, and it was first used in clinical practice in the United States in the mid 1800s. Since that time, it has become a frequently used anesthetic gas. It is known for its relative safety, but it is not without potential adverse effect, as this case report demonstrates. Ni-trous oxide irreversibly oxidizes vitamin B_{12}, making it inactive as a coenzyme. This has been thought to lead to decreased DNA synthesis in the embryo and teratogenicity. The specific case report that I have chosen describes the neurologic deterioration and death of a child with a novel inherited enzyme deficiency. The authors suggest that nitrous oxide be avoided in these patients, even if the diagnosis is not certain.

M. Wood, MD, FRCA

The Effects of Common Airway Maneuvers on Airway Pressure and Flow in Children Undergoing Adenoidectomies
Bruppacher H, Reber A, Keller JP, et al (Univ Children's Hosp Beider Basel, Basel, Switzerland; Fachtechnische Hochschule, Oensingen, Switzerland; Univ of Washington, Seattle; et al)
Anesth Analg 97:29-34, 2003   6–7

Background.—Children with normal upper airway structures having elective procedures under general anesthesia may require airway maneuvers such as chin lift (CL), jaw thrust (JT), and continuous positive airway pressure (CPAP) to achieve airway patency. Although all these airway maneuvers increase the glottic opening size, JT with or without CPAP, relieves airway obstruction in patients with tonsillar and adenoidal hyperplasia, but CL does not improve it and may make it worse. It was theorized that airway patency is not improved by CL because it does not address obstruction proximal to the oropharynx but JT does by clearing the airway below the soft palate. By using pressure-tip catheters to determine the obstruction site in patients seen for adenoidectomy, local pressure measurements were obtained and compared.

Methods.—Sevoflurane was used for anesthesia in 16 children, aged 2 to 9 years, scheduled to undergo elective adenoidectomy to relieve snoring with troubled breathing, apnea, or both. None had pulmonary disease, craniofacial dysmorphism, chest or spine deformities, or neuromuscular disorders. After induction of anesthesia, a custom-built 5F silicone catheter mounted with 2 micro pressure transducers was advanced transnasally into the esophagus; correct catheter positioning was where the proximal transducer was at the level of the middle pharyngeal constrictor muscle just below the uvula.

During spontaneous breathing, simultaneous measures were obtained of the flows and pressures in the mask, oropharynx, and esophagus. In addition, maximal pressure differences during inspiration (ΔP) were determined, reflecting inspiratory pressure amplitude measured at the mask (P_{ma}), oropharynx (P_{op}), and esophagus (P_{es}).

CL and JT maneuvers were performed randomly, with and without CPAP, as follows: At baseline, the anesthesiologist held the mask against the face and applied gentle pressure without chin support; in CL, the chin was lifted at the inferior border of the mental protuberance by using the left hand until there was close contact between the upper and lower rows of teeth without mandibular protrusion; with JT, the mouth was opened by displacing the jaws at the mandibular angles using both hands, moving upward and anteriorly; and during CPAP, the popoff valve of the circle system was closed and a pressure of 5 cm H_2O was applied to BL, CL, and JT.

Results.—At baseline, the observed $\Delta P_{ma} - P_{es}$ was 12.3 cm H_2O. All airway maneuvers reduced this measure as a result of declines in $\Delta P_{ma} - P_{op}$ and $\Delta P_{op} - P_{es}$ in all interventions except CL, when $\Delta P_{ma} - P_{op}$ remained similar. Minute ventilation and maximal inspiratory peak flow increased significantly with JT with and without CPAP.

Conclusion.—Partial or total obstruction is often noted in anesthetized children who are to undergo adenoidectomies. Of the airway maneuvers done to maintain airway patency and improve tidal breathing values, JT with or without CPAP effectively decreases obstruction of the upper airway. Although the tidal breathing pattern was significantly influenced by all the maneuvers, CL without CPAP did not improve oral airway patency.

▶ This study clearly defines a clinical issue that most of us have observed in our practice, that is, that a CL often fails to adequately relieve airway obstruction while a properly preformed JT is much more effective. By dividing airway obstruction into proximal to the oropharynx and distal to the oropharynx and measuring pressures in those areas, it is easy to understand the often observed lack of improvement with a chin lift when obstruction in the mouth is not improved

S. Black, MD

Predictors of Red Cell Transfusion in Children and Adolescents Undergoing Spinal Fusion Surgery

Meert KL, Kannan S, Mooney JF (Wayne State Univ, Detroit)
Spine 27:2137-2142, 2002 6–8

Background.—Major blood loss is a frequent occurrence in spinal fusion in children and adolescents. Several conservation methods are used routinely during spinal fusion procedures, such as patient positioning to avoid compression, controlled hypotensive anesthesia, acute normovolemic hemodilution, epinephrine infiltration of paravertebral tissues, application of fibrin sealant to decorticated bone, and intraoperative and postoperative infusion of shed blood. However, red cell replacement is frequently necessary in these patients, even with these blood conservation techniques. The preoperative identification of patients at increased risk of red cell transfusion would allow more specific use of interventions designed to control excessive bleeding during spinal fusion. Clinical predictors of allogeneic and autologous red cell transfusion were identified in children and adolescents undergoing spinal fusion surgery.

Methods.—A retrospective review was conducted of medical records of all patients who underwent posterior spinal fusion surgery at a single institution from July 1999 to June 2001. Logistic and stepwise multiple regression analyses were performed to identify predictors of allogeneic and autologous red cell transfusion intraoperatively and postoperatively.

Results.—A total of 107 patients (42% males; median age, 13.7 years) were identified (Table 1). The median intraoperative blood loss in these pa-

TABLE 1.—Demographics, Surgical Variables, and Transfusion Requirements (N = 107)

Variable	Number (%)	Median (Range)
Sex (male)	45 (42)	
Age (y)		13.7 (1-20)
Weight (kg)		45 (9-85)
Preoperative medications		
Anticonvulsants	9 (8)	
Antibiotics	21 (20)	
Nonsteroidal antiinflammatory agents	9 (8)	
Preoperative donation of autologous blood	19 (18)	
Amount of autologous blood donated (units)	2 (1-4)	
Cobb angle (degrees)		61 (30-148)
Number of vertebrae fused		13 (4-20)
Anatomic location		
Cervicothoracic	4 (4)	
Thoracic	12 (11)	
Thoracolumbar	66 (62)	
Thoracolumbosacral	23 (21)	
Lumbosacral	2 (2)	
Bone graft site		
Rib	45 (42)	
Iliac	18 (17)	
Vertebrae	20 (19)	
Duration of surgery (h)	7.6 (3.0-14.4)	
Amount of hemodilution (mL/kg)	8.5 (3.5-13)	
Amount of scavenged blood infused (mL/kg)	8 (1.5-44)	
Use of postoperative drains	50 (47)	
Blood loss (mL/kg)		
Intraoperative		22 (4-72)
Postoperative		0 (0-52)
Transfusions		
Allogeneic packed red blood cells	63 (59)	
Autologous packed red blood cells	14 (13)	
Fresh frozen plasma	13 (12)	
Platelet concentrate	3 (3)	
Cryoprecipitate	2 (2)	
Amount of transfusions (mL/kg)		
Allogeneic red blood cells		17 (3-65)
Autologous red blood cells		7 (4-19)
Fresh frozen plasma		10 (8-57)
Platelet concentrate		11 (8-12)
Cryoprecipitate		2 (1-3)

Note: The amount of autologous blood donated and the amounts of hemodilution, scavenged blood, and other blood products received exclude those patients who did not undergo these interventions.

(Courtesy of Meert KL, Kannan S, Mooney JF: Predictors of red cell transfusion in children and adolescents undergoing spinal fusion surgery. *Spine* 27:2137-2142, 2002.)

tients was 22 mL/kg (range, 4.4-72 mL/kg). Blood transfusion was performed in 63 patients (59%) who received a median of 17 mL/kg (range, 3-65 mL/kg) of allogeneic packed red blood cells. In addition, 14 patients (13%) received 7 mL/kg (range, 4-19 mL/kg) of autologous red cells donated preoperatively. Independent predictors of a greater number of allogeneic red blood cells infused were underlying muscular disease, lower body weight, and a higher number of vertebrae fused. The amount of autologous blood donated preoperatively was found to be predictive of the number of autologous red cells transfused.

Conclusions.—Children and adolescents with underlying neuromuscular disease undergoing spinal fusion surgery frequently require allogeneic red cell transfusion. These patients may be less capable of donating autologous blood before surgery. New therapeutic approaches to reduction of blood loss and transfusion requirements are needed in these patients.

An Autologous Blood Donation Program for Paediatric Scoliosis Patients in Hong Kong
Lo KS, Chow BFM, Chan HT, et al (Duchess of Kent Children's Hosp, Sandy Bay, Hong Kong)
Anaesth Intensive Care 30:775-781, 2002   6–9

Background.—Many blood conservation techniques are available for patients undergoing corrective surgery for scoliosis. Among these techniques, autologous blood transfusion offers many advantages. This approach eliminates the blood-borne transmission of viruses, prions, and parasites and avoids immune-mediated reactions, immunosuppression, and allo-immunizations. However, autologous blood transfusion does not eliminate the risk of clerical error, bacterial contamination, and many other non–immune-mediated reactions. Preoperative autologous blood donation (PABD) programs have been previously described. A systematic review has reported that PABD decreased exposure to allogeneic blood but increased the exposure to any blood transfusion. The efficacy, safety, and patient satisfaction with a PABD program for children and teenagers undergoing corrective surgery for scoliosis were determined.

Methods.—A retrospective review was conducted of patients who required corrective spinal surgery for scoliosis at 1 institution in Hong Kong and who participated in the PABD program at that institution. Safety was defined by the frequency and type of adverse reactions. Efficacy was assessed on the basis of patient compliance with the autologous blood donation schedule; the desired versus actual yield of donated blood; usage, wastage, and sufficiency of PABD blood; and failure of the program. Program failure was defined as the inability of a patient to finish the program because of complications or cancellation or the need for allogeneic blood.

Results.—From a total of 77 patients identified, 45 patients donated the requested amount of blood. It was found that these 45 compliant patients had been requested to donate fewer units of blood compared with noncompliant patients (mean, 4.0 vs 4.6 units, respectively). Two patients had surgery delayed, which made the collected autologous blood unavailable. An association was observed between the extent of the surgical procedure and the need for allogeneic blood transfusion. Overall, 6.5% of donated units of blood were discarded. No major complications were reported, and 93% of patients reported satisfaction with the program.

Conclusions.—In the setting of careful patient selection and good interdepartmental coordination, PABD seems to be safe and effective in pediatric patients undergoing extensive corrective surgery for scoliosis.

▶ In these 2 articles (Abstracts 6–8 and 6–9), transfusion requirements in children undergoing scoliosis correction were reviewed. In the Meert et al article (see Abstract 6–8), preoperative predictors for intraoperative transfusion were identified: neuromuscular disease, low body weight, and number of levels involved in the surgical procedure. In both studies, intraoperative blood loss was found to be high: up to 40% of the estimated blood volume, and the majority of patients required transfusion intraoperatively. In the Lo et al study (see Abstract 6–9), preoperative donation of autologous blood was encouraged in all willing patients, regardless of age or weight. In their study, only 16% of patients required allogeneic blood products compared with 59% in the Meert et al study, in which only a small portion of patients participated in PABD. From these articles, it is clear that children and adolescents undergoing scoliosis correction could benefit from a program of PABD in terms of reduced exposure to allogeneic blood products. From the Lo et al study, it seems that success depends on good education, communication, and coordination of a program starting 1 to 2 months before surgery.

S. Black, MD

Efficacy of Aprotinin in Children Undergoing Craniofacial Surgery
D'Errico CC, Munro HM, Buchman SR, et al (Univ of Michigan, Ann Arbor; Children's Hosp, Columbus, Ohio)
J Neurosurg 99:287-290, 2003   6–10

Background.—Aprotinin is a serine protease inhibitor that has been in use for more than 70 years in numerous clinical settings, including acute pancreatitis, adult respiratory distress syndrome, trauma, and septic shock. Aprotinin has been studied for use in several procedures that have potential for large blood loss, such as orthotopic liver transplants in adults and children, total hip arthroplasty, spinal fusion, and nonbypass thoracic procedures. In recent years, the performance of craniofacial surgery in infants has become more extensive, and complete reshaping of the cranial vault is associated with a high risk of excessive blood loss. The efficacy of aprotinin in reducing the need for blood transfusion was determined in children undergoing reconstructive craniofacial surgery.

Methods.—A total of 39 patients (mean age, 1.2 ± 1.2 years) were enrolled in this prospective, randomized, placebo-controlled, double-blind study (Table 1). Two demographically similar groups were given 240 mg/m^2 IV aprotinin over 20 minutes followed by 56 mg/m^2/h or equal infusions of saline (placebo).

Results.—Patients in the aprotinin group received less blood per kilogram of body weight than did patients in the placebo group (32 ± 25 mL/kg vs 52 ± 34 mL/kg). Patients in the aprotinin group also experienced less change in

TABLE 1.—Demographic Summary of 39 Patients Who Underwent Craniofacial Surgery

Variable	Aprotinin	Placebo	Total
		Patient Group	
no. of patients	18	21	39
median age (yrs)	1.4 ± 1.1	0.76 ± 0.5*	1.2 ± 1.2
sex (% M/F)	64/36	61/39	64/36
weight (kg)	10.3 ± 3.2	11.2 ± 15.2	10.9 ± 1.4
ASA classification			
1	9	10	18
2	8	10	17
3	1	1	2
hematocrit level (%)			
preop	33.2 ± 3.9	33.2 ± 3.1	33.2 ± 3.4
lowest	22.3 ± 4.8	18.5 ± 2.7*	20.3 ± 4.3
postop	28.2 ± 5.9	31.4 ± 7.3	30.0 ± 6.8
duration of surgery (min)	480 ± 84	463 ± 77	471 ± 80
surgical procedure			
cranial vault reshaping	6	12	18
frontal orbital advancement	3	0	3
combined	9	9	18

*$P < .05$.

Abbreviation: ASA, American Society of Anesthesiologists physical status classification.

(Courtesy of D'Errico CC, Munro HM, Buchman SR, et al: Efficacy of aprotinin in children undergoing craniofacial surgery. *J Neurosurg* 99:287-290, 2003.)

hematocrit levels during surgery. The blood loss during surgery was judged to be significantly less than usual in the aprotinin group (Table 2). In addition, the aprotinin group had reduced requirements for blood transfusions in the first 3 postoperative days. No adverse events were observed in either the aprotinin or the placebo group.

Conclusions.—Blood transfusion requirements in pediatric patients undergoing craniofacial reconstruction seem to be reduced by infusion of aprotinin. The reduction in blood transfusion requirements led, in turn, to a reduction in the risks associated with exposure to banked blood components.

▶ The use of aprotinin to decrease intraoperative blood loss and transfusion in recent years has been extending to a wide variety of procedures. Initially reserved for repeat cardiac procedures with potentially life-threatening hemorrhage, it is now used for procedures from liver transplants to major joint sur-

TABLE 2.—Surgeons' Assessments of the Operative Field in 39 Patients Who Underwent Craniofacial Surgery

Assessment	Aprotinin	Placebo
	Patient Group (%)	
no. of patients	18	21
drier than expected	69*	26
as expected or wetter than expected	31	74

*$P < .05$.

(Courtesy of D'Errico CC, Munro HM, Buchman SR, et al: Efficacy of aprotinin in children undergoing craniofacial surgery. *J Neurosurg* 99:287-290, 2003.)

gery. In most cases, it is reported to be effective in decreasing blood loss, transfusion requirements, or both without significant complications, either from allergic reactions or thromboembolic complications. In this article, it was demonstrated to reduce the volume of red blood cell transfusion reported on a milliliter-per-kilogram basis in children undergoing complex craniofacial reconstruction. These procedures (depending on their complexity, of course) may be associated with large perioperative blood loss and transfusion requirements for sometimes 100% or more of the child's estimated blood volume. In this study, the use of aprotinin decreased the volume of transfused red cells by approximately 40%, and no significant difference was found in the transfusion of other products. This is, indeed, a clinically and statistically significant difference. Decreasing exposure to banked blood products is of potential benefit to these patients. Given the relatively small size of this study—39 patients, the incidence of uncommon but serious complications and their impact on outcomes cannot be defined. Given the expanding use of aprotinin to a wide variety of procedures, the likelihood of encountering patients with prior exposure and a significantly increased risk of serious allergic reactions to aprotinin will increase.

S. Black, MD

A Retrospective Review of Three Antibiotic Prophylaxis Regimens for Pediatric Cardiac Surgical Patients
Maher KO, VanDerElzen K, Bove EL, et al (Univ of Michigan, Ann Arbor)
Ann Thorac Surg 74:1195-1200, 2002   6–11

Introduction.—It is well accepted that antibiotic prophylaxis (AP) should be started before surgery. Yet the optimal duration of prophylaxis postoperatively is not clear for pediatric patients undergoing cardiac surgery. Several trials of adult surgical patients indicate that continuing prophylactic antibiotics for 48 hours or less postoperatively may be optimal. Data from the most recent survey of 43 pediatric cardiac surgical centers reported AP protocols: antimicrobial prophylaxis was continued by 29 (67%) centers if a thoracostomy tube was present and by 31 (72%) of centers if a mediastinal tube was present. The experience with more than 4000 pediatric surgical patients at the University of Michigan (Ann Arbor) was examined to investigate antibiotic prophylaxis regimens.

Methods.—Infections were divided into 2 groups: superficial incisional and deep incisional/mediastinitis. A modification of the Center for Disease Control and Prevention definition for surgical site infections (SSIs) was used. (1) A superficial incisional SSI must meet these criterion: Infection occurs within 30 days after surgery and involves only skin and subcutaneous tissue of the incision. (2) Deep incisional SSI must meet these criterion: Infection occurs within 30 days postoperatively if no implant is left in place or within 1 year if implant is left in place and the infections seems to be associated with the surgical procedure and involves deep soft tissue (eg, fascial and muscle layers) of the incision. (3) Mediastinitis/organ space SSI must meet the following criterion: Infection occurs within 30 days postoperatively if no implant is left in place or within 1 year if implant is in place and the infection seems to be associated with the surgical procedure and infection involves any part of the body, excluding the skin incision, fascia, or muscle layers, that is opened or manipulated during surgery.

Three antibiotic prophylaxis protocols were serially used during a 6-year period: Protocol 1 (n = 786): cefazolin was administered preoperatively and continued as long as thoracostomy tubes or central venous catheters were present. Protocol 2 (n = 1095): cefazolin was ceased 48 hours postoperatively, regardless of the presence of tubes or catheters. Protocol 3 (n = 2039): cefazolin was continued as long as thoracostomy tubes, and not central venous catheters, were present. Vancomycin and gentamicin was administered postoperatively in patients with an open chest wound until chest closure. The incidence of SSIs and unrelated bloodstream infections were retrospectively determined (the latter for both cardiac medical and surgical patients) for all 3 protocols.

Results.—The SSIs for 100 surgeries for protocols 1, 2, and 3, were 2.04, 6.58, and 1.67, respectively ($P < .05$ for protocol 2 vs protocols 1 and 3). Patients with an open chest had a higher incidence of SSI (18.8% for protocol 2 and 9.3% for protocol 3). The rate of bloodstream infections per 1000 patient-days for protocols 1, 2, and 3, respectively, were 2.18, 6.51, and 5.02 ($P < .05$ for protocol 1 vs protocols 2 and 3).

Conclusion.—The provision of antibiotic prophylaxis for as long as thoracostomy tubes are in place many diminish the rate of SSI (relative to discontinuing antibiotics sooner).

▶ This study sheds light on an important clinical question: What is the appropriate duration of prophylactic antibiotics in the perioperative period for pediatric patients undergoing correction of congenital cardiac defects? It is a retrospective review of a large number of patients. Because of its retrospective nature it is possible that other unrecognized changes in practice led to the change in infection rate attributed to the antibiotic regimen. However, because the first and third regimens, which both include coverage with antibiotics throughout the period the thoracostomy tube is in place, were the ones associated with the lowest infectious risk, it seems likely the differences are related to the antibiotic regimen rather than improvement in perioperative infection-prevention techniques over time. The importance of SSIs is clear; they result in readmission of more than half the patients in whom they develop.

M. F. Trankina, MD

Adverse Events After Protamine Administration Following Cardiopulmonary Bypass in Infants and Children

Seifert HA, Jobes DR, Have TT, et al (Univ of Pennsylvania, Philadelphia)
Anesth Analg 97:383-389, 2003   6–12

Introduction.—The assorted clinical presentations of protamine reactions have implicated a variety of physiologic mediators. Attempts to identify a sole immune mechanism have produced inconsistent results. Risk factors for serious reactions to protamine in adults include previous reactions to the drug, allergies to other medications, allergies to fish, and previous exposure to IV protamine or protamine-containing insulin preparations. Risk factors for protamine reactions may be different in children. The incidence of and risk factors for adverse events (AEs) in infants and children after IV administration of protamine after cardiopulmonary bypass (CPB) were examined in a retrospective cohort investigation.

Methods.—All relevant anesthesia records from a 3-year period were evaluated to identify AEs after protamine administration. The AEs were grouped according to 3 criteria: (1) a reduction in systemic mean arterial blood pressure (MAP) of at least 25% baseline or of at least 10% and necessitating treatment with inotropes, vasopressors, or reinstitution of CPB; (2) an increase in right atrial or central venous pressure of at least 10% from baseline linked with a reduction in MAP of at least 10% or needing any intervention; and (3) noncardiogenic pulmonary edema, as evidenced by any reduction in oxygen saturation necessitating an increase of inspired oxygen concentration, ventilatory rate, tidal volume, or ventilating pressures. Bronchospasm was also considered a relevant AE. The events had to occur within 30 minutes after administration of protamine and had to last for a minimum of 5 minutes. Protamine was administered as a bolus in all patients. These potential confounders were evaluated: year of surgery, type of surgery, ASA physical status, elective versus emergency surgery, surgeon, anesthesiologist, history of fish allergy, use of volatile anesthetics, duration of CPB, use of circulatory arrest, use of inotropes or vasopressors after CPB but before protamine administration, administration of IV calcium after CPB but before protamine, and histamine H1 or H2 receptor blockade before surgery.

Results.—Of 1249 anesthesia records, no episodes of isolated or hypotensive-related right-sided cardiac failure or acute pulmonary dysfunction were recorded. Median patient age at the time of surgery was 208 days (range, 0-5799 days). The rate of systemic hypotension after protamine administration ranged between 17.6% (95% confidence interval [CI], 1.11%-2.65%) and 2.88% (95% CI, 2.03%-3.97%) depending on the strictness of case definition. Unadjusted univariate analyses with the primary case definition revealed that female sex, smaller heparin dose, larger protamine dose, and no administration of modified ultrafiltration were linked with statistically significant increases in the risk of AEs. In multivariate analysis, female sex, larger protamine dose, and smaller heparin dose were significantly linked with the risk of AEs by the primary case definition.

Conclusion.—The incidence of AEs after protamine administration during surgeries on children younger than 16 years is similar to that for adults. Female sex, larger protamine doses, and smaller heparin dose were independent risk factors for severe events in children.

▶ Protamine administration to reverse heparin after CPB has long been known to be associated with complications including hypotension, pulmonary edema, pulmonary hypertension, and right heart failure. In this large retrospective study incidence and risk factors for protamine adverse reactions in pediatric patients are reported. While the incidence is similar to that reported in adults, the risk factors, not surprisingly, are different. Female sex, higher protamine dose, and lower heparin dose all were associated with a higher risk for hypotension after protamine. It would be interesting to see if a smaller dose of protamine in female pediatric patients would result in adequate reversal of heparin while perhaps lowering the risk for hypotension.

M. F. Trankina, MD

7 Head Injury and Neuroanesthesia

Patient Age and Outcome Following Severe Traumatic Brain Injury: An Analysis of 5600 Patients
Hukkelhoven CWPM, Steyerberg EW, Rampen AJJ, et al (Erasmus Med Ctr, Rotterdam, The Netherlands; Univ of Virginia, Charlottesville; Univ of California, San Diego; et al)
J Neurosurg 99:666-673, 2003   7–1

Background.—In systemic diseases, such as a subarachnoid hemorrhage, traumatic brain injury (TBI), and dementia, increasing age is associated with a worse outcome. TBI is a significant health and socioeconomic problem throughout the world and the leading cause of death and disability in younger patients in more economically developed countries. It is unclear whether there are critical age thresholds in TBI, and the strength of the association has not previously been investigated across large series. The strength and shape of the relationship between age and outcome in TBI was assessed by evaluation of the 6-month mortality rate and unfavorable outcomes based on the Glasgow Coma Scale.

Methods.—The character of the association between age and TBI outcome was examined in 4 prospective series with a total of 2664 patients. All patients had a closed TBI and were of adult age; 96% of patients were younger than 65 years. The strength of the association was evaluated in a meta-analysis of individual patient data for the same 2664 patients and aggregate data on 2948 patients from studies of TBI published from 1980 to 2001, which yielded a total of 5612 patients. Univariate and multivariate logistic regression analyses were performed.

Results.—There was an increase with age in the proportions of mortality and unfavorable outcomes, at 21% and 39%, respectively, among patients under age 35 years versus 52% and 74%, respectively, for patients older than age 55 years. The association between age and both mortality and unfavorable outcome was continuous and could be described by a linear term and expressed statistically by a linear and quadratic term. The use of age thresholds in that analysis resulted in a considerable loss of information. The strength of the association (expressed as an odds ratio per 10 years of age) was 1.47 for death and 1.49 for unfavorable outcome in univariate analysis

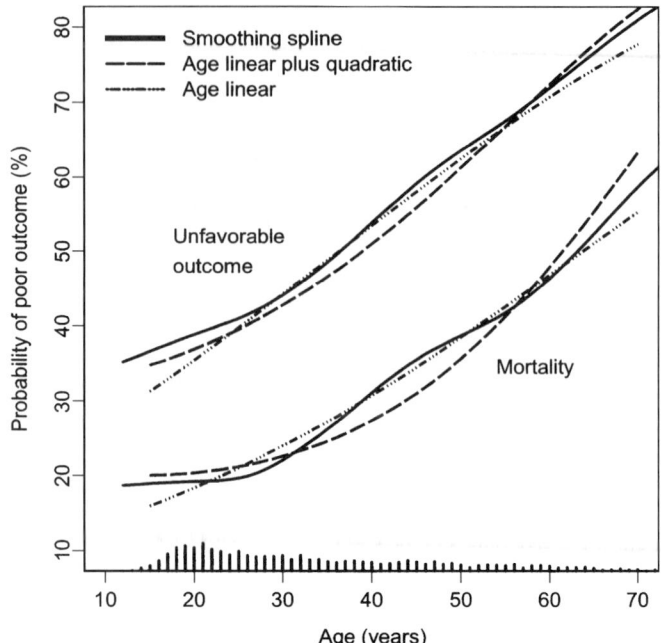

FIGURE 1.—Graph demonstrating the univariable association between age and 6-month outcome in 2664 patients with severe traumatic brain injuries. Age was described as a continuous linear term (age linear), an age linear plus quadratic term, and a smoothing spline. The vertical strokes at the base of the graph indicate the age distribution. For ease of interpretation, the probability scale is presented in this figure rather than the logistical log-odds scale generally used in logistic regression models. A linear association on the log-odds scale corresponds to a sigmoid curve on the probability scale. Model variables for age linear (age per 10 years) were as follows: logit (mortality) = −2.18 + 0.34 * age and logit (unfavorable outcome) = −1.34 + 0.37 * age. Model variables for age linear plus age quadratic (age per 10 years) were as follows: logit (mortality) = −1.26 − 0.18 * age + 0.06 * age^2 and logit (unfavorable outcome) = −0.77 + 0.03 * age + 0.04 * age^2. (Courtesy of Hukkelhoven CWPM, Steyerberg EW, Rampen AJJ, et al: Patient age and outcome following severe traumatic brain injury: An analysis of 5600 patients. *J Neurosurg* 99:666-673, 2003.)

and 1.39 and 1.46, respectively, in multivariate analysis (Fig 1). The odds for a poor outcome were increased by 40% to 50% for every 10 years of age.

Conclusions.—These findings demonstrate a continuing association between older age and worsening outcomes after TBI. It is, therefore, disadvantageous to define the effect of age on outcome discretely when estimation of a prognosis or adjustment for confounding variables is made.

▶ It has long been recognized that increasing age is associated with a worse outcome after a severe TBI, but this article points out important issues. First, the effect of age is continuous rather than there being a cutoff age at which the outcome changes dramatically. Instead, with each 10 years of life, the chance of death or a poor neurologic outcome increases by about 50%. This is important as we consider the prognosis of our own patients and as we look at trials investigating new treatment strategies. In addition, not only does the chance of survival decrease with increasing age but the fewer people who survive are also less likely to do well as age increases. Finally, it seems that the increased morbidity and mortality after a head injury with increasing age is not likely due to other coexisting conditions but to the greater vulnerability of the aging brain to injury.

S. Black, MD

Sex-Related Differences in Patients With Severe Head Injury: Greater Susceptibility to Brain Swelling in Female Patients 50 Years of Age and Younger

Farin A, Deutsch R, Biegon A, et al (Univ of California, San Diego; Lawrence Berkeley Natl Lab, Berkeley, Calif)

J Neurosurg 98:32-36, 2003   7–2

Background.—Most victims of severe head injury (70% to 80%) are male, and several studies have reported evidence for sex-related differences and gonadal hormone effects on the incidence, outcome, and treatment response of neurologic disorders in the case of Alzheimer disease, stroke, epilepsy, and multiple sclerosis. Several analyses of the influence of sex on the outcome of traumatic brain injury have produced conflicting results, which may be a function in part of the small number of females included in clinical studies of severe head injury.

The largest controlled clinical trial of brain injury to date was recently completed. Its findings regarding the effects of female gonadal hormones on fluid balance and the high frequency of idiopathic intracranial hypertension in premenopausal female patients were the impetus for the present study in which the influence of sex and age on factors affecting outcome in patients with severe head injury were examined.

Methods.—Data from the prospective international trial of tirilazad mesylate for patients with head injury were retrospectively evaluated. The study included 957 patients, of whom 23% were female. All of the patients were between the ages of 15 and 79 years, and all presented with Glasgow Coma Scale scores of 3 to 8, with evidence of structural brain damage or subarachnoid hemorrhage on the initial CT scan. Comparisons between male and female patients were made regarding the frequency of several recognized risk factors, including swelling of the brain, intracranial hypertension, systemic hypotension, advanced age, subarachnoid hemorrhage, and injury severity and dichotomized Glasgow Outcome Scale scores obtained 6 months after injury.

Results.—Overall, brain swelling and intracranial hypertension were found with significantly greater frequency in female versus male patients (35% vs 24%, and 39% vs 31%, respectively). The highest rates were observed for female patients under age 51 years (38% vs 24% and 40% vs 30%, respectively, for male patients under 51 years of age). This effect was found to be independent of Glasgow Coma Scale scores, which did not differ between male and female patients. Outcomes tended to be worse for female patients younger than 50 years, but the difference was not statistically significant.

Conclusion.—Female patients with severe head injury, particularly pre-menopausal patients aged 50 years or younger, are significantly more likely than male patients with comparable injury severity to experience brain swelling and intracranial hypertension. It is suggested that younger women may benefit from more aggressive monitoring and treatment of intracranial hypertension.

▶ Interesting findings added to a complicated debate. Gonadal hormones may inhibit premenopausal females ability to compensate with significant traumatic brain injury but may have neuroprotective benefits long term (a 7% reduction in Glasgow Outcome Score at 6 months compared to males in this study). No matter the potential benefit, the message here seems to be to anticipate more brain swelling and intracranial hypertension and have a low threshold for more aggressive treatment in this patient population.

J. D. Lang, Jr, MD

Placement of Intracranial Pressure Monitors by Non-Neurosurgeons

Harris CH, Smith RS, Helmer SD, et al (Univ of Kansas, Witchita; Via Christi Regional Med Ctr, Wichita, Kan)
Am Surg 68:787-790, 2002   7–3

Background.—Maintenance of adequate cerebral perfusion is of critical importance in the treatment of patients with closed head injury. The cerebral perfusion pressure is defined as the difference between the mean arterial pressure and the intracranial pressure (ICP), and placement of an intracranial monitor is required for determination of the cerebral perfusion pressure and continuous monitoring of ICP. Historically, the insertion of such monitoring devices has been performed by neurosurgeons; however, others, including general surgeons, have successfully inserted simple ICP monitors. The efficacy of ICP monitor placement was evaluated, and the complication rates for placement of ICP monitors by general surgery residents, trauma surgeons, and staff neurosurgeons were compared.

Methods.—A retrospective review was conducted of the medical records of trauma patients with cerebral injury who required insertion of parenchymal ICP monitors between January 1994 and January 1999. Placement of monitors was performed by staff neurosurgeons, trauma surgeons, and general surgery residents. The residents received appropriate training in the placement of ICP monitors. Medical records were examined for demographic variables including age, gender, mechanism of injury, admission Glasgow Coma Score, and Injury Severity Score; duration of ICP monitoring; and complications.

Results.—A total of 157 monitors were placed in 146 patients with intracranial injury. Surgical residents inserted 87 ICP monitors without neurosurgical or trauma attending surgeons at the bedside and 43 monitors with immediate supervision by general surgeons or neurosurgeons. A total of 26 ICP monitors were placed without the participation of residents, and 1 monitor was placed without the involvement of a resident or neurosurgeon. No major technical complications, episodes of intracranial hemorrhage, or infectious complications were encountered.

Conclusion.—Insertion of simple ICP monitors by non-neurosurgeons has the potential for improving the care of patients with brain injury in geographic areas that are underserved by neurosurgeons. It is proposed that insertion of simple parenchymal ICP monitors should be considered a core skill for trauma surgeons and should be included in surgical residency training.

▶ A clear demonstration that procedures once thought exclusive to a certain specialty can, in fact, be safely performed by others. I would propose that anesthesiology-trained intensivists in an ICU environment that is target-rich with neurosurgery cases and/or head trauma should be taught this skill as well.

J. D. Lang, Jr, MD

The Effects of Large-Dose Propofol on Cerebrovascular Pressure Autoregulation in Head-Injured Patients

Steiner LA, Johnston AJ, Chatfield DA, et al (Addenbrooke's Hosp, Cambridge, England)
Anesth Analg 97:572-576, 2003   7–4

Background.—Propofol is often administered for sedation and control of increased intracranial pressure (ICP) in patients with head injuries. It has been shown in the literature that propofol infusion will preserve or improve cerebrovascular pressure autoregulation in healthy individuals. Pressure au-

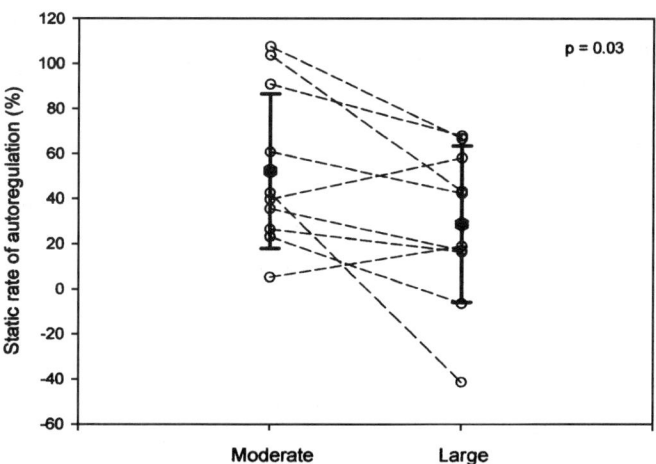

FIGURE 1.—Static rate of autoregulation at a moderate and a large dose of propofol. Individual data from 10 patients are presented. The *hexagon and error bars* represent mean ± SD. (Courtesy of Steiner LA, Johnston AJ, Chatfield DA, et al: The effects of large-dose propofol on cerebrovascular pressure autoregulation in head-injured patients. *Anesth Analg* 97(2):572-576, 2003.)

TABLE 1.—Hemodynamic Variables

	Propofol Moderate (2.3 ± 0.4 μg/mL)		Propofol Large (4.3 ± 0.4 μg/mL)	
	CPP 1	CPP 2	CPP 1	CPP 2
CPP (mm Hg)	69 ± 4	86 ± 4	69 ± 4	87 ± 5
ICP (mm Hg)	16.0 ± 2.5	15.8 ± 3.7	15.6 ± 3.3	15.8 ± 5.1
FVm (cm/s)	70 ± 21	79 ± 25	62 ± 22*	73 ± 27†

Note: All data are mean ± SD.
*P < .01 compared with CPP 1 at the moderate propofol target concentration.
†P < .05 compared with CPP 2 at the moderate propofol target concentration. All other comparisons did not reach significance.
Abbreviations: CPP, Cerebral perfusion pressure; ICP, intracranial pressure; FVm, averaged mean flow velocity from both middle cerebral arteries.
(Courtesy of Steiner LA, Johnston AJ, Chatfield DA, et al: The effects of large-dose propofol on cerebrovascular pressure autoregulation in head-injured patients. *Anesth Analg* 97(2):572-576, 2003.)

toregulation is an important prognostic factor in patients with head injuries because a strong association exists between dysautoregulation and impaired outcomes. The effect of an increase in the plasma propofol concentration on pressure autoregulation in patients with head injuries was examined.

Methods.—The study group was composed of 10 patients (7 men, 3 women) with a median age of 35 ± 12 years. The median Glasgow Coma Scale score at admission was 7 (range, 3-9). The pattern of injury was classified as an evacuated mass lesion in 8 patients and diffuse injury II in 2 patients. Target-controlled infusions were used to determine the static rate of autoregulation at moderate (2.3 ± 0.4 μg/mL) and large (4.3 ± 0.04 μg/mL) target concentrations of plasma propofol. Doppler measurements from the middle cerebral artery were obtained at cerebral perfusion pressures of 70 and 85 mm Hg at each propofol concentration.

Results.—The middle cerebral artery flow velocities at the larger propofol concentration were significantly lower than those at the moderate concentration, and no concurrent increase in the arteriojugular difference in oxygen content occurred (Fig 1). This finding was compatible with maintained flow–metabolism coupling. However, a significant decrease was found in the static rate of autoregulation, from 54% ± 36% to 28% ± 35% (Table 1).

Conclusions.—The cerebrovascular effects of propofol in patients with head injuries seem to be different from the effects in healthy individuals. Caution is urged in the administration of large doses of propofol in patients with head injuries because the potential exists to increase the vulnerability of the injured brain to secondary trauma.

▶ This article points out another reason for caution in the use of propofol for sedation in patients with head injuries. Not long after its introduction, propofol in higher doses was shown to be associated with decreases in mean arterial pressure that exceeded decreases in ICP. This led to decreases in cerebral perfusion pressure, which, in some patients, was below the cerebral autoregulatory level. In these severely head-injured patients, the higher dose of propofol was associated with worsening of cerebral autoregulation. As the authors point out, impaired autoregulation is associated with a worse outcome. I would agree that interventions impairing autoregulation should be avoided—or undertaken with awareness of their risk–benefit ratio. However, it is possible that impaired autoregulation is a marker of a worse injury rather than a cause of a worse outcome. It may be that like ICP (in which elevated ICP is associated with a worse outcome, but measures lowering ICP, such as barbiturates, do not improve the outcome), treatments that alter autoregulation may not alter the outcome.

S. Black, MD

Intubation After Cervical Spinal Cord Injury: To Be Done Selectively or Routinely?
Velmahos GC, Toutouzas K, Chan L, et al (Univ of Southern California, Los Angeles)
Am Surg 69:891-894, 2003   7–5

Background.—More than 10,000 individuals have cervical spinal cord injuries (CSCIs) in the United States each year, at a cost of more than $1 million per patient. The mortality in patients with high CSCIs ranges from 20% to 50%. Compromise of respiratory functioning in patients with CSCIs may result in acute respiratory failure and the need for intubation and mechanical ventilation. It is unknown whether intubation should be offered preemptively in all patients with CSCIs or selectively on the basis of signs of acute respiratory failure. There are risks associated with both decisions: waiting may exacerbate the neurologic injury, whereas preemptive intubation may cause unnecessary intubation-related morbidity. The role of routine early intubation in patients with CSCIs was evaluated.

Methods.—A review was conducted of the medical records of 68 patients with CSCIs. Univariate and multivariate analyses were used to identify independent risk factors for the need for intubation.

Results.—Of the 68 patients evaluated, 50 (74%) required intubation and 27 (40%) had pneumonia. Among patients with CSCIs above the level of C5, 87.5% required intubation compared with 61% of patients with CSCIs at C5–C8. Among patients with complete quadriplegia, 90% required intubation compared with 48.5% of patients with incomplete quadriplegia or paraplegia. A total of 31 patients were seen without overt signs of acute respiratory failure on admission; among these patients, 13 (42%) later had decompensation and were later intubated up to 53 hours after admission. Six of these patients developed pulmonary complications associated with the emergent intubation. Three independent risk factors for the need for intubation were identified: Injury Severity Score greater than 16, CSCI higher than C5, and complete quadriplegia. The combination of the latter 2 risk factors resulted in intubation in 21 of 22 patients (95%).

Conclusions.—Most patients with CSCIs require intubation. Intubation should be offered routinely and early in patients with CSCIs above C5 because delays may result in otherwise preventable morbidity.

▶ As pointed out in this retrospective study, patients with CSCIs and neurologic impairment are highly likely to require intubation during their hospitalization. It is well-known that intubation alone may predispose a patient to pulmonary infectious complications, and we are all conscious of the importance of avoiding unnecessary prophylactic intubation or mechanical ventilation. These authors define a high-risk group of patients—those with cord injuries at or above C5 and/or complete quadriplegia—that most likely will require intubation. In addition, they clearly show that emergent intubation in the setting of acute trauma and a cord injury is potentially associated with a significantly increased risk of morbidity. This is demonstrated by complications occurring in nearly 50% of patients intubated after respiratory decompensation developed in the first day or days after trauma. Their recommendations seem prudent: to seriously consider prophylactic intubation for all patients with cord injuries above C5, complete quadriplegia, or both.

C. Black, MD

Cardiovascular Responses to Endotracheal Intubation in Patients With Acute and Chronic Spinal Cord Injuries
Yoo KY, Jeong SW, Kim SJ, et al (Chonnam Natl Univ Med School, Gwangju, South Korea)
Anesth Analg 97:1162-1167, 2003   7–6

Background.—An increased heart rate and blood pressure are usually associated with laryngoscopy and tracheal intubation, in part, because of a reflex sympathetic discharge. However, in patients with spinal cord lesions, the sympathetic nervous system may be differentially affected according to the level of the injury, while the parasympathetic system may remain intact. Initially, cardiovascular responses may transiently decrease after a spinal cord injury; patients with acute quadriplegia often manifest low blood pressure. However, paroxysmal hypertension may occur in the later stage of quadriplegia as a result of an increase in adrenoreceptor functioning and/or a loss of descending inhibitory control. Thus, it would appear that injury to the spinal cord may alter cardiovascular responses to intubation as a function of both time elapsed from the injury and the level of the injury. Whether the cardiovascular responses to intubation change as a function of the time elapsed in patients with spinal cord injuries was determined.

Methods.—A total of 106 patients with traumatic complete spinal cord injuries were divided into early and chronic groups on the basis of time elapsed since injury (ie, < and > 4 weeks after injury) and into groups with quadriplegia or paraplegia, according to the level of the injury. A control group of 25 patients with no spinal cord injuries were also examined. The

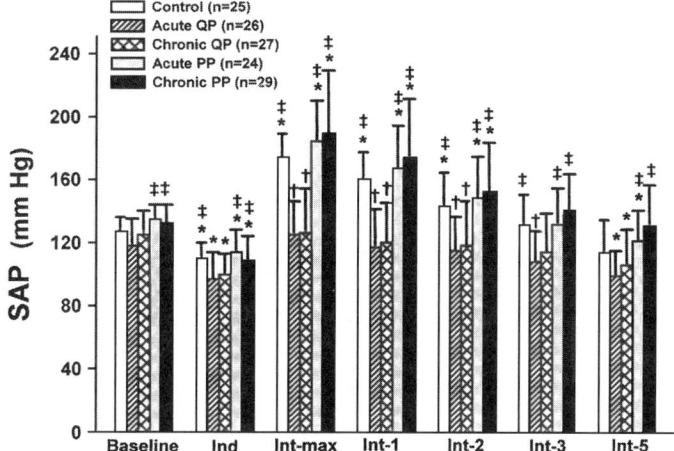

FIGURE 1.—Systolic arterial blood pressure (SAP) before and after endotracheal intubation in spinal cord-injured and control patients. Values are mean ± SD (n = number of patients). *$P < .05$ versus baseline; †$P < .05$ versus the control group; ‡$P < .05$ versus the acute QP group. *Abbreviations: acute QP,* Patients with acute quadriplegia; *chronic QP,* patients with chronic quadriplegia; *acute PP,* patients with acute paraplegia; *chronic PP,* patients with chronic paraplegia; *Ind,* 1 minute after induction; *Int-max,* maximum response within 1 minute after intubation; *Int-1 -2, -3, and -5,* responses at 1, 2, 3, and 5 minutes after intubation. (Courtesy of Yoo KY, Jeong SW, Kim SJ, et al: Cardiovascular responses to endotracheal intubation in patients with acute and chronic spinal cord injuries. *Anesth Analg* 97(4):1162-1167, 2003.)

main outcome measures were systolic arterial blood pressure, heart rate, and plasma concentrations of catecholamines.

Results.—The systolic arterial blood pressure was not affected by intubation in either the acute or the chronic quadriplegic group but was significant-

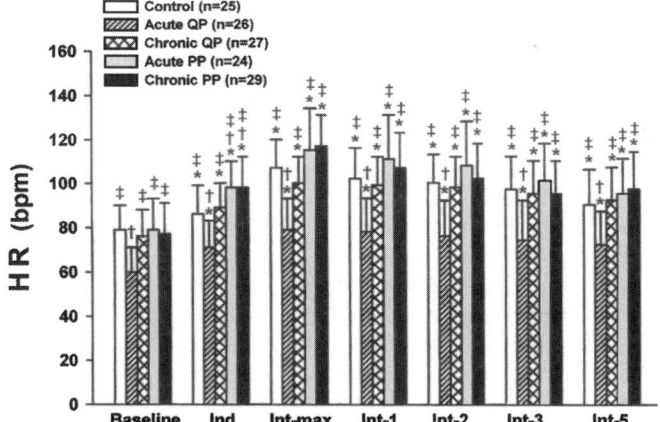

FIGURE 2.—Heart rate (HR) before and after endotracheal intubation in spinal cord-injured and control patients. Values are mean ± SD (n = number of patients). *$P < .05$ versus baseline; †$P < .05$ versus the control group; ‡$P < .05$ versus the acute QP group. *Abbreviations: acute QP,* Patients with acute quadriplegia; *chronic QP,* patients with chronic quadriplegia; *acute PP,* patients with acute paraplegia; *chronic PP,* patients with chronic paraplegia; *Ind,* 1 minute after induction; *Int-max,* maximum response within 1 minute after intubation; *Int-1 -2, -3, and -5,* responses at 1, 2, 3, and 5 minutes after intubation.(Courtesy of Yoo KY, Jeong SW, Kim SJ, et al: Cardiovascular responses to endotracheal intubation in patients with acute and chronic spinal cord injuries. *Anesth Analg* 97(4):1162-1167, 2003.)

TABLE 2.—Incidence of Adverse Effects in Spinal Cord-Injured and Control Patients

Variable	Control ($n = 25$)	Acute QP ($n = 26$)	Chronic QP ($n = 27$)	Acute PP ($n = 24$)	Chronic PP ($n = 29$)
Hypertension	16	1*	2*	20	21
Hypotension	1	9*	9*	1	1
Tachycardia (HR > 120 bpm)	3	0	2	6	14*
Bradycardia (HR < 60 bpm)	2	12*	2	1	3
Dysrhythmia	2	1	2	4	4

*$P < .05$ versus the control group.

Abbreviations: acute QP, Patients with acute quadriplegia; *chronic QP*, patients with chronic quadriplegia; *acute PP*, patients with acute paraplegia; *chronic PP*, patients with chronic paraplegia; *HR*, heart rate.

(Courtesy of Yoo K Y, Jeong S W, Kim S J, et al: Cardiovascular responses to endotracheal intubation in patients with acute and chronic spinal cord injuries. *Anesth Analg* 97(4):1162-1167, 2003.)

ly increased in both the acute and the chronic paraplegic groups (Fig 1). Heart rate was significantly increased in all groups, but the degree of change was less in the acute quadriplegic group than in other groups (Fig 2). Plasma concentrations of catecholamines were increased in every group but the acute quadriplegic group. The magnitude of this increase in catecholamines was attenuated in the chronic quadriplegic group, accentuated in the acute paraplegic group, and similar in the chronic paraplegic group when compared with the control group. No difference was found among the groups in the incidence of arrhythmias (Table 2).

Conclusions.—It seems that the cardiovascular and catecholamine response in patients who undergo endotracheal intubation may change as a function of the time elapsed since the spinal cord injury and the level of the injury.

▶ This study clearly defines the different hemodynamic response to a brief laryngoscopy and intubation after induction of general anesthesia in patients with acute and chronic spinal cord injuries. There are several important clinical implications. First, even though patients with acute quadriplegia are more likely to have bradycardia, they do show mild increases in heart rate with intubation, which is in contrast to the further decreases in heart rate with tracheal suctioning that have been reported in the same type of patients. Second, there is no hypertensive response to laryngoscopy and intubation in the quadriplegic patients, which alters the drugs we may need to give at induction. Not surprisingly, the quadriplegic patients are more likely to become significantly hypotensive after induction. Third, with regard to the paraplegic patients, their hemodynamic responses are similar to those in patients without spinal cord injuries, with the important exception that it may be exaggerated in the patients with chronic paraplegia. These patients are more likely to develop tachycardia and severe hypertension. These observations are important to anesthesiologists as we plan our induction sequence in these patients.

S. Black, MD

Serum Neuron-Specific Enolase Predicts Outcome in Post-Anoxic Coma:
A Prospective Cohort Study
Meynaar IA, Oudemans-van Straaten HM, Wetering J, et al (Reinier de Graaf
Gasthuis, Delft, The Netherlands; Onze Lieve Vrouwe Gasthuis, Amsterdam;
Isala Klinieken, Zwolle, The Netherlands; et al)
Intensive Care Med 29:189-195, 2003   7–7

Background.—When cardiopulmonary resuscitation (CPR) is successful and spontaneous circulation is restored, most patients will be comatose as a result of postanoxic encephalopathy. Many of these patients will not regain consciousness and will subsequently die or remain in a permanent vegetative state. It is important for several reasons to differentiate between comatose patients after CPR who have no chance of regaining consciousness and those who may regain consciousness. Whether serial serum neuron-specific enolase (NSE) can be used to make this differentiation was investigated.

Methods.—This observational cohort study was conducted in an 18-bed general ICU. The study group was composed of 110 comatose patients admitted to the ICU after CPR. Serum NSE was measured at admission and daily for 5 days in survivors. The patients received full intensive treatment until recovery or the absence of cortical response to somatosensory evoked potentials more than 48 hours after CPR-proved irreversible coma.

Results.—Of the 110 patients admitted, 34 regained consciousness, of whom 5 died in hospital. The remaining 76 patients did not regain consciousness and 72 died in hospital. Serum NSE at 24 hours and 48 hours after CPR was significantly higher in patients who did not regain consciousness. None of the patients with a serum NSE level greater than 25.0 µg/L at any time regained consciousness. The addition of SNE to the Glasgow Coma Scale score and somatosensory evoked potentials increased the predictability of a poor neurologic outcome from 64% to 76%.

Conclusion.—High serum NSE in comatose patients at 24 and 48 hours after cardiopulmonary resuscitation predicts a poor neurologic outcome. The addition of NSE to the Glasgow Coma Scale score and somatosensory evoked potentials increases the predictability of neurologic outcome.

▶ A potentially nice serum marker that can be used for prognostication. This is a NSE that can be elevated under a variety of circumstances (stroke and intracerebral hemorrhage). If other corroborating data can be generated in other studies, clinical utilization in cases like this (patient's postcardiopulmonary resuscitation) may not be too far off.

J. D. Lang, Jr, MD

Incidences of Venous Air Embolism and Patent Foramen Ovale Among Patients Undergoing Selective Peripheral Denervation in the Sitting Position

Girard F, Ruel M, McKenty S, et al (Hôpital Notre-Dame, Montreal; Washington Univ, St Louis)
Neurosurgery 53:316-320, 2003   7–8

Background.—Venous air embolism (VAE) is a potentially fatal complication. Its incidence and severity in patients undergoing selective peripheral denervation in the sitting position have not been definitively determined. The incidence and severity of VAE, the incidence of paradoxical air embolism, and the occurrence of patent foramen ovale were established.

Methods.—Data on 342 patients were analyzed in this retrospective review. All had had selective peripheral denervation at one center between 1988 and 2001. Cases of patent foramen ovale were detected by transesophageal echocardiography.

Findings.—Seven patients had VAE, for an incidence of 2%. On a 5-point scale, VAE severity was 2 for 3 patients, 3 for 3, and 4 for 1 (see scale in original article). None of the patients died. Patent foramen ovale was detected in 5.2% of the 96 transesophageal echocardiographic examinations. The 5 affected patients underwent surgery in the prone or park bench position. There were no cases of paradoxical air embolism.

Conclusion.—These authors report a very low incidence of VAE and recommend that detection of a patent foramen ovale should prompt a change in position for this surgery.

▶ These authors report an incidence of VAE of 2% in patients undergoing selective peripheral denervation for spasmodic torticollis in the sitting position. That incidence is low and similar to the incidence reported in other smaller series.[1]

Of concern is that only 40% of the patients were monitored with precordial Doppler. The authors suggest that this lack of routine Doppler monitoring is unlikely to miss many patients with VAE because the volume of air infused to trigger diagnosis by changes in end-tidal CO_2 is not much greater than the volume required to trigger diagnosis with Doppler. This is likely not a valid argument in the clinical environment, especially in a retrospective study.

It is likely that end-tidal CO_2 was recorded certainly no more often than every 5 to 15 minutes. An episode of VAE could easily occur between these recording points. The high sensitivity of end-tidal CO_2 monitoring referred to by the authors comes from animal experiments in which the end-tidal CO_2 is monitored continuously. Therefore, it is likely that episodes of VAE were missed in the 60% of patients not monitored with precordial Doppler.

The fact that 57% of patients who experienced VAE had significant hemodynamic changes also suggests that many minor episodes of VAE occurred undetected. Prior to routine use of precordial Doppler in sitting craniotomies, VAE was an uncommon but dangerous complication. After use of Doppler monitoring was routine, VAE was diagnosed commonly but rarely caused clin-

ically significant hemodynamic events.[2] The more conservative recommendation might be to routinely use Doppler rather than, as the authors suggest, to
routinely place a central line.

S. Black, MD

References

1. Lobato EB, Black S, DeSoto H: Venous air embolism and selective denervation for torticollis. *Anesth Analg* 84:551-553, 1997.
2. Black S, Ockert DB, Oliver WC, et al: Outcome following posterior fossa craniotomy in sitting vs. horizontal positions. *Anesthesiology* 69:49-56, 1988.

Venous Air Embolism During Awake Craniotomy In a Supine Patient
Balki M, Manninen PH, McGuire GP, et al (Univ of Toronto)
Can J Anesth 50:835–838, 2003   7–9

Background.—Venous air embolism (VAE) is a well-documented complication of procedures involving an operative field above the level of the heart.
A nonfatal case of intraoperative VAE, with unusual clinical features, occurring during an awake craniotomy was reported.

> *Case Report.*—A 61-year-old man, was scheduled for excision of a
> dominant hemisphere brain tumor. His medical history included di-
> abetes and hypertension. Airway assessment, physical examination,
> and laboratory values were all normal. An awake craniotomy in the
> supine position was scheduled for cortical mapping before tumor re-
> section. An hour after surgery had begun, during dural opening, the
> patient started to cough continuously. This was followed by tachyp-
> nea, hypoxia, and a decline in end-tidal carbon dioxide (Fig). Except
> for transient hypertension, cardiovascular variables remained stable
> during this episode. Airway obstruction and low cardiac ouput were
> excluded. Standard treatment for VAE was initiated, and the patient
> recovered without further complications.

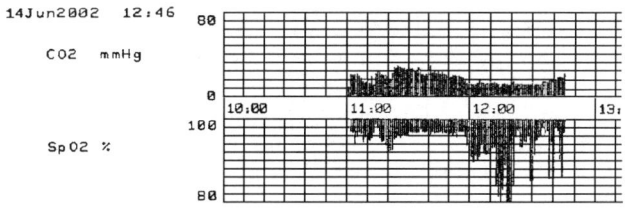

FIGURE.—Intraoperative tracing of the end-tidal carbon dioxide and oxygen saturation (*Sp* O2). At the
time of the suspected venous air embolism, there was a decrease in end-tidal carbon dioxide from 28 to 16 mm
Hg. (Courtesy of Balki M, Manninen PH, McGuire GP, et al: Venous air embolism during awake craniotomy
in a supine patient. *Can J Anesth* 50:835-838, 2003.)

Conclusion.—This case of VAE was seen with unusual clinical features. Early diagnosis of VAE is important for effective management.

▶ This case report is an important reminder that the risk for VAE continues to be present. With the dramatic decrease in the use of the sitting position for neurosurgical procedures, both the occurrence of VAE and our awareness of the potential for VAE have decreased. The greatest likelihood for morbidity and mortality from VAE continues to be in situations where the diagnosis of VAE is not suspected. As the use of awake craniotomies continues to increase, we should expect an increase in episodes of VAE.

The traditional sensitive monitors for VAE may be less sensitive or less likely to be used in the awake patient. Capnography via nasal cannula in the spontaneously breathing patient may be less reliable. Transesophageal echocardiography is not an option. Precordial Doppler should be as effective in the awake as asleep neurosurgical patient. However, the constant Doppler tones tend to be irritating to a neurosurgical team not accustomed to Doppler use, and this problem could be a substantial impediment to its use during awake procedures.

J. Black, MD

The Efficacy and Safety of Aprotinin for Hemostasis During Intracranial Surgery

Palmer JD, Francis JL, Pickard JD, et al (Southampton Gen Hosp, England; Addenbrooke's Hosp, Cambridge, England; Florida Hosp, Orlando)
J Neurosurg 98:1208-1216, 2003   7–10

Background.—Aprotinin has been evaluated for efficacy in reducing intraoperative bleeding in several recent studies. It has been shown that aprotinin is associated with reduced blood loss after prostate surgery and cardiac and liver surgery. In addition, topical aprotinin has been used to reduce the risk of rebleeding in brain tumor surgery in a large, uncontrolled series. However, no randomized, prospective studies of the use of aprotinin in neurosurgery have been performed. The safety and efficacy of prophylactic high-dose IV aprotinin for the reduction of intraoperative blood loss in the neurosurgical population were determined.

Methods.—This randomized, double-blind, placebo-controlled study involved a total of 100 patients in parallel groups in 2 regional neurosurgical departments. All patients had a preoperative diagnosis of intracranial meningioma or vestibular schwannoma subsequently confirmed on histologic studies. The patients were all older than 18 years, not pregnant, and without a history of bleeding diathesis, previous exposure to aprotinin, or ingestion of antiplatelet or anticoagulant medications within the 2 weeks before surgery. Aprotinin was administered in doses of 30,000 kallikrein-inhibiting units (KIU)/kg body weight at induction of anesthesia, and infusions of 10,000 KIU/kg/h continued to the completion of surgery or a maximum of 8 hours. The main outcome measures were intraoperative blood loss, blood

TABLE 2.—Intraoperative Blood Loss in 90 Assessable Patients Who Underwent Neurosurgery With or Without Aprotinin

Blood Loss	Meningioma			VS		
	Aprotinin	Placebo	P Value	Aprotinin	Placebo	P Value
overall						
geo mean ± geo SD	546 ± 3.51	1093 ± 2.67		242 ± 2.56	243 ± 2.55	
no. of patients	30	26		17	17	
at Center 1						
geo mean ± geo SD	568 ± 4.18	1262 ± 2.64		233 ± 3.51	236 ± 3.47	
no. of patients	21	19		7	8	
at Center 2						
geo mean ± geo SD	493 ± 1.95	741 ± 2.65		248 ± 2.12	251 ± 1.62	
no. of patients	9	7		10	9	
overall log						
LSM ± SE	6.23 ± 0.22	6.92 ± 0.24	0.028*	5.48 ± 0.25	5.49 ± 0.25	0.97†
overall based on LSM of log transformed data						
geo mean ± geo SE	508 ± 1.25	1014 ± 1.27		240 ± 1.28	243 ± 1.28	

*Significant at a probability level of .05.
†Not significant.
Abbreviations: VS, Vestibular schwannoma; *Geo,* geometric; *LSM,* least-squares mean.
(Courtesy of Palmer JD, Francis JL, Pickard JD, et al: The efficacy and safety of aprotinin for hemostasis during intracranial surgery. *J Neurosurg* 98:1208-1216, 2003.)

transfusion, the Glasgow Outcome Scale score, and the Index of Independence. All patients underwent screening for deep vein thrombosis and were assessed with the Mini-Mental State Examination.

Results.—Intraoperative blood loss was reduced with aprotinin, from 1014 mL (geometric mean) with placebo to 508 mL with aprotinin (Table 2). Patients with schwannomas had lower blood loss than those with meningiomas and aprotinin did not alter blood loss. Blood transfusion was not an outcome measure in this study; however, 37 units of blood were used in 11 patients in the aprotinin group compared with 58 units in 13 patients in the placebo group. No significant differences were found between the groups in terms of thrombotic risk or other outcome measures.

Conclusions.—While aprotinin use resulted in decreased estimated blood loss, the authors did not recommend its routine use in meningioma resection. Rather they recommended considering prophylactic aprotinin in patients with tumors expected to be associated with greater than usual intraoperative bleeding or in situations making transfusion more difficult, contraindicated, or associate greater risks.

► This prospective, randomized trial demonstrates that aprotinin can decrease blood loss during a craniotomy for meningioma resection, a procedure known to be associated with a relatively high blood loss compared with resection of other common intracranial tumor types. In addition, it demonstrates that no complications were associated with its use, at least in a relatively small series. However, as the authors note, it does not lead to a decrease in the percentage of patients requiring transfusions or a reduction in cost; rather, in this series, an increase in cost occurred. The authors' concerns and recommendations seem sound. Aprotinin is a possible adjunct in patients undergoing procedures likely to have higher than usual blood loss (eg, for large meningiomas involving intracranial vessels, hemangioblastomas or reoperations for vascular tumors) or in patients with other concerns regarding transfusions, such as Jehovah's Witnesses or patients with antibodies to red blood cell antigens. Its routine use for craniotomies does not seem to be cost-effective and may lead to sensitization of patients to aprotinin, which would increase their risk of anaphylaxis should the drug be administered in other clinical situations with more proven benefit.

S. Black, MD

Prevention of Thromboembolism After Neurosurgery for Brain and Spinal Tumors
Carman TL, Kanner AA, Barnett GH, et al (Cleveland Clinic Found, Ohio)
South Med J 96:17-21, 2003   7–11

Background.—Patients undergoing surgery for primary and metastatic brain tumors are at particular risk for venous thromboembolism (VT) because of the hypercoagulability associated with malignancy and invasive neurologic procedures. There are also risk factors such as prolonged anesthesia, paresis, and extended immobility. The significant risk of deep vein thrombosis (DVT), combined with a pulmonary embolism–related mortality rate of 33% to 58% after surgery for brain tumors, indicates the need for aggressive prophylaxis against VT. The goal of this prophylaxis is the reduction in incidence of DVT and thus a reduction in the morbidity and mortality associated with pulmonary embolism. The purpose of this study was to identify current trends in perioperative VT prophylaxis use by practicing neuro-

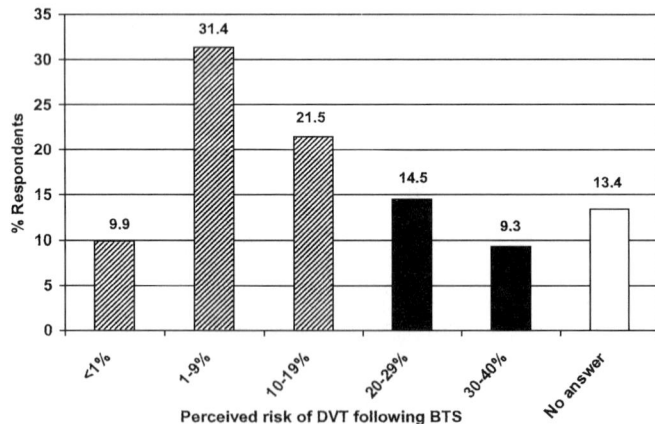

FIGURE 1.—Respondents' perceived risk of deep venous thrombosis (*DVT*) after brain tumor surgery (*BTS*) in the absence of prophylaxis. *Solid bars* represent the most correct estimate of risk to the patient, 20% to 40%. (Reprinted with permission from the *Southern Medical Journal* courtesy of Carman TL, Kanner AA, Barnett GH, et al: Prevention of thromboembolism after neurosurgery for brain and spinal tumors. *South Med J* 96:17-21, 2003.)

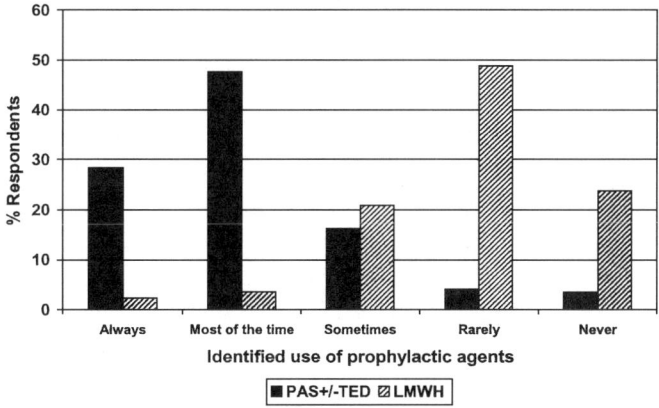

FIGURE 4.—Respondents' indication of their use of pneumatic anti-embolism stocks (*PAS*) with or without the addition of thromboembolism deterrence stocking (*TED*) as the sole form of prophylaxis after brain tumor surgery and their use of low molecular weight heparin (*LMWH*) for prophylaxis. (Reprinted with permission from the *Southern Medical Journal* courtesy of Carman TL, Kanner AA, Barnett GH, et al: Prevention of thromboembolism after neurosurgery for brain and spinal tumors. *South Med J* 96:17-21, 2003.)

surgeons and to investigate the relationship between VT risk awareness and the use of prophylaxis.

Methods.—A confidential survey was conducted of 590 neurosurgeons in the United States. The survey assessed DVT risk awareness and the patterns of use for thromboprophylaxis among these surgeons.

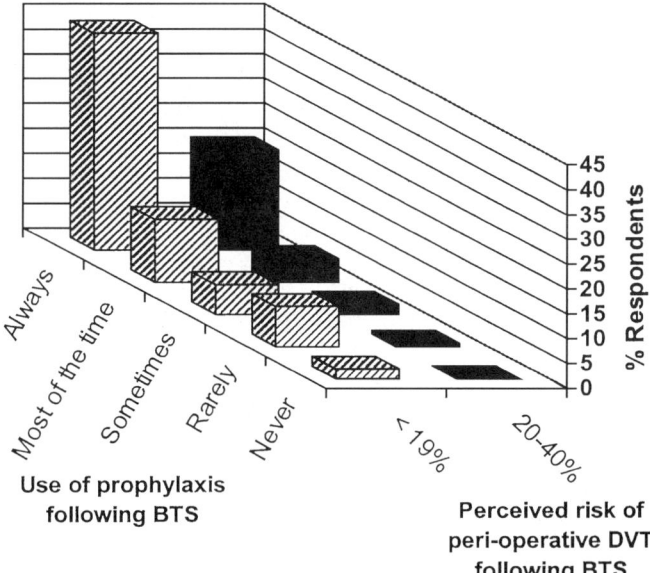

FIGURE 5.—Comparison of the respondents' perceived risk of perioperative deep venous thrombosis (*DVT*) after brain tumor surgery (*BTS*) with their indicated use of prophylaxis after BTS. (Reprinted with permission from the *Southern Medical Journal* courtesy of Carman TL, Kanner AA, Barnett GH, et al: Prevention of thromboembolism after neurosurgery for brain and spinal tumors. *South Med J* 96:17-21, 2003.)

Results.—A total of 172 neurosurgeons responded (Fig 1). Of these, 108 (63%) respondents underestimated the risk of DVT after brain tumor surgery. After operating on patients who had brain or spinal tumors, 81.4% and 78.5% of respondents, respectively, reported using DVT prophylaxis. After surgery for patients with brain tumors, 76.2% of respondents reported using solely mechanical methods of prophylaxis for these patients "always" or "most of the time (Figs 4 and 5)."

Conclusion.—There is a tendency among neurosurgeons in the United States to underestimate the risk of DVT associated with brain tumor surgery and to use mechanical thromboprophylaxis, despite the availability of effective pharmacologic antithrombotic drugs. A greater understanding of the risk of thrombosis in these patients and additional clinical studies to address safety may increase the use of prophylaxis and the perceived safety of antithrombotics for patients undergoing surgery for brain and spinal tumors.

▶ This interesting survey serves to remind us that brain tumor patients are in a high risk group for postoperative DVT. Although this is well known, the practice of most neurosurgeons does not include pharmacologic prophylaxis as is currently routinely used for other high-risk patient groups such as total joint replacement patients. The authors suggest this is due to the frequent underestimation of the risk for DVT they observed in this survey. It is equally likely due to the risk for significant neurologic morbidity associated with a coagulopathy in neurosurgical patients.

The morbidity for excessive bleeding at the operative site is considerably different after joint replacement. While studies have been reported indicating no significant increase in postoperative bleeding with postoperative initiation of anticoagulation after neurosurgical procedures, more needs to be done.[1] To change the current practice of neurosurgeons, more studies need to be completed confirming the safety of pharmacologic DVT prophylaxis.

S. Black, MD

Reference

1. Agnelli G, Piovella F, Buoncristiani P, et al: Enoxaparin plus compressive stockings compared with compressive stockings alone in the prevention of venous thromboembolism after elective neurosurgery. *N Engl J Med* 339:80-85, 1998.

Intraoperative Neurophysiologic Detection of Iatrogenic C5 Nerve Root Injury During Laminectomy for Cervical Compression Myelopathy
Fan D, Schwartz DM, Vaccaro AR, et al (Surgical Monitoring Associates, Bala Cynwyd, Pa; Thomas Jefferson Univ, Philadelphia)
Spine 27:2499-2502, 2002   7–12

Background.—The incidence of postoperative C5 nerve root palsy is reported to range from 0% to 12.9% for laminectomy and from 2.5% to 14.9% for laminoplasty. C5 nerve root palsy may not be detected even in the presence of intraoperative neuromonitoring with conventional upper extremity mixed nerve or dermatomal somatosensory-evoked potentials (SSEPs) or transcranial motor-evoked potentials, which are usually recorded from hand muscles. The effectiveness of a modified monitoring technique, which consisted of combined simultaneous application of both transcranial electric motor-evoked potentials (TceMEPs) and spontaneous electromyography (spEMG), in the intraoperative detection of early C5 nerve root palsy was evaluated.

Methods.—A retrospective review and prospective studies were conducted of the intraoperative neuromonitoring data from 200 patients who underwent cervical laminectomy for myelopathy between 1998 and 2000. The retrospective review included 132 patients who were monitored with conventional techniques, including ulnar and posterior tibial nerve SSEPs, C5–C7 dermatomally evoked potentials, and TceMEPs from hand and leg muscles. The remaining 68 patients underwent prospective studies, including TceMEPs and spEMG with the use of deltoid and biceps muscles.

Results.—Among the patients in the retrospective study, 6 of 132 were seen postoperatively with C5 nerve root palsy showing unilateral deltoid muscle paralysis, despite unremarkable conventional SSEPs, dermatomally evoked potentials, and TceMEPs from hand and leg muscles. In the prospective group of patients, 2 of 68 experienced postoperative iatrogenic C5 nerve root injuries. Impending C5 nerve root injuries were identified successfully in the 2 patients who manifested significant changes in deltoid and biceps TceMEPs and spEMG, which averted more serious consequences in these patients. No false-negative or false-positive results occurred.

Conclusions.—Intraoperative deltoid and biceps TceMEPs and spEMG monitoring should be considered in any patient in whom a risk of iatrogenic C5 nerve root injury exists during surgery.

▶ Isolated C5 nerve root injury can cause significant functional impairment after cervical spine procedures involving C5 and, as reported in this article, can occur in up to 10% to 15% of patients. In the retrospective portion of this study, the C5 injury was undetected by a combination of upper and lower extremity SSEPs, mixed dermatomal-evoked potentials, and motor-evoked potentials (recorded from the hand). This is not surprising as conventional SSEPs are known to be insensitive to isolated root injuries. Likewise, dermatomal SSEPs have also been reported to be insensitive. Finally, motor-evoked potential recordings from hand muscles would not be expected to detect a C5 injury. Simply adding spontaneous EMG recordings for the prospective patients detected all cases of C5 injury intraoperatively. The motor-evoked potentials recorded from deltoid electrodes allowed evaluation of the functional integrity of the nerve after the EMG discharges were noted during the surgical stress on the C5 nerve root. It is likely that adding deltoid EMG monitoring, which is technically easier, in neurophysiologic monitoring laboratories having less experience with motor-evoked potential monitoring would be equally effective in the detection of surgical trespass of the C5 root.

S. Black, MD

Levels of Anti-Inflammatory Cytokines and Neurological Worsening in Acute Ischemic Stroke

Vila N, Castillo J, Dàvalos A, et al (Instituto Investigaciones Biomédicas August Pi i Sunyer, Barcelona; Santiago de Compostela; Hospital Universitario Doctor Josep Trueta, Girona, Spain; et al)
Stroke 34:671-675, 2003   7–13

Background.—One third of patients with acute ischemic stroke are at risk for early neurologic worsening, which is associated with increased mortality and long-term functional disability. The basic mechanisms that underlie this phenomenon are not completely understood; however, biochemical factors have been proposed. Ischemic brain injury is characterized by acute local inflammatory response, which is mediated by cytokines. Increased production of proinflammatory cytokines and chemokines has been detected in experimental models of brain ischemia as well as in patients with acute stroke; increased levels of proinflammatory cytokines are related to a greater extent of cerebral infarct and poorer clinical outcome in patients with ischemic stroke.

Experimental models have shown that ischemic tissue damage can be reduced with a variety of anti-inflammatory agents, including interleukin (IL)-10 and IL-4. The implications of IL-10 and IL-4 in the setting of deteriorating ischemic stroke were assessed.

Methods.—A total of 231 patients with ischemic stroke who were hospitalized within the first 24 hours after stroke onset were included in this study. Neurologic worsening was defined when the Canadian Stroke Scale score dropped at least 1 point in the first 48 hours after admission. Anti-inflammatory cytokines were assayed in plasma obtained at admission.

Results.—The condition of 83 patients (35.9%) worsened within the first 48 hours after onset of stroke. Significantly lower concentrations of IL-10 were found in patients with neurologic worsening; however, IL-4 levels were similar in patients with or without deterioration. Multivariate analysis showed that lower plasma concentrations of IL-10 were associated with clinical worsening. This association was independent of hyperthermia, hyperglycemia, or neurologic condition on admission. On further analysis, it was determined that early worsening was associated with lower IL-10 plasma levels in patients with subcortical infarcts or lacunar stroke but not in patients with cortical lesions.

Conclusion.—The anti-inflammatory cytokine IL-10 is associated with the early clinical course of patients with acute ischemic stroke, particularly for patients with small-vessel disease or subcortical infarctions.

▶ This study is important and brings to light the yin and yang of proinflammatory and anti-inflammatory biomolecules and their clinical consequences. It also gives therapeutic insight in that an agent, such as recombinant IL-10, may be efficacious in patients with acute ischemic stroke who have potentially devastating injury. Such a trial is hopefully being designed.

J. D. Lang, Jr, MD

Clinical Significance of Elevated Troponin I Levels in Patients With Nontraumatic Subarachnoid Hemorrhage

Deibert E, Barzilai B, Braverman AC, et al (Washington Univ, St Louis)
J Neurosurg 98:741-746, 2003   7–14

Background.—Aneurysmal subarachnoid hemorrhage (SAH) affects about 30,000 persons per year in the United States. Some patients have electrocardiographic abnormalities, regional or focal wall-motion abnormalities on echocardiography, or increased creatine kinase-MB (CK-MB) concentrations, which may result in concerns about cardiac ischemia and may therefore delay appropriate treatment. The ability of cTnI to predict left ventricular dysfunction on echocardiograms was compared with that of CK-MB in patients with nontraumatic SAH.

Methods.—Forty-three patients with nontraumatic SAH were included in the study. Electrocardiograms and echocardiograms were obtained, and CK-MB and cTnI concentrations were measured serially. Patients known to have coronary artery disease were excluded from the analysis. Patients with increased enzyme concentrations and abnormal findings on echocardiography were further assessed for coronary artery disease.

Findings.—Levels of cTnI were increased in the first 24 hours after hemorrhage in 28% of patients. Echocardiographic evidence of left ventricular dysfunction was seen in 7 of 12 patients, all of whom had a return to baseline function on follow-up examinations. The sensitivity of cTnI was 100% in detecting left ventricular function in patients with SAH, compared with 29% for CK-MB.

Conclusion.—An increased cTnI concentration is a good indicator of left ventricular dysfunction in patients with SAH. In this series, cardiac dysfunction was reversible and thus should not preclude operative interventions or heart donation. More aggressive hemodynamic monitoring may be needed until cardiac function normalizes.

► This study again addresses the important issue of identifying those patients after SAH with cardiac dysfunction. As abnormal ECG is common after SAH and cardiac dysfunction is uncommon, but occasionally clinically significant, identifying those patients in whom cardiac dysfunction has developed post SAH has great clinical impact. Clearly, from this study and others, troponin levels are a highly reliable indicator and if troponin levels are not elevated, it is likely that no further workup needs to be done. It is very interesting to note that even though many of these patients had risk factors for coronary artery disease, none had evidence of significant disease. Finally, the complete recovery of cardiac function postoperatively is a common—and encouraging—finding.

S. Black, MD

8 Critical Care Medicine

Adult Critical Care Medicine

Variability in Surgical Caseload and Access to Intensive Care Services
McManus ML, Long MC, Cooper A, et al (Harvard Med School, Boston; Boston Univ; Boston School of Public Health)
Anesthesiology 98:1491-1496, 2003   8-1

Background.—When the demand for a service varies, resource allocation can be inadequate. Because health care is an area of variable demand, when the occupancy of a hospital is high, crowding, staff overload, and unmet patient needs result because of the downsizing of the care delivery system. Pediatric tertiary hospitals operate as a safety net in caring for children who are seriously ill, providing specialized services that are unavailable elsewhere. ICUs that are crowded may block the flow of patient care. The nature and impact of variability on hospital practices and the quality of medical care were assessed by applying variability methodology to investigate the relationships between fluctuations in demand and volume and access to critical care services.

Methods.—All of the requests received over the course of 1 year for admission to the ICU of a large urban children's hospital were assessed. The nature of the request and the patient's final disposition were noted. Staff intensive care specialists classified the various data. Daily variability of requests was analyzed and matched to the unit's ability to care for the increased patient load.

Results.—Over the course of 1 year, 1978 requests for admission were received. Scheduled surgical procedures accounted for 47% of the requests, while unscheduled medical or surgical emergencies were involved in the remainder. Although the day-to-day demand for intensive care services varied considerably, full unit operations showed no significant interruptions. The average daily census was 15.2, for an overall average occupancy of 85%.

Patients stayed an average of 3.8 days; the stays of scheduled patients averaged 2.0 days, and those of emergency patients averaged 4.9 days. Scheduled requests accounted for more of the variability in the system than unscheduled ones. An extremely high correlation was noted between scheduled surgical requests and refusals of admission. Factors found to explain the number of rejections included day of the week, number of admissions, and a

115

lagged effect representing cumulative admissions over 1 to 6 days, or a length-of-stay effect.

Conclusion.—When resources are limited, variability must be managed to avoid adverse effects on the efficiency and effectiveness of complex systems such as the health care system. The variability in the scheduled surgical case-load contributed more than that in the unscheduled cases and presents the opportunity to reduce a source of stress on the system. If variability is not addressed, access to care and overall responsiveness to emergencies will be impaired.

▶ This study hits home! Unfortunately, we are constantly dealing with ICU beds operating at a high capacity, thus leading to patients being placed off-service or denied access from outlying hospitals. Additional problems of growing concern are delays in recovery room discharges, resulting in case delays and, unfortunately, the occasional case cancellation. This counterintuitive approach of controlling "artificial variability" (scheduled surgical cases) deserves study, since such strategies as increasing staffing or rationing are mere quick fixes with no long term benefits and either further deny services or increase costs. Operating room committees all over this nation should evaluate this novel insight.

J. D. Lang, Jr, MD

Accepting Critically III Transfer Patients: Adverse Effect on a Referral Center's Outcome and Benchmark Measures
Rosenberg AL, Hofer TP, Strachan C, et al (Univ of Michigan, Ann Arbor; Veterans Affairs Ann Arbor Healthcare System, Mich)
Ann Intern Med 138:882-890, 2003   8–2

Background.—Purchasers, providers, and the federal government have relied on a variety of benchmarking methods for comparison of outcomes, quality, and costs of health care. However, common benchmarking methods applied to clinical performance rarely, if ever, account for admission source, and, in particular, the effect of a patient transfer from 1 medical facility to another. The small biases that exist in comparisons of observed versus expected deaths can have a significant effect on how high-quality institutions compare with peer hospitals. The ICU is an ideal setting for the study of the effect of a patient's transfer from another hospital, as the ICU has the most sophisticated and validated set of case-mix measures available. This study investigated the extent of bias in benchmarking outcomes when performance measures do not account for the greater severity of illness in transfer patients.

Methods.—A total of 4579 consecutive admissions for 4208 patients in the medical ICU (MICU) at 1 tertiary care university hospital were included in this prospective cohort study. The main outcome measures were the

MICU and hospital lengths of stay, MICU readmission, and hospital mortality rates.

Results.—In comparison with directly admitted patients, MICU patients transferred from another hospital had significantly higher Acute Physiology Scores at admission and discharge. Transfer patients had a 38% longer stay in the MICU, a 41% longer hospital stay, and 2.2 times greater likelihood of hospital mortality, even after full adjustment for case mix and severity of illness. With identical efficiency and quality, a referral hospital with a 25% MICU transfer rate compared with another with a 0% transfer rate would be penalized by 14 excess deaths per 1000 admissions when a benchmarking program adjusts only for case mix and severity of illness and not for the source of admission.

Conclusion.—The acceptance of transfer patients can have an adverse effect on the efficiency and quality benchmarks of the referral institution. There is a need to account for this phenomenon in benchmarking and profiling efforts beyond ICUs, or referral centers may have an incentive to refuse care to patients who would benefit from transfer to their institution.

▶ This gives an interesting caveat concerning the effects on benchmarking. It is known that ICU-to-ICU transfers carry a significant mortality, but taking this into consideration and profiling the data in a way that reflects more on the admitting institution rather than on the accepting institution seems appropriate. Other recommendations are offered in this article to assist in avoiding decrease in quality benchmarks. Another interesting finding in this study is that no mortality differences existed between floor-to-ICU admissions versus ICU-to-ICU transfers. I didn't see a breakdown on how many of those floor-to-ICU admissions were "bounce backs."

J. D. Lang, Jr, MD

Critically Ill Patients Readmitted to Intensive Care Units—Lessons to Learn?
Metnitz PGH, Fieux F, Jordan B, et al (Université Paris VII; Univ of Vienna; Hosp de St António dos Capuchos, Lisboa, Portugal)
Intensive Care Med 29:241-248, 2003   8–3

Background.—The challenges facing modern intensive care are not only medical but ethical and economic as well, creating a need for evaluation of the quality of care delivered. Because intensive care is a costly area of health care and accounts for a significant portion of a hospital's budget, there is pressure to reduce costs by discharging patients as early as possible to reduce their length of stay in the intensive care unit. However, this strategy may not always be beneficial and may in fact increase the number of premature discharges, exerting a negative effect on outcome. Increased readmission rates to the ICU have repeatedly been associated with premature discharges. The risk factors for critically ill patients who were readmitted to an ICU during their hospital stay were evaluated.

Methods.—A total of 15,180 patients discharged from 30 medical, surgical, and mixed ICUs in Austria over 2 years were included in this prospective, multicenter cohort study. Data on clinical characteristics, Simplified Acute Physiology Score II, Logistic Organ Dysfunction system, Simplified Therapeutic Intervention Scoring System, length of ICU stay, ICU mortality, and hospital mortality were analyzed.

Results.—A total of 780 patients (5.1%) were readmitted; the risk of dying during the hospital stay was 21.7%, compared with 5.2% for those not readmitted. Among mechanically ventilated patients, the time between extubation and discharge during the first ICU stay was significantly shorter for patients who were readmitted than for nonreadmitted patients (median, 1 day vs 2 days). Readmitted patients were in greater need of organ support on the day of their first ICU discharge, with more patients still in need of ventilatory, cardiovascular, and renal support compared with nonreadmitted patients.

Conclusion.—The results of this study support the view that there is a group of patients who are at higher risk of readmission to the ICU. At their first ICU discharge, these patients were seen with residual organ dysfunction, which was associated with an increased risk for readmission. It appears that optimizing organ functions before discharge from the ICU could reduce the rates of readmission.

▶ A very large study confirms our suspicions that patients readmitted to the ICU have significantly increased mortality (4-fold in this study). With the pressures being placed on ICUs in large tertiary care centers, there may be a tendency to discharge patients too quickly in order to efficiently utilize (or what we think is efficient utilization) the ICU for other patients, say from the emergency department or operating room. Findings interesting to me were that many patients in the study were actually discharged the day that either ventilatory support or vasoactive drugs had been discontinued. Also, another interesting finding was that the readmission rate was significantly increased when patients were discharged from the ICU in the evening, indicating that these patients may have been discharged because of a bed shortage. Thus, the patient with the greatest need gets the bed.

J. D. Lang, Jr, MD

Comparison of Point-of-Care Versus Central Laboratory Measurement of Electrolyte Concentrations on Calculations of the Anion Gap and the Strong Ion Difference
Morimatsu H, Rocktäschel J, Bellomo R, et al (Austin and Repatriation Med Centre, Heidelberg, Australia)
Anesthesiology 98:1077-1084, 2003   8–4

Background.—Based on the electrolyte measurements taken in critically ill patients, clinicians can calculate the anion gap (AG) and the strong ion difference (SID), which help in determining acid-base status, adding information that can influence clinical decision making. Point-of-care testing may allow bedside determinations of arterial blood gases, blood glucose and potassium, hemoglobin, and hematocrit. However, discrepancies between the bedside values and those determined in the central laboratory have been detected, indicating that the technology used may be limited. Three hundred simultaneous paired blood samples from critically ill patients were obtained by both point-of-care technology and standard central laboratory technology, with the results compared for determining plasma sodium, potassium, and chloride concentrations as well as AG and SID values.

Methods.—The 300 patients had a mean age of 60.2 years and a mean Acute Physiology and Chronic Health Evaluation II score of 17.9. The AG and SID values were calculated from data from the blood gas and electrolyte analyzer for point-of-care measurements as well as the automated blood biochemistry analyzer in the central hospital laboratory. The measures of plasma sodium, potassium, and chloride concentrations were obtained simultaneously and also compared.

Results.—The point-of-care measurements were as follows: mean plasma sodium concentration, 138.3 mM; mean plasma potassium concentration, 4.21 mM; and mean plasma chloride concentration, 103.4 mM. The central laboratory testing measurements were 140.4 mM for sodium, 4.20 mM for potassium, and 102.4 mM for chloride. Significant differences were noted in the calculated AG from the 2 different techniques, which yielded 17.6 mEq/L for central laboratory measurements and 14.5 mEq/L for point-of-care measurements. The mean difference for the calculated AG was 3.1 mEq/L.

Significantly different SID apparent values were also obtained, with a mean SID apparent value of 40.7 mEq/L for point-of-care measurements and 43.7 mEq/L for central laboratory measurements. Of the 300 patients, 78 had an abnormally high AG determined by the central laboratory technology, but point-of-care measurements only identified 36 of these. Four patients had elevated AG measurements by point-of-care technology yet were found to have normal results on central laboratory analysis.

The difference in AG between the 2 technologies was over 5 mEq/L for 83 patients, over 7 mEq/L for 33 patients, and over 10 mEq/L for 5 patients. The median sodium and calcium concentrations were significantly less when 1 mL instead of 3 mL of blood was used. When plasma instead of whole blood was used, sodium, calcium, and chloride concentrations obtained by point-of-care methods differed significantly from those determined by the central laboratory.

Conclusion.—Significant differences in the sodium and chloride concentrations were obtained using a point-of-care blood gas and electrolyte analyzer versus a central laboratory automated biochemical analyzer. The AG value, calculated SID apparent value, and individual electrolyte values were significantly different based on these measurements and may have clinical relevance. With the move to obtain more and more measurements at bedside, clinicians need to be aware of these discrepancies.

▶ More and more perioperative areas are moving to point-of-care testing. While I believe the results of this study are important, the statistical significance doesn't reach the threshold of clinical significance, in general, in this case. In most critically ill patients, following AGs can be misleading no matter the technique. For instance, in the hypoalbuminemic patient, loss of a negative ion like albumin allows patients to have an AG acidosis without the AG. Very few decisions are going to be made on a single value. One always has to have clinical suspicion and, in general, other corroborating data before therapeutic decisions are made about acid-base and electrolyte perturbations. With that said, the study is important because it allows us to better understand the limitations of our newer technologies.

J. D. Lang, Jr, MD

Critically Ill Patients With Severe Acute Respiratory Syndrome
Lapinsky SE, for the Toronto SARS Critical Care Group (Univ of Toronto; et al)
JAMA 290:367-373, 2003   8–5

Background.—Severe acute respiratory syndrome (SARS) produces an acute respiratory illness that leads to critical illness in 23% to 32% of patients. The health care system has been strained by the influx of SARS patients and the concerns related to quarantine and SARS infection among health care workers (HCWs). Understanding SARS-related critical illness is required to plan more effectively for the care needed. The epidemiology, clinical characteristics, and outcomes at 28 days for SARS patients who are critically ill were outlined, with an estimate of the impact accompanying SARS transmission from critically ill patients to HCWs.

Methods.—The medical records of 38 adult patients with SARS-related critical illness were reviewed retrospectively. All had been admitted to ICUs in the Toronto area. Daily data collection was undertaken for the first 7 days in the ICU, with 28 days of follow-up.

Results.—One hundred ninety-six patients had probable or suspected SARS, with 38 (19%) developing critical illness. Eighteen percent of the patients were HCWs. Patients ranged in age from 39.0 to 69.6 years (median, 57.4 years), with a predominance of older non-HCWs seen in the critically ill group. In addition, the critically ill patients were more likely to have co-morbid conditions such as diabetes.

Eighty-two percent of the critically ill patients met the diagnostic criteria for acute respiratory distress syndrome, with 29 patients (15% of all SARS patients) requiring mechanical ventilation. Over the first 7 days in the ICU, 34% of the ventilated patients suffered barotrauma, 37% developed cardiovascular dysfunction, 21% hepatic dysfunction, and 11% renal dysfunction.

Eight days was the median time between the onset of symptoms and admission to the ICU; 19 days was the median time from symptom onset to death. At 28 days, mortality was 34% of the total number of patients and 45% of those requiring mechanical ventilation. At 28 days, 6 patients were still requiring mechanical ventilation. At 8 weeks, mortality for those requiring mechanical ventilation was 52%, while the overall mortality rate was 39%, with 3 patients still requiring mechanical ventilation.

Poor outcome occurred in patients of older age, with a history of diabetes mellitus, with tachycardia on admission, or with elevated creatine kinase levels. Patients who required ICU care tended to have bilateral radiographic lung infiltrates at a higher rate than other patients. ICU patients transmitted SARS to HCWs on 2 occasions. As a result, 10-day closures of 35 critical care beds in a tertiary care university medical-surgical ICU (38% of those in Toronto) were required; 38 concurrent bed closures (33% of the Toronto community medical-surgical ICU bed capacity) also occurred because of ICU SARS transmission and quarantine of HCWs.

Conclusion.—A high proportion of the patients who had probable or suspected SARS developed critical illness requiring care in an ICU. While the median time from symptom onset until death was 19 days, many deaths occurred after the follow-up time of 28 days. Older age, preexisting diabetes mellitus, tachycardia on admission, and elevated creatine kinase levels were associated with higher mortality rates. Because HCWs tended to be younger than other SARS patients, they were less likely to die. Half of the SARS patients who required mechanical ventilation died. In addition, the critical care resources of the region were significantly strained by the outbreak.

Acute Respiratory Distress Syndrome in Critically Ill Patients With Severe Acute Respiratory Syndrome

Lew TWK, Kwek T-K, Tai D, et al (Tan Tock Seng Hosp, Singapore; Alexandra Hosp, Singapore)
JAMA 290:374-380, 2003   8–6

Background.—Over 8000 individuals worldwide have been infected with severe acute respiratory syndrome (SARS) since the index case in November 2002. Two thirds of these cases were reported in China. About 25% of patients with SARS progress to acute lung injury (ALI)/acute respiratory distress syndrome (ARDS), and the mortality is high. Tan Tock Seng Hospital was designated for the intake and isolation of suspected and probable SARS cases, with nearly all critically ill SARS patients treated in a single dedicated SARS ICU. The clinical characteristics and outcomes of 46 critically ill patients with probable SARS treated over 13 weeks were outlined.

Methods.—The 46 adult patients admitted to the ICU with symptoms and signs consistent with ALI/ARDS constituted 23% of the 199 patients hospitalized for SARS. Their cases were reviewed retrospectively to determine the clinical spectrum and outcomes of these individuals, with the main outcome being mortality 28 days after symptom onset.

Results.—Overall 28-day mortality was 10.1% of the 199 patients and 37% of those admitted to the ICU. At 13 weeks, the mortality rates were 13.6% and 52.2%, respectively. Seventy-five percent of the deaths resulted from complications related to severe ARDS, multiorgan failure, thromboembolic complications, or septicemic shock and occurred late in the disease's course. ARDS characteristics included ease of de-recruitment of alveoli and poor airway secretion, bronchospasm, or dynamic hyperinflation.

Patients who recovered early (within 14 days of onset) had a shorter course of ALI, with fraction of inspired oxygen requirements peaking on the eighth day of illness (median), which coincided with the day of ICU admission. Early recovery was linked to lower Acute Physiology and Chronic Health Evaluation II scores and higher baseline ratios of partial pressure of oxygen, compared with other patients. Those in the intermediate recovery group had improved oxygenation and pulmonary compliance after 5 days (median) of mechanical ventilation; those with late recovery had a protracted, severe course of ARDS, had the most complications, and needed the most interventions and treatment. Despite maximal supportive therapy, the survival in patients who had a protracted course of ARDS with complications was low.

Conclusion.—The clinical findings for patients with SARS who developed ALI and ARDS were characterized by ease of de-recruitment of alveoli and a finding of poor airway secretion, bronchospasm, or dynamic hyperinflation. Complications occurred often and required maximal supportive therapy, but mortality was still high.

▶ "New" diseases such as SARS, ebola, and hanta virus require anesthesiologists to become a quick study, as they will be requested to care for these patients in need for initial stabilization in areas such as the emergency department and for both acute and longitudinal care in the ICU. Knowledge about the disease and prevention precautions are paramount for both patient and HCW. Both of these studies (Abstracts 8–5 and 8–6) reveal that mortality is high, and that progression to ALI and ARDS is common. Interesting was that the epidemiology was similar between Canada and Singapore. A difference was that no HCWs in Singapore developed SARS versus 74 in Canada. Patients with SARS that progressed to ARDS were more difficult to ventilate and oxygenate then non-SARS patients with ARDS. One interesting bit of information regarding treatment was that patients with ARDS trended toward a better outcome if treated with immunoglobulin and steroids.

J. D. Lang, Jr, MD

Impact of Randomized Trial Results on Acute Lung Injury Ventilator Therapy in Teaching Hospitals
Weinert CR, Gross CR, Marinelli WA (Univ of Minnesota, Minneapolis; Hennepin County Med Ctr, Minneapolis, Minn)
Am J Respir Crit Care Med 167:1304-1309, 2003   8–7

Background.—Mechanical ventilation is a life-saving therapy for patients with acute lung injury (ALI). Many studies have been conducted to determine the optimal support method for these patients. It has been shown that reducing tidal volumes administered to these patients is the only intervention that has been shown to decrease mortality. Many medical advances are introduced slowly into clinical practice; however, it has been assumed that clinicians at teaching hospitals are early adopters of advances in medical practice. Whether the very low tidal volume strategy is in fact being adopted by clinicians at teaching hospitals was investigated.

Methods.—Trends in ventilatory prescription were examined in 398 patients with acute lung injury who were treated between 1994 and 2001 at 3 teaching hospitals. Changes in tidal volume were modeled in 2 ways. First, visual inspection was performed of a scatter plot of tidal volume over time fitted with a smoothed line by a locally weighted least-squares method. Second segmented models were used to test whether the observed breakpoint in the smoothed line was detectable statistically. To describe the evolution of the ventilatory prescription during the early ALI period, day 1 positive end-expiratory pressure was compared with day 3 values. Days 1 and 3 clinician-set tidal volumes were also compared.

Results.—No change in tidal volumes was noted until late 1998, when volumes started to slowly decline at the rate of 48.0 mL/y. In the 2 years after the results were released from a large trial that showed the superiority of 6 mL/kg tidal volume therapy over 12 mL/kg, tidal volumes of 651 ± 128 mL/kg or 10.1 ± 1.9 mL/kg were prescribed. Postintubation tidal volumes were minimally reduced during the subsequent 2 days of mechanical ventilation. Hospital category, male sex, and onset of disease before May 1999 were associated with higher volumes, and lung injury severity was inversely associated with higher volumes.

Conclusion.—Clinicians practicing at the teaching hospitals involved in this report have not rapidly adopted low tidal volume ventilation which may reduce mortality in patients with acute lung injury.

▶ A telling study by one of the most progressive pulmonary centers in the United States, demonstrating that despite powerful clinical evidence, incorporating low tidal volume ventilation into ones clinical acumen occurs slowly. In my opinion, this is where ICU design and protocols should pay tremendous dividends by ensuring that certain strategies are adhered to and cannot be undermined by nonintensivists. From this study I was unable to ascertain this.

J. D. Lang, Jr, MD

Injurious Mechanical Ventilation and End-Organ Epithelial Cell Apoptosis and Organ Dysfunction in an Experimental Model of Acute Respiratory Distress Syndrome

Imai Y, Parodo J, Kajikawa O, et al (Univ of Toronto; Univ Health Network, Toronto; Seattle Veterans Administration Med Ctr; et al)
JAMA 289:2104-2112, 2003   8–8

Background.—The acute respiratory distress syndrome (ARDS) has a mortality rate of at least 30%. The most common cause of death in patients with ARDS is dysfunction of other organs, or multiple organ dysfunction syndrome (MODS). MODS is often irreversible and the mortality associated with this syndrome ranges from 60% to 98%. At present, there is no effective treatment for or means of preventing MODS. However, a decline in MODS has been reported recently in clinical trials in which patients with ARDS were treated with a protective ventilatory strategy. The hypothesis that an injurious ventilatory strategy may cause end-organ epithelial cell apoptosis and organ dysfunction was investigated.

Methods.—In a rabbit model, 24 animals with acid-aspiration lung injury were ventilated by injurious or noninjurious ventilatory strategies. For the in vitro phase of the experiment, rabbit epithelial cells were exposed to plasma from the in vivo study. Finally, plasma samples from human patients included in a prior randomized, controlled trial of a lung protective strategy were analyzed. The main outcome measures were biochemical markers of liver and renal dysfunction in the in vivo animal study; induction of apoptosis in LLC-RK1 renal tubular cells in the in vitro animal study; and correlation of plasma creatinine and soluble Fas ligand in the in vivo human study.

Results.—In the in vivo animal study, the injurious ventilatory strategy was associated with an increased rate of epithelial cell apoptosis in the kidney (mean, 10.9% vs 1.86%) and villi of the small intestine (6.7% vs 0.97%), compared with the lung protective strategy. Biochemical markers indicative of renal dysfunction were elevated in vivo. In the in vitro experiments, the Fas:Ig, a fusion protein that blocks Fas ligand, attenuated induction of apoptosis in vitro. A significant correlation was observed between changes in soluble Fas ligand and changes in creatinine in the patients with ARDS.

Conclusion.—Mechanical ventilation can result in epithelial cell apoptosis in the kidney and small intestine, accompanied by biochemical evidence of organ dysfunction. The findings of this study may provide a partial explanation for the high rate of MODS among patient with acute respiratory distress syndrome and the decrease in morbidity and mortality in ARDS patients who are treated with a lung protective strategy.

▶ This study represented the initial paper published in the "Translational Medical Research" section of *JAMA*. It adds considerable legitimacy to the literature that reports that adhering to a protective strategy of mechanical ventilation in the setting of lung injury lessens the chances of extra-pulmonary organ dysfunction. Organ systems that appeared to be particularly vulnerable in this study were the kidneys and small intestine. These organs are vulnerable for multiple reasons, including proinflammatory mediator release from the lung itself as a result of inappropriate ventilator settings which caused volutrauma and recruitment-derecruitment injury, and also adverse hemodynamic consequences that could have been encountered in the "injurious" ventilator strategy groups.

J. D. Lang, Jr, MD

High-Frequency Oscillatory Ventilation for Acute Respiratory Distress Syndrome in Adults: A Randomized, Controlled Trial
Derdak S, and Multicenter Oscillatory Ventilation for Acute Respiratory Distress Syndrome Trial (MOAT) Study Investigators (Wilford Hall Med Ctr, San Antonio, Tex; et al)
Am J Respir Crit Care Med 166:801-808, 2002   8–9

Background.—Mechanical ventilation for patients with acute respiratory distress syndrome (ARDS) may result in further injury to the lung and may contribute to the systemic inflammatory response of these patients. High-frequency oscillatory ventilation (HFOV) is a ventilation strategy that in theory accomplishes all the objectives of protective lung ventilation. Observational studies of HFOV in patients with ARDS have shown improvements in oxygenation and suggest better outcomes when it is applied early in the course of ARDS. The safety and effectiveness of HFOV were compared with those of conventional ventilation in adults with ARDS.

Methods.—A total of 148 adults with ARDS were enrolled in this multicenter, randomized, controlled trial and were assigned to either HFOV (75 patients) or conventional ventilation (73 patients).

Results.—The applied mean airway pressure was significantly higher in the HFOV group compared with the conventional ventilation group in the first 72 hours. There was early (less than 16 hours) improvement in partial pressure of arterial oxygen/fraction of inspired oxygen in the HFOV group compared with the conventionally ventilated group; however, this difference was not sustained beyond 24 hours. The oxygenation index decreased similarly over the first 72 hours in the 2 groups. The mortality rate at 30 days was 37% in the HFOV group and 52% in the conventional ventilation group. At day 30, 36% of patients were alive in the HFOV group compared with 31% of patients in the conventional ventilation group. No significant differences between the groups were observed in hemodynamic variables, oxygenation failure, ventilation failure, barotraumas, or mucus plugging.

Conclusion.—High-frequency oscillation is a safe and effective ventilatory method for the treatment of ARDS in adults.

▶ A strong statement supporting the use of HFOV in patients suffering from ARDS. A comparison trial comparing HFOV with a "protective" strategy is warranted. One other caveat is this: In order for benefits of HFOV to be appreciated, respiratory therapists, nursing personnel, house staff, and faculty must have an intimate knowledge of this unique approach to ventilation strategy.

J. D. Lang, Jr, MD

Dose-Response Characteristics During Long-term Inhalation of Nitric Oxide in Patients With Severe Acute Respiratory Distress Syndrome: A Prospective, Randomized, Controlled Study

Gerlach H, Keh D, Semmerow A, et al (Vivantes-Klinikum Neukoelln, Berlin; Univ Hosp Charité-Virchow, Berlin; Ernst-von-Bergmann Hosp, Potsdam, Germany; et al)

Am J Respir Crit Care Med 167:1008-1015, 2003   8–10

Background.—Inhaled nitric oxide (NO) has been found to significantly reduce pulmonary hypertension and intrapulmonary shunt in adult patients with acute respiratory distress syndrome (ARDS), thus improving systemic oxygenation. However, early retrospective studies showed that continuous application of high-dose inhaled NO (10 ppm or more) did not improve clinical outcome. It has subsequently been found that the individual effect of inhaled NO is dose dependent and varies interindividually. The effects of long-term, high-dose (10 ppm) inhaled NO on systemic oxygenation and pulmonary vascular resistance was characterized in adult patients with ARDS. It was postulated that the individual response, or sensitivity of the pulmonary vasculature for exogenous NO, might change during long-term inhaled NO therapy.

Methods.—Forty patients with ARDS were included in this prospective, randomized study. Dose-response characteristics during long-term inhaled NO therapy were examined. The patients were randomly assigned to conventional therapy (control) or continuous treatment with 10 ppm of inhaled NO until weaning. Dose-response curves of partial pressure of arterial oxygen (PaO_2)/fraction of inspired oxygen (FIO_2) versus the inhaled NO dose were measured at regular intervals.

Results.—Before treatment, peak improvement in PaO_2/FIO_2 was obtained at 10 ppm for both control and NO-treated patients. After 4 days of treatment, the dose-response curve of the NO-treated patients was left-shifted, with a peak response at 1 ppm. At higher doses (10 and 100 ppm) there was deterioration of oxygenation, and in several patients the response to inhaled NO disappeared entirely. This effect was not observed in the control group. Inhaled NO was not found to have an effect on the duration of mechanical ventilation or duration of stay in the ICU.

Conclusion.—Long-term inhaled NO with constant doses of 10 ppm yields increased sensitivity after several days and does not permit reduction of ventilation parameters. Thus, the findings of previous trials of inhaled NO in patients with ARDS should be interpreted with care. These previous trials relied on constant NO concentrations, which might have become over-doses, causing deterioration of oxygenation after several days.

▶ A wonderfully conducted study that evaluated the dose-response effects on inhaled NO in patients suffering from ARDS. This study should stimulate a reevaluation of how we deliver inhaled NO to this patient population. With this study demonstrating higher PaO_2/FIO_2 ratios on 1 ppm and actual deterioration in the same index with escalating concentrations, more work is warranted in investigating the multitude of mechanisms that contribute to this result and whether this dose-response observed by Gerlach et al is reproducible and demonstrates benefit with a larger patient number. The reduction in extracorporeal membrane oxygenation, in itself, is a significant observation in this adult population. Reducing patients' exposures to strategies such as those reduce complications and costs.

J. D. Lang, Jr, MD

Treatment of Acute Respiratory Distress Syndrome With Recombinant Surfactant Protein C Surfactant
Spragg RG, Lewis JF, Wurst W, et al (Univ of California, San Diego; San Diego Veterans Affairs HealthCare System, Calif; Univ of Western Ontario, London, Canada; et al)
Am J Respir Crit Care Med 167:1562-1566, 2003   8–11

Background.—Acute respiratory distress syndrome (ARDS) is characterized by marked edema of the lung, which results in progressive impairment of gas exchange, atelectasis, and decreased lung compliance. The function of the lung surfactant system is impaired in patients with ARDS, and this impairment may be a contributing factor to atelectasis and decreased pulmonary compliance. The rationale that supports the use of exogenous surfactant in the treatment of patients with ARDS is derived from several observations and is the result of several clinical trials. The efficacy of a recombinant surfactant protein C–based surfactant as a treatment for ARDS was evaluated.

Methods.—In this phase I/II trial, a total of 40 patients were prospectively randomly assigned to either standard therapy or standard therapy plus 1 or 2 doses of exogenous surfactant 4 times over 24 hours.

Results.—Administration of the surfactant was well tolerated. There was no significant treatment benefit associated with surfactant treatment. Bronchoalveolar lavage of treated patients at 48 hours demonstrated the presence of exogenous surfactant components, but there was no evidence of improved surface tension–lowering function. In addition, interleukin-6 concentrations were significantly lower in the treated patients compared with the values in the control group, a finding that was consistent with an anti-inflammatory treatment effect. Lavage fluid obtained at 120 hours did not indicate the presence of exogenous surfactant.

Conclusion.—These findings provide evidence of the safety of administration of recombinant surfactant protein C surfactant to patients with acute lung injury. Future studies might be designed to utilize larger surfactant doses and a longer dosing schedule.

Treatment With Bovine Surfactant in Severe Acute Respiratory Distress Syndrome in Children: A Randomized Multicenter Study

Möller JS, and the Surfactant ARDS Study Group (Winterberg 1, Saarbrücken, Germany; et al)

Intensive Care Med 29:437-446, 2003   8–12

Background.—Acute respiratory distress syndrome (ARDS) is still associated with high mortality in children. The enforcement of standardized ventilation protocols and a decline in the incidence of multiple trauma and sepsis have led to a continuous decrease in severe ARDS incidence in children. However, mortality has remained high in children with profound hypoxemia and severe underlying conditions such as immunosuppression, so many other therapies, in addition to those that are aimed at preventing barotrauma and volutrauma, have been reported. Whether bovine surfactant administered to children with severe ARDS will improve oxygenation was investigated.

Methods.—Nineteen patients were included in a single-center study, which was then followed by a multicenter randomized trial involving 35 patients in a comparison of surfactant with a standardized treatment algorithm. All of the patients were born after 44 weeks' gestation and were under age 14 years. All had been admitted for at least 4 hours, ventilated for 12 to 120 hours, and were without heart failure or chronic lung disease. A dose of 100 mg/kg bovine surfactant was administered intrathecally under continuous ventilation and PEEP as soon as the partial pressure of arterial oxygen (PaO_2)/fraction of inspired oxygen (FIO_2) ratio dropped to less than 100 for 2 hours.

A second equivalent dose was allowed within 48 hours. The primary end point was PaO_2/FIO_2 at 48 hours, and the secondary end points were PaO_2/FIO_2 at 2, 4, 12, and 24 hours, survival, survival without rescue, days on ventilation, and analysis of subgroups to identify patients who might benefit from the administration of surfactant.

Results.—In the pilot study, the PaO_2/FIO_2 increased by a mean of 100 at 48 hours. A higher PaO_2/FIO_2 ratio was observed in the surfactant group 2 hours after the first dose (58 from baseline vs 9 from baseline in the control group), and at 48 hours, there was a trend toward a higher ratio (38 vs 22 from baseline). The surfactant group had a significantly lower rate of rescue therapy. A second surfactant dose was administered to 11 patients with no effect on outcome criteria. A significant difference in PaO_2/FIO_2 in favor of surfactant at 48 hours was observed in the subgroup with an initial PaO_2/FIO_2 ratio higher than 65 and in patients without pneumonia.

Conclusions.—Oxygenation is improved immediately after administration of surfactant therapy in patients with severe ARDS. However, this improvement is sustained only in those patients who do not have pneumonia and who have an initial PaO_2/FIO_2 ratio higher than 65.

▶ The surfactant replacement dilemma continues! These studies (Abstracts 8–11 and 8–12) demonstrate the difference between the adult and pediatric literature. Our group was a part of the Spragg et al study (Abstract 8–11). The methods were good, as was the product. However, no difference in primary or secondary end points was observed. One positive is that no detrimental effects were observed. Dosing (inadequate) in adults seems to be pervasive throughout previous trials, coupled with poor distribution in the distal airways. These constraints seem minimal, especially in the neonate or toddler, as oxygenation in mild to moderate disease generally increases and allows for "less aggressive" ventilation to take place. As a potential remedy in adults, some current surfactant trials are employing bronchoscopically assisted delivery to the lobar segments to ensure surfactant delivery. This, coupled with increased dosing and increased frequency for longer intervals, may show more promise.

J. D. Lang, Jr, MD

Single Dexamethasone Injection Increases Alveolar Fluid Clearance in Adult Rats

Noda M, Suzuki S, Tsubochi H, et al (Tohoku Univ, Sendai, Japan)

Crit Care Med 31:1183-1189, 2003   8–13

Background.—The epithelial Na+ channels and Na+/K+-adenosine triphosphatase (ATPase) in alveolar epithelium play a significant role in the absorption of excessive fluid from the alveolar space. Intact alveolar fluid clearance (AFC) is vital not only in clearing fluid from the lungs at birth and keeping the alveolar space relatively free of fluid for adequate gas exchange, but also pathologically in opposing the accumulation of intra-alveolar fluid accumulation in acute lung injury at birth. There have been many attempts to stimulate AFC. Whether single dexamethasone injection at therapeutic doses would modulate lung epithelial Na+ channels and Na+/K+-ATPase and increase alveolar fluid clearance in adult rats was investigated.

Methods.—A total of 138 adult male Sprague-Dawley rats were included in this controlled laboratory study. The rats were intraperitoneally injected with dexamethasone at a dose ranging from 0.02 to 2.0 mg/kg and were allowed free access to food and water. AFC was determined by measuring the increase in albumin concentration in the lung instillate solution.

Results.—There was a significant increase in AFC at 48 and 72 hours after dexamethasone treatment. The effect of dexamethasone was dose dependent. Increased AFC was associated with a faster recovery from hypoxemia, which was induced by filling the alveolar space with instillate solution. This increase in AFC was inhibited by amiloride and ouabain. On quantitative reverse transcriptase–polymerase chain reaction, dexamethasone treatment increased lung β-epithelial Na+ channel mRNA levels. There was also a slight increase in the expression of γ-epithelial Na+ channel mRNA. However, α-epithelial Na+ channel mRNA levels did not differ from control levels. The levels of α1- or β1-Na+/K+-ATPase mRNA were unchanged 72 hours after dexamethasone treatment. However, lung Na+/K+-ATPase hydrolytic activity was increased at 48 and 72 hours after dexamethasone treatment.

Conclusion.—Single dexamethasone injection at a therapeutic dose can modulate lung epithelial Na+ channels and Na+/K+-ATPase and increase the clearance of alveolar fluid, which accelerates recovery from pulmonary edema.

▶ AFC-enhancing therapies should be a part of any strategy when formulating a therapeutic plan in a patient suffering from pulmonary edema. This study evaluated single-dose dexamethasone and found that AFC was enhanced via Na+ channel stimulation and Na+/K+-ATPase activity. The AFC peaked at 72 hours and was also associated with improved oxygenation. There is speculation as to how dexamethasone works, but most probably dexamethasone possesses some mineralocorticoid activity. Type II alveolar cells, the cells where the apical and basolateral Na+ channels reside, are responsive to mineralocorticoid activity. The exact dosing in humans; route of administration; side effects; and effect on patients with lung injury, where the air-blood barrier may be disrupted, deserves study.

J. D. Lang, Jr, MD

The Cuff Leak Test to Predict Failure of Tracheal Extubation for Laryngeal Edema

De Bast Y, De Backer D, Moraine J-J, et al (Free Univ of Brussels, Belgium)
Intensive Care Med 28:1267-1272, 2002   8–14

Background.—Endotracheal intubation may be attended by local complications, such as mechanical lesions and biochemical reactions at the interface between the plastic or silicone tube material and the mucosa of the upper airway. The incidence of these complications has declined with the use of more flexible polyvinyl chloride tubes that generate less pressure on the anatomical structures, and with the use of high-volume, low-pressure cuffs that cause fewer mucosal lesions. Laryngeal edema secondary to endotracheal intubation manifests as respiratory distress and inspiratory whistling (stridor), and may require early reintubation. No sure method exists for identifying patients at risk of severe laryngeal edema before extubation. However, the absence of a leak around an endotracheal tube before extubation may be predictive of laryngeal edema. The usefulness and predictive value of the cuff leak test to identify those patients who will require early reintubation for laryngeal edema were evaluated.

Methods.—The study included 76 patients who were intubated endotracheally for more than 12 hours. The best cutoff value that could predict the need for reintubation for significant laryngeal edema was determined, and the patients were then divided into 2 groups on the basis of this cutoff value.

Results.—Reintubation for laryngeal edema was required in 8 (11%) of 76 patients. Patients requiring reintubation had smaller leaks than the other patients, and the best cutoff value for gas leak was 15.5%. Among the 51 patients in the high-leak group, only 2 (3%) patients required reintubation. In the low-leak group, 6 (24%) of 25 patients required reintubation. The cuff leak test had a sensitivity of 75%, a positive predictive value of 25%, and a negative predictive value of 96.1%. The classification had an accuracy of 72.4%.

Conclusions.—A gas leak around the endotracheal tube that is greater than 15.5% can be used as a screening test to reduce the risk of reintubation for laryngeal edema.

▶ This is a useful study for the practicing intensivist. The study is not devoid of limitations but gives us another screening tool to assist in minimizing re-intubations, at least in the adult patient population in a medical-surgical ICU setting. Reintubation is a serious matter in the ICU as it increases attributable mortality rates via several mechanisms, most notably by increasing pneumonia rates. However, in this specific patient population, extubation failure due to laryngeal edema my lead to increased morbidity and mortality rates by way of difficulty in reestablishing an airway. This value (15.5%) tested prospectively in a larger number of patients seems like a very worthy clinical project.

J. D. Lang, Jr, MD

Development of a Continuous Renal Replacement Program in Critically Ill Patients

Gilbert RW, Caruso DM, Foster KN, et al (Arizona Burn Ctr, Phoenix, Ariz)
Am J Surg 184:526-533, 2002   8–15

Background.—Among the many challenges facing critically ill patients is the development of acute renal failure, which affects 4% to 7% of ICU patients. If the patient can tolerate the hemodynamic and metabolic stress of intermittent hemodialysis or peritoneal dialysis, these methods can effectively manage acute renal failure, but this is often not the case. Continuous renal replacement therapy (CRRT) offers a number of advantages over hemodialysis and peritoneal dialysis but has not been widely used in hospitals because it is more complex, requires specially trained nurses and physicians, carries significant start-up and maintenance costs, and has a history of low reimbursement. All of the costs required to start up a new CRRT program and to determine whether the hospital is receiving adequate reimbursement were assessed, along with an evaluation of the impact on patient outcomes.

Methods.—The latest CRRT equipment and an innovative hands-on CRRT training program were used to create a specialized CRRT team. New revenue charge codes were created and existing ones updated to track costs and reimbursement. The financial records of patients having CRRT were evaluated retrospectively for hospital cost to perform the procedure, total hospital billing to the payer, revenue 881 from CRRT charged to the payer, total charges and reimbursement on the account, percentage of reimbursement received, collected revenue, and who paid.

Results.—The total cost for the development and initiation of the CRRT program was $79,622.80. The 39 patients who had CRRT therapy from April 2000 to February 2002 ranged in age from 1 day to 85 years, and their treatment times were 10 to 1140 hours. Mortality was 59%. Combining the 36 complete patient accounts available, the total hospital bill was $13,960,312.23; hospital reimbursement was $6,018,501.00. The total cost for CRRT, including nursing and supplies, was $222,323.98, for which the hospital billed $656,090.63. A profit of $437,678.50 could have been realized, but because of noncompliance with charge capture at the nursing level, a substantial number of nursing hours and supplies were not accounted for.

The actual billing by the hospital was $386,794.32 and total reimbursement was $165,779.86, for a net loss of $56,544.12. Just over 47% of the patients had private insurance or workman's compensation, while nearly 53% had Medicare, state or federally funded Medicaid, or paid the bill themselves. A net profit of $10,294.12 was seen regarding the 21 burn patients receiving CRRT, but net losses from other patients were $42,564 (exfoliative disorder patients), $11,967.78 (surgical patients), $5978.25 (trauma patients), $3934.79 (pediatric/neonatal patients), and $2392.85 (cardiology patients).

Conclusion.—For all patients except those with burns, the CRRT program showed a loss of revenue. However, CRRT programs improved patient care by providing dialysis for patients otherwise unable to tolerate the procedure. The hospital administration and CRRT staff must collaborate in initiating and maintaining a CRRT program to ensure that it is comprehensive, provides a higher standard of patient care, ensures continued education, includes quality management initiatives, and provides at least revenue-neutral reimbursement.

▶ A study worthy of note because of the routine use of CRRT in the ICU and because of its purported advantages. As with many other evolving technologies, having the appropriate infrastructure in place to ensure efficient use falls short, thus undermining the potential advantages gained by its use. With CRRT the same holds true. Device malfunction, dialysate changes, and flow-related issues with vascular access occur not infrequently and, if not attended to promptly, undercut benefits accrued by both the patient and hospital. Many systems never consider additional personnel for "in-house" coverage because they automatically equate that to increased costs. This study did not prove cost-benefit because of inadequacies elsewhere. But if one assumes appropriate billing practices, the probabilities of cost- benefit coupled with enhanced patient care is a win-win situation where all benefit.

J. D. Lang, Jr, MD

Immunologic and Hemodynamic Effects of "Low-Dose" Hydrocortisone in Septic Shock: A Double-Blind, Randomized, Placebo-Controlled, Crossover Study

Keh D, Boehnke T, Weber-Cartens S, et al (Humboldt Univ, Berlin; Vivantes Klinikum Neukoelln, Berlin, Germany)

Am J Respir Crit Care Med 167:512-520, 2003   8–16

Background.—Results in recent randomized, controlled trials have indicated that prolonged (5 days or more) administration of low doses of hydrocortisone (240 to 300 mg/d) as compared with higher doses (up to 40 g/d) over a shorter time (1 to 2 days) improves shock reversal in patients with early or late septic shock. However, little is known regarding the immunologic effects of continuously infused low doses of hydrocortisone in septic shock. Specifically, protection from overshooting inflammatory response must be balanced with the risk of aggravated immunosuppression, which has gained increasing importance in understanding of sepsis pathophysiology and multiple organ failure.

Low doses of glucocorticoids are increasingly used as adjunctive therapy for stabilization of blood pressure in septic shock patients, so an understanding of immune reactions is important for the identification of possible risks associated with this therapeutic approach. The effects of hydrocortisone on the balance between proinflammation and anti-inflammation were evaluated.

Methods.—Forty patients with septic shock were randomly assigned in a double-blind, cross-over study to receive either the first 100 mg of hydrocortisone as a loading dose and 10 mg per hour until day 3 or placebo followed by the opposite medication until day 6.

Results.—Infusion of hydrocortisone was accompanied by an increase in mean arterial pressure and systemic vascular resistance and a decline of heart rate, cardiac index, and norepinephrine requirement. A reduction of plasma nitrite/nitrate indicated inhibition of nitric oxide formation and correlated with a reduction of vasopressor support. The inflammatory response, endothelial and neutrophilic activation, and anti-inflammatory response were attenuated. Human leukocyte antigen-DR expression was only slightly depressed in peripheral blood monocytes, while in vitro phagocytosis and the monocyte-activating cytokine interleukin-12 increased. Hemodynamic and immunologic rebound effects were induced by the withdrawal of hydrocortisone.

Conclusion.—Low-dose hydrocortisone therapy in patients with septic shock is capable of restoring hemodynamic stability. The immunologic response to stress is modulated in an antiinflammatory rather than immunosuppressive manner.

▶ This study of significant sophistication further defines the hemodynamic and immunomodulatory influences of "low dose" hydrocortisone in patients suffering from septic shock. A very interesting point brought to light by this study was the reduction in nitric oxide production, which probably contributed significantly to the reduction in norepinephrine. Other studies have focused on increased adrenergic receptor density and/or responsiveness.

J. D. Lang, Jr, MD

Deactivation of Norepinephrine by Peroxynitrite as a New Pathogenesis in the Hypotension of Septic Shock
Takakura K, Xiaohong W, Takeuchi K, et al (Fukui Med Univ, Japan)
Anesthesiology 98:928-934, 2003   8–17

Background.—Vascular hyporeactivity to catecholamines is a limiting factor in the successful treatment of hypotension in patients with septic shock and results in a high mortality rate. The precise mechanisms of vascular hyporeactivity have not been clearly discerned, but large amounts of nitric oxide (NO) and superoxide anion appear to be involved in the hyporeactivity. The inducible isoform of NO synthase has been identified in many tissues, including the vascular endothelium, smooth muscle, and myocardium. NO is reactive with superoxide anion in formation of the potentially toxic NO metabolite, peroxynitrite ($ONOO^{-1}$). Whether $ONOO^{-1}$ decreases the vasocontractile activity of norepinephrine was investigated.

Methods.—Norepinephrine was treated with $ONOO^{-1}$ of 3-morpholinosydonimine-N-ethyl-carbamine (SIN-1), an $ONOO^{-1}$ producer, in a 5×10^2 M sodium phosphate buffer solution at pH 7.4, and absorbance of the product was measured spectrophotometrically at 295 and 370 nm. This pretreated norepinephrine was then administered to isolated rat thoracic aortas, and contractions were observed in functional experiments. The rate constant between norepinephrine and $ONOO^{-1}$ was determined by means of a competition assay with cysteine in functional experiments. Finally, norepinephrine pretreated with $ONOO^{-1}$ was administered IV into anesthetized rats to measure blood pressure.

Results.—Norepinephrine pretreated with $ONOO^{-1}$ was confirmed spectrally as oxidized norepinephrine. Pretreated norepinephrine was observed to decrease its vasocontractile force in an $ONOO^{-1}$ concentration–dependent manner. The decrease in its force was lower at pretreatment with $ONOO^{-1}$ in a lower pH buffer. A rate constant for the $ONOO^{-1}$-norepinephrine reaction was 6×10^2 M/S. Norepinephrine incubated with SIN-1 was observed to decrease its vasocontractile force in an incubation time–dependent fashion. There was no significant change in arterial blood pressure in anesthetized rats after administration of norepinephrine pretreated with $ONOO^{-1}$.

Conclusion.—These findings indicate that norepinephrine was oxidized and deactivated by $ONOO^{-1}$. This deactivation may provide at least a partial explanation for the hyporeactivities of vasoconstriction to norepinephrine in patients in septic shock.

▶ A very provocative study that continues to "chip away" at the mechanisms leading to hypotension in patients suffering from septic shock.

J. D. Lang, Jr, MD

Effect of Increasing Norepinephrine Dosage on Regional Blood Flow in a Porcine Model of Endotoxin Shock
Treggiari MM, Romand J-A, Burgener D, et al (Univ Hosp, Geneva; Sahlgren's Univ Hosp, Göteborg, Sweden)
Crit Care Med 30:1334-1339, 2002   8–18

Background.—Catecholamines are used in the treatment of septic shock to counteract systemic hypotension when fluid resuscitation has not succeeded in restoring sufficient arterial blood pressure. Norepinephrine is administered for the restoration and maintenance of an adequate systemic and organ perfusion pressure, and it has been suggested that norepinephrine may improve blood pressure, urine output, and even splanchnic perfusion. This study evaluated the effect of a norepinephrine-induced differential increase in mean arterial pressure on splanchnic and renal perfusion in a porcine model of volume-resuscitated endotoxic shock.

Methods.—This prospective, controlled, acute interventional study was conducted at an animal research laboratory and included 14 landrace pigs, of which 7 were treated with norepinephrine and 7 were used as endotoxemic controls. Norepinephrine was administered to reverse hypotension in 7 fluid-resuscitated pigs which had been anesthetized with α-chloralose and equipped with flow probes around the portal vein and renal artery. Renal and jejunal mucosal layer Doppler flowmetry and jejunal tonometry were used to perform measurements before 2-hour endotoxin infusion and at the end of each increased level of mean arterial pressure.

Results.—Increasing the mean arterial pressure with norepinephrine by 10 mm Hg provided significant increases in cardiac output, systemic oxygen extraction, and portal venous blood flow; stabilized metabolic acidosis; and showed a tendency toward restoration of renal and jejunal mucosal flows to preshock levels. An increase of 20 mm Hg in mean arterial pressure further improved cardiac output and oxygen delivery but without improving portal vein, renal artery, or jejunal mucosal blood flows.

Conclusion.—Administration of norepinephrine to increase mean arterial pressure by 10 mm Hg in an acute model of volume-resuscitated endotoxic shock resulted in the improvement of systemic and regional perfusion. However, the administration of norepinephrine to increase mean arterial pressure by 20 mm Hg did not result in increased renal and splanchnic blood flow despite enhancing cardiac output.

▶ The debate on which vasoactive agent is superior in patients with distributive shock rages on. Norepinephrine has emerged as the vasopressor of choice in this setting.[1] Data are continuing to accrue demonstrating norepinephrine's ability to improve global hemodynamics but also improve focal perfusion to vulnerable vital organ systems. "Leave 'em dead" with Levophed may be dead itself?

J. D. Lang, Jr, MD

Reference

1. Sharma VK, Dellinger RP: The international sepsis forum's controversies in sepsis: my initial vasopressor agent in septic shock is norepinephrine rather than dopamine. *Crit Care* 7:3-5, 2003.

Effects of Preoperative Oral Carbohydrates and Peptides on Postoperative Endocrine Response, Mobilization, Nutrition and Muscle Function in Abdominal Surgery
Henriksen MG, Hessov I, Dela F, et al (Aarhus Univ, Denmark; Univ of Copenhagen)
Acta Anaesthesiol Scand 47:191-199, 2003   8–19

Background.—The "nulla per os" (NPO) regimen from the midnight prior to surgery has become a universal practice despite contemporary reports of much faster emptying of clear fluids from the stomach than had previously been believed. This practice has remained largely unchallenged until recently. New research has suggested that NPO may not only be unnecessary and unpleasant but may actually be harmful. At present, surgery is followed by a long-lasting state of relative peripheral insulin resistance, which is reduced by the administration of glucose infusion or oral carbohydrate-rich drinks immediately before surgery instead of fasting. This study investigated whether oral carbohydrate or carbohydrate with peptide drinks preoperatively instead of fasting would improve postoperative voluntary muscle strength; nutritional intake and ambulation; decrease postoperative fatigue, anxiety, and discomfort; and reduce the endocrine response to surgery.

Methods.—A total of 48 patients were randomly assigned to 1 of 3 groups to receive 2 × 400 mL of carbohydrate-rich drinks (intervention groups) or to fast overnight with only water. One intervention group was given a carbohydrate drink, and the other received a carbohydrate/peptide drink. The main outcome measures were voluntary grip and quadriceps strength, body composition, pulmonary function, Visual Analogue Scale score of 8 parameters of well-being, muscle biopsies and insulin, glucagon, insulin-like growth factor–1, and free fatty acids. These were measured before and after the operation. Immediate oral nutrition and early enforced mobilization were included in the basic postoperative regimen for all groups.

Results.—The significant postoperative decrease in glycogen synthase activity in the muscle biopsies typically seen in patients who are NPO before surgery was reduced in the intervention groups. In combination, the intervention groups had a less reduced quadriceps strength after 1 week (-10% vs -16%) and 1 month (-5% vs -13%). There were minor alterations in the endocrine response to surgery, with no difference between groups, and there were no differences between the groups in terms of ambulation time, nutritional intake, or subjective measures of well-being.

Conclusion.—A significant decrease in glycogen synthase activity, a rate-limiting enzyme in glucose storage, occurs in patients who fast overnight before undergoing major abdominal surgery. This decline could be reduced by providing carbohydrate-rich drinks. The findings of this study may have clinical importance for muscle function.

▶ An intriguing study addressing presurgical ingestion of variations in nutritional substrate content on metabolic, muscular, and emotional indexes in the postoperative setting after abdominal surgery. The study was too small to make any definitive statement but is a great first-step. A large, randomized, controlled trial with the appropriate statistical power should be undertaken to assess how dietary manipulation preoperatively can affect postoperative outcome. It is areas such as these where potential savings of lives and costs can be made. If a low-cost intervention up front can be made and translated into decreased ICU stays and susceptibility to nosocomial infection and increased emotional well-being, it should be aggressively supported and pursued. I was a little surprised that pancuronium, a neuromuscular blocker demonstrated to contribute to postoperative pulmonary complications, was used in all of the patients (even the octogenarians). In the next study, the methods might benefit from altering the anesthetic technique.

J. D. Lang, Jr, MD

Use of Capnometry to Verify Feeding Tube Placement

Araujo-Preza CE, Melhado ME, Gutierrez FJ, et al (Staten Island Univ, NY)
Crit Care Med 30:2255-2259, 2002   8–20

Background.—Although a 2-step protocol and several other clinical methods have been recommended in an attempt to verify proper placement, there continue to be case reports of complications, morbidity, and mortality related to feeding tube placement. Among the complications of feeding tubes are pneumothorax, atelectasis, pleural effusion, bronchopleural fistula, hydrothorax, empyema, mediastinitis, pneumonitis, esophageal perforation, and pneumonia. Placement of the feeding tube is evaluated by several different methods, none of which are completely reliable. The effectiveness of capnometry (carbon dioxide monitoring) for verification of gastric placement of a stylet-guided nasogastric tube was investigated in intubated, mechanically ventilated patients.

Methods.—This prospective, descriptive study was conducted in a medical-surgical ICU, a coronary care unit, and a chronic ventilator unit and enrolled a total of 53 adult patients receiving mechanical ventilation and enteral feedings. After insertion of the feeding tube to a length of 30 cm and before the first radiograph was obtained, the end-tidal carbon dioxide detector was attached to the proximal end of the feeding tube. The detector was left in place for 1 minute and was observed for a change in color.

The detector is originally purple and will change color to tan, or even yellow, on contact with carbon dioxide. If the end-tidal carbon dioxide remained purple, it was interpreted as gastrointestinal placement. Conversion to tan or yellow would have indicated airway placement. The first chest radiograph was obtained to confirm observations made with the detector. The feeding tube was advanced, and a final chest radiograph verified its position below the diaphragm.

Results.—No carbon dioxide was detected in 52 of 53 placements. Positioning in the gastrointestinal tract was confirmed by the 2-step procedure. The technique was 100% specific, and there were no false-positive findings. One of the placements was found to be in the trachea. Carbon dioxide was appropriately detected with the end-tidal carbon dioxide detector, indicating no false negative findings. For verification of sensitivity, 20 placements were made directly into the trachea through an endotracheal tube. Carbon dioxide was detected in all 20 placements.

Conclusion.—Capnometry is a safe method for verification of proper placement of the feeding tube, and thus the first chest radiograph can be safely eliminated. The use of capnometry for verification of feeding tube placement can reduce the time and cost of this procedure.

▶ Depending on whether you're a postpyloric or gastric feeding person, this study may be of use. Using the capnograph as a tool for other duties seems a worthy cause. All the described methods for placing feeding tubes have their limitations. And certainly instilling enteral feeds and other substances directly into the lung is unforgivable. We are trying this technique in our ICU. An important point that I took from the study was that when the investigators intentionally placed the feeding tube in the trachea (on 20 occasions), carbon dioxide was detected colorimetrically, and this also occurred with the 1 accidentally placed feeding tube. Fluoroscopy is expensive and time consuming and obviously has radiation hazards. One should refer directly to the study methodology on how to connect the capnometer to the feeding tube.

J. D. Lang, Jr, MD

Decreased Mortality and Infectious Morbidity in Adult Burn Patients Given Enteral Glutamine Supplements: A Prospective, Controlled, Randomized Clinical Trial
Garrel D, Patenaude J, Nedelec B, et al (Hôtel-Dieu Montreal; Institut Armand-Frappier, Pointe Claire, Quebec)
Crit Care Med 31:2444-2449, 2003   8–21

Background.—Glutamine (G) is an important energy source for immune cells and the intestinal epithelium, a major nitrogen carrier from muscles to the digestive tract and immune system in severe trauma, and a precursor to nucleotides. Animal studies have indicated that G has a protective effect on intestinal mucosa and inhibits bacterial and endotoxin translocation from the intestinal lumen to the bloodstream. Enteral G supplements have been shown to reduce morbidity caused by infection in trauma patients, but their effect in burn patients is unknown. Whether enteral G supplements can ameliorate morbidity caused by infection, length of care required, and protect the health of the immune system in patients with burns was evaluated.

Methods.—Forty-five adults had severe, full-thickness burns and were being treated in a burn center. Enteral nutrition was given by a nasoenteral tube inserted under endoscopic guidance into the third portion of the duodenum; the rate was 30 mL/h, with increases every 12 hours until 120 mL/h had been given (depending on patient tolerance). Parenteral nutrition was begun within 48 hours of admission. Two groups were formed, with 1 receiving 4.3 g of G every 4 hours for a total of 26 g/d and the other an isonitrogenous control mixture consisting of aspartic acid, asparagine, and glycine given in 50 mL of sterile water through the feeding tube. The evaluation lasted until healing occurred. Length of care required, incidence of positive blood cultures (PBCs), and mortality were noted. Measurements of phagocytosis by circulating polymorphonuclear cells were obtained every 3 days.

Results.—Three patients died within 72 hours and a fourth could not receive enteral nutrition and amino acid supplementation for the first 10 days; these 4 patients were excluded. The 2 groups did not differ with respect to energy and protein intake, resting energy expenditure, nitrogen balance, insulin received, urinary cortisol excretion, or blood glucose level. No deaths occurred in the G group after 72 hours; in the control group, 8 patients died, a rate reflecting that noted for this type of patient at the burn center. No differences were found between groups in terms of length of care, number of surgical operations, or time from admission to first surgery. Control patients had PBCs at a rate 3 times that of the glutamine group (19% vs 7.5%), and more control subjects had PBCs for over 2 days. None of the G patients had PBCs for *Pseudomonas aeruginosa*, while 6 of the control group did. Plasma levels of G were similar in the 2 groups, and the incidence of wound infection and severity of respiratory disease did not differ between the groups, suggesting that the effect of G is local.

Conclusion.—The higher rate of PBCs among burn patient control subjects compared with the G group resembles data found for trauma patients. G may be protective against *P aeruginosa*, in that none of those receiving it had positive cultures for this organism. Because it is a glutathione precursor, G may be particularly effective in the intestinal mucosa, possibly protecting intestinal immune function. Burn patients may benefit from improved intestinal barrier function, particularly the competence of the intestinal immune system since mortality is linked to systemic infection with burns. The decreased mortality in G patients may be related to its administration (route and regimen). This should be investigated further.

▶ This is an important study in a patient population that we commonly care for. The topic of nutrition in the critically ill patient is schizophrenic to say the least. This study added something to the clinical evidence. All the positive effects observed in the study seemed to result from positive local gastrointestinal effects, not systemic benefits. When compared to other studies, differences in this study were dosing (higher), enteral administration (vs parenteral), and bolus administration (vs continuous infusion). An interesting twist would have been additional limbs with Oxepa only and Oxepa plus glutamine. This study should stimulate a larger multicenter trial.

J. D. Lang, Jr, MD

Hyperglycemia Exacerbates Muscle Protein Catabolism in Burn-Injured Patients
Gore DC, Chinkes DL, Hart DW, et al (Univ of Texas, Galveston)
Crit Care Med 30:2438-2442, 2002   8–22

Introduction.—The factors that adversely affect wound healing in severe burn injury include hyperglycemia and muscle protein catabolism. A loss of lean body mass has been found to correspond with significant increases in infection rates and a prolonged need for mechanical ventilation. Adult patients with burns over more than 40% of their body surface area were studied retrospectively for a possible association between severity of hyperglycemia and the rate of protein loss from muscle.

Methods.—The study included data from 29 patients (mean age, 31 years) and an average body mass index of 25.8. All were cared for in a similar manner with early excision of the burn wound, autografting, use of broad-spectrum antibiotics, and enteral feeding. Indirect calorimetry and phenylalanine net balance measurements were taken 5 to 7 days after a débridement and grafting procedure. Patients were stratified according to plasma glucose values: normal (plasma glucose ≤ 130 mg/dL), mildly hyperglycemic (plasma glucose, 130-200 mg/dL), and severely hyperglycemic (plasma glucose ≥ 200 mg/dL).

Results.—Patients in the 3 categories of plasma glucose values were similar in age, body weight, body size, extent of burn injury, nutritional intake, and percentage on a ventilator. Platelet count, however, was significantly lower in the severely hyperglycemic group than in the normal glucose group. Severe hyperglycemia was also associated with significantly higher arterial concentrations of phenylalanine and a significantly greater net efflux of phenylalanine from the leg. The 3 groups were similar in resting energy expenditure and respiratory quotient.

Conclusion.—Hyperglycemia was associated with an increased rate of muscle protein catabolism in these severely burned patients. This increase was apparent in the greater net efflux of phenylalanine from the leg in patients with severe hyperglycemia. A link may be present between resistance of muscle to the action of insulin and both glucose clearance and muscle protein catabolism.

▶ This study suggests a potential mechanism of why "tight" glucose control increases survival rates for the critically ill patient. This study was small, but demonstrated metabolic benefits (less protein catabolism) when glucose concentrations were kept at 130 mg/dL or less. A larger trial in this same population with these 3 classifications of hyperglycemia would be interesting. Focus should be on wound healing, phagocyte function, platelet function, phenylalanine balance, sepsis rates (especially recurrence) and mortality rates.

J. D. Lang, Jr, MD

Paresis Acquired in the Intensive Care Unit: A Prospective Multicenter Study
De Jonghe B, for the Groupe de Réflexion et d'Etude des Neuromyopathies en Réanimation (Centre Hospitalier de Poissy-Saint-Germain en Laye, Poissy, France; et al)
JAMA 288:2859-2867, 2002   8–23

Introduction.—ICU-acquired neuromuscular disorders have been reported in prospective observational trials based on electrophysiologic or histologic findings. The clinical incidence of ICU-acquired neuromuscular disorders in patients recovering from severe illness has not been determined. A prospective cohort investigation was performed between March 1999 and June 2000 at 3 medical and 2 surgical ICUs in 4 hospitals in France to evaluate the clinical incidence, risk factors, and outcome of ICU-acquired paresis (ICUAP) during recovery from a critical illness in the ICU. The electrophysiologic and histologic patterns in these patients were assessed.

Methods.—All consecutive patients in the ICU without preexisting neuromuscular disorders who underwent mechanical ventilation for 7 or more days underwent daily screening for awakening. The first day a patient was considered awake was labeled day 1. Patients with severe muscle weakness on day 7 were regarded as having ICUAP. The primary outcome measures were incidence and duration of ICUAP, risk factors for ICUAP, and the comparative duration of mechanical ventilation between patients with ICUAP and control subjects.

Results.—The incidence of ICUAP was 25.3% (95% confidence interval [CI], 16.9%-35.2%) among 95 patients with satisfactory awakening. All patients with ICUAP had a sensorimotor axonopathy. Of these, all who underwent a muscle biopsy had specific muscle involvement not associated with nerve involvement. The median duration of ICUAP after day 1 was 21 days; the mean duration of mechanical ventilation after day 1 was significantly longer in patients with those without ICUAP (18.2 vs 7.6 days; $P = .03$). Independent predictors of ICUAP were female gender (odds ratio [OR], 4.66; 95% CI, 1.19-18.30), number of days with dysfunction of 2 or more organs (OR, 1.28; 95% CI, 1.11-1.49), duration of mechanical ventilation (OR, 1.10; 95% CI, 1.00-1.22), and administration of corticosteroids (OR, 14.90; 95% CI, 3.20-69.80) before day 1.

Conclusion.—ICUAP was common during recovery from critical illness and was linked with a prolonged duration of mechanical ventilation. Corticosteroids may also have a role in the development of ICUAP.

▶ This study dovetails nicely with the Herridge et al article on ARDS (Abstract 1–16). Both have demonstrated a high incidence of acquired muscular complications during episodes of critical illness. This study, again like Herridge et al, has implicated corticosteroids as being contributory. Interestingly, ICUAP seems fairly forgiving (most had resolved by 9 months, 50% by 3 weeks) contrasted with patients 12 months after recovering from the acute respiratory distress syndrome, who still had significant muscular problems. These findings should prompt physicians to carefully weigh the risks and benefits of corticosteroid use in critically ill patients.

J. D. Lang, Jr, MD

Pediatric Critical Care Medicine

Nature of Conflict in the Care of Pediatric Intensive Care Patients With Prolonged Stay
Studdert DM, Burns JP, Mello MM, et al (Harvard School of Public Health, Boston; Children's Hosp, Boston; Brigham and Women's Hosp, Boston)
Pediatrics 112:553-558, 2003   8–24

Background.—Care for critically ill children requires that families make important decisions about treatment while experiencing grief, stress, and fatigue. Clinicians must perform highly demanding procedures, provide ongoing prognostic updates for and educate family members, assist in coping, and help determine what must be done. All of this is done in a volatile environment where conflict can erupt.

Previous investigations have focused on conflict over end-of-life decisions for adult patients. This frame of reference is limited in 3 ways as follows: (1) Decisions about life-sustaining treatment can trigger disputes in the ICU; however, disputes can arise in many other circumstances; (2) Pediatric care may differ markedly from that for adults; and (3) ICU disputes are not limited to relationships between the clinician and the family; disputes may occur among clinicians and within families. The frequency, types, sources, and predictors of conflict in prolonged-stay PICU situations were assessed.

Methods.—The 110 patient participants were admitted over 11 months and had PICU stays over 8 days. Clinicians included intensive care physicians and nurses who had provided care. Data came from medical charts, hospital administrative databases, and a chart abstraction tool documenting whether the clinician discussed with the family withholding or withdrawing life-sustaining treatments. Conflicts were prospectively identified via interviews of the treating physicians and nurses just after the patient's enrollment and 7 days later, at PICU discharge or at the child's death, whichever occurred first.

Conflict was defined as a dispute, disagreement, or difference of opinion about patient care that involved more than 1 person and required a decision or action. Among these were disputes over the major goals of therapy or expected outcomes or decisional paralysis. Six primary sources of team/family disagreements, 5 sources of intrateam disputes, and 3 sources of intrafamilial disputes were identified.

Results.—Among 51 patients, 55 conflicts occurred; thus, almost half of the patients represented at least 1 conflict over intensive care. In 60% (33 cases), the conflict was team/family, in 38% (21) it was intrateam, and in the rest it was intrafamilial. Overall 20% of conflicts were between PICU team members and surgical specialists. Of team/family conflicts, 48% involved poor communication, 39% unavailability of parents/guardians to discuss options and make decisions, and 39% disputes over the care plan.

Clinicians reported preferences in life-sustaining care as a major source of conflict in less than half of care plan disputes. Of intrateam conflicts, 38% resulted from poor communication and 33% from disagreements over the care plan; only 1 of these latter areas involved life-sustaining care. Patient factors linked to a greater likelihood of conflict were nonwhite race and Medicaid insurance coverage; those linked to less likelihood of conflict were private health insurance and Catholic religion. On multivariate analysis, Medicaid insurance was the only strong independent risk factor for conflict in the PICU.

Conclusion.—Conflicts arising in caring for critically ill children have a distinct nature. Most pit clinicians against family members, with a third between clinicians—usually intensive care physicians and surgical specialists. Data on PICU conflict resemble those with adult patients concerning communication breakdown as causative. However, PICU care appears especially susceptible to conflict, with rates of both team/family and intrateam conflict about 50% higher than with adults. Also, conflict over life-sustaining treatments, are less prominent sources of conflict in pediatric critical care. However, the unavailability of decision makers increases conflict in pediatric cases, most likely because the clinicians depend on parents' input for day-to-day decision making.

Among Medicaid-insured patients, the odds of conflict were 5 to 8 times higher than among privately insured patients. Factors identified as contributors to conflict include lower educational levels, parental unavailability, and less trust in providers and satisfaction with medical care among persons of lower socioeconomic status. Information about the source of conflicts should prompt interventions such as ethics consultations and family meetings to avoid problems.

▶ In this study, the authors identified types of conflicts and factors predicting the occurrence of conflicts in pediatric patients with prolonged (defined as > 8 days) PICU stay. The incidence of some conflict regarding patient care was quite high. Unlike adult patients, it was infrequently related to withdrawal of support or end-of-life issues. Somewhat surprisingly, severity of illness was not related to likelihood for development of conflicts. In fact, in the multivariant analysis, only Medicaid insurance coverage was associated with increased likelihood of conflicts. Many of these conflicts are related to failure of communications and unavailability of the patients' families for discussions regarding care. It seems likely that system changes to address each of these issues could result in improved communication and decreased conflicts.

S. Black, MD

Cost-Effectiveness of Inhaled Nitric Oxide in Near-Term and Term Infants With Respiratory Failure: Eighteen- to 24-month Follow-up for Canadian Patients

Jacobs P, Finer NN, Fassbender K, et al (Univ of Alberta, Edmonton, Canada; Inst of Health Economics, Edmonton, Alta, Canada; Univ of California, San Diego; et al)
Crit Care Med 30:2330-2334, 2002   8–25

Background.—Inhaled nitric oxide (NO) is effective in improving oxygenation for several conditions in newborn infants with severe respiratory distress who are candidates for the use of extracorporeal membrane oxygenation (ECMO). There has been a significant increase in the use of ECMO since the 1980s and, although it has been shown to be effective in reducing mortality, ECMO is an expensive technology that has not been shown to reduce overall hospital costs during the initial hospitalization. A cost-effectiveness analysis was performed, on the basis of 18 to 24 months of follow-up, on the use of inhaled NO versus oxygen in near-term and term infants with severe respiratory failure who were referred for consideration for ECMO.

Methods.—This cost-effectiveness analysis was performed in conjunction with a randomized, controlled trial conducted by the Canadian Inhaled Nitric Oxide Study Group for patients with severe respiratory distress. The patients were cared for in Canadian regional neonatal ICUs, and follow-up was based on standard care.

Patients were randomly assigned to inhaled NO or oxygen. If their condition deteriorated, they qualified for ECMO; however, not all qualified patients received ECMO. Standard care was provided after hospital discharge. Costs included in the analysis were those for initial hospitalization and standard medical services above routine care and developmental services received until follow-up. Outcome measures included mortality rate, clinical outcomes, and a variety of neurodevelopmental indicators.

Results.—There were no significant differences in costs between interventions. Infants who received inhaled NO generally fared better than those who received oxygen, but the only significant variable was the incidence of seizure disorders (2.7% for NO vs 22.6% for oxygen). Inhaled NO was the preferred intervention on the basis of economic considerations.

Conclusion.—These findings support the use of inhaled NO in near-term and term infants having respiratory care.

▶ A study in the pediatric population demonstrating that inhaled NO is not cost prohibitive. This, of course, is different in the adult patient population (in the United States), as the FDA has only approved it for pediatric use. Thus, it can only be used in off-label fashion. This has forced us to utilize alternative agents in our adult patient population (sildenafil, inhaled epoprostanol, inhaled milrinone) with pulmonary hypertension and/or reduced PaO_2/FIO_2 ratios.

J. D. Lang, Jr, MD

Altered Neutrophil Function in the Neonate Protects Against Sepsis-Induced Lung Injury

Calkins CM, Bensard DD, Partrick DA, et al (Univ of Colorado, Denver; Children's Hosp of Denver)
J Pediatr Surg 37:1042-1047, 2002   8–26

Background.—Acute lung injury and subsequent acute respiratory distress syndrome are a significant cause of morbidity and mortality in both pediatric and adult ICUs. The outcome in acute respiratory distress syndrome is influenced by a number of factors, including the nature of the precipitating condition and the degree to which multiorgan failure occurs. Neutrophils (PMNs) are well-known effectors of lung injury after sepsis. The accumulation of PMNs in the lung is dependent on a complex cascade of events, including the local production of chemokines. It has been shown that neonates are protected from lung injury after zymosan-induced sepsis. The hypothesis that this protection is caused by either altered PMN function or diminished lung chemokine production in neonates compared with adults was investigated.

Methods.—Sepsis was induced in neonatal and adult rats through an intraperitoneal injection of zymosan. The animals were killed after 24 hours, and the lungs were examined for PMN accumulation and function, chemokine production, and lung injury.

Results.—The septic neonates were protected from pulmonary edema, while the septic adult animals were not. There was an increase in both lung PMN number and chemokine production in both septic neonate and adult animals when compared with vehicle-treated animals. PMN function was significantly decreased in neonates when compared with adults.

Conclusion.—PMN function and lung injury in septic neonatal rats were diminished in comparison with those of adult septic rats, despite equivalent lung PMN accumulation and chemostatic protein production. The neonates may have a relative degree of protection from sepsis-induced lung injury caused by immature PMN function.

▶ Intriguing study! With increases in neonatal lung PMNs and chemokines, it was surprising that lung myeloperoxidase (MPO) activity, thus lung wet/dry weight ratios, was significantly decreased in the neonatal compared to the adult (rat) lungs. Lung homogenates were used to measure MPO activity. More sophisticated methods to assess MPO location and the process of MPO translocalization will be pivotal in elucidating the potential mechanisms responsible for these findings. Are the PMNs being modified prior to passing into the pulmonary circulation? These findings could have therapeutic ramifications.

J. D. Lang, Jr, MD

9 Other Perioperative Patient Care Issues

Knowledge and Practice Regarding Prophylactic Perioperative Beta Blockade in Patients Undergoing Noncardiac Surgery: A Survery of Canadian Anesthesiologists
VanDenKerkhof EG, Milne B, Parlow JL (Queen's Univ, Kingston, Ont, Canada)
Anesth Analg 96:1558-1565, 2003   9–1

Introduction.—Barriers to the practice of evidence-based medicine include issues of translation and implementation of research to clinical practice. Canadian anesthesiologists were surveyed to ascertain their knowledge and practices associated with prophylactic perioperative β-blockade, a therapy widely addressed in the literature that has the potential for a significant positive effect on patient outcome.

Findings.—Questionnaires were mailed to 1234 members of the Canadian Anesthesiologists' Society. The overall rate of response was 54%. Of these, 95% of respondents were aware of the perioperative β-blocker literature; 93% of this group agreed that β-blockers were beneficial in patients with known coronary artery disease. Fifty-seven percent related that they always or usually administered prophylactic β-blockers in patients with known coronary artery disease (Fig 2); 34% of the regular users continued therapy beyond the early postoperative period. Only 9% of respondents indicated that a formal protocol existed at their institution.

Conclusion.—It appears that barriers to the translation of research to practice were not linked to a lack of awareness of the current best evidence. With regard to perioperative β-blockers, controversies within the literature, along with practical considerations, may be greater barriers to implementation of best evidence.

► Many anesthesiologists recognize the importance of perioperative β-adrenergic blockade in anesthetic practice. However, given same day admission policies and current hospital practice, it is not easy to translate good practice into everyday anesthesia. This article describes the barriers. It is important because this is one of the few therapeutic interventions that anesthesiologists perform which affect events outside the operating room.

M. Wood, MD, FRCA

A

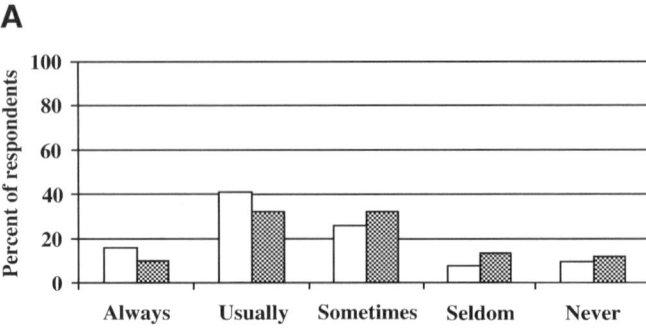

B

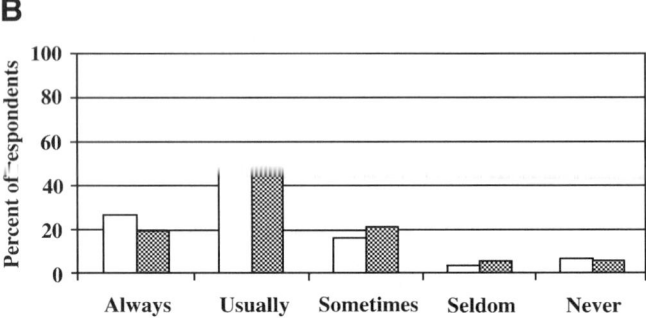

FIGURE 2.—Frequency of β-blocker use among anesthesiologists who indicated that they were aware of the β-blocker literature. Data presented represent responses to the question How often do you use prophylactic β-blockers as a routine part of perioperative care in at-risk patients? **A,** Data represent all 534 anesthesiologists who indicated awareness of the literature. *White columns* represent responses regarding patients with known coronary artery disease (CAD); *hatched columns* represent responses regarding patients with 2 or more risk factors for CAD. **B,** *White columns* represent frequency of β-blocker use among 296 anesthesiologists who strongly agreed that perioperative β-blockers have an effect on postoperative outcomes in patients with known CAD; *hatched columns* represent frequency of β-blocker use among 200 anesthesiologists who strongly agreed that perioperative β-blockers have an effect on postoperative outcomes in patients with 2 or more risk factors for CAD. (Courtesy of VanDenKerkhof EG, Milne B, Parlow JL: Knowledge and practice regarding prophylactic perioperative beta blockade in patients undergoing noncardiac surgery: A survey of Canadian anesthesiologists. *Anesth Analg* 96:1558-1565, 2003.)

Perioperative Management of Patients Receiving Oral Anticoagulants: A Systematic Review

Dunn AS, Turpie AGG (Mount Sinai School of Medicine, New York; McMaster Univ, Hamilton, Ont, Canada)
Arch Intern Med 163:901-908, 2003   9–2

Introduction.—There is no consensus regarding the optimal management of patients receiving oral anticoagulants (OACs) who undergo surgery or invasive procedures. A systematic review and synthesis of the English language literature that addresses the perioperative management and outcomes of patients receiving long-term OAC therapy was performed.

Methods.—A MEDLINE search of English language clinical trials from January 1966 to June 2001 was conducted. The Cochrane Collaborative database was also searched. References from both searches were examined for pertinent trials.

Results.—Thirty-one articles were included. The quality of the trials examined was generally poor. There were no randomized controlled trials and the duration of follow-up was usually not stated. Twenty-nine thrombolic events were reported in 1868 patients (1.6%; 95% confidence interval [CI], 1.0%-2.1%), including 7 strokes (0.4%; 95% CI, 0%-0.7%). Thrombolic event rates by management strategy were 0.4% (1/237) for continuation of OAC, 0.6% (6/996) for discontinuation of OAC treatment without administration of IV heparin, 0% (0/166), for discontinuation of OAC therapy with IV heparin administration, 0.6% (1/180) for discontinuation of OAC therapy with administration of low molecular weight heparin, and 8.0% (21/263) for unspecific or vague strategies. Major bleeding while receiving therapeutic OAC was unusual for dental procedures (0.2% [4/2014]), arthrocentesis (0% [0/32]), cataract surgery (0% [0/203]), and upper endoscopy or colonoscopy with or without biopsy (0% [0/111]).

Conclusion.—Most patients can undergo dental procedures, arthrocentesis, cataract surgery, and diagnostic endoscopy without the need to change their anticoagulation regimen. For invasive and surgical procedures, oral anticoagulation should be withheld and treatment should be individualized. Current literature is limited in its ability to help select an optimal anticoagulant regimen.

▶ I chose this article because a review of this topic is timely, and many of us are struggling to define protocols for our own hospitals. The editorial[1] that accompanies this systematic, evidence-based literature review reminds us of the authors' statement, "It is not possible to draw firm conclusions on the relative efficacy and safety of different management strategies using the available literature..." However, many patients receive OACs, and a decision plan is required when they undergo surgery.

M. Wood, MD, FRCA

Reference

1. Ansell JE: The perioperative management of warfarin therapy (editorial). *Arch Intern Med* 163:881-883, 2003.

Physiologic Effects of Intravenous Fluid Administration in Healthy Volunteers
Holte K, Jensen P, Kehlet H (Hvidovre Univ Hosp, Denmark)
Anesth Analg 96:1504-1509, 2003   9–3

Background.—The optimal dose regimens for perioperative IV fluid administration have not often been based on scientific evidence, so there are large variations in practice. It was hypothesized that a fluid infusion could have adverse effects on organ function. Subjects underwent preoperative fasting, were given an intraoperatively relevant amount of fluid infused over a 3-hour period in the morning, and were hospitalized for 24 hours; no surgery was actually performed. The subjects were aged 59 to 67 years because most surgical patients are 60 years or older. The specific effects evaluated were pulmonary function, exercise capacity, 24-hour weight gain, and balance function.

Methods.—The study followed a prospective, double-blinded, cross-randomized format and was designed to mimic the typical perioperative course after minor to moderate surgery. The 12 healthy volunteers received infusions of lactated Ringer's solution 40 mL/kg (median, 2820 mL) or 5 mL/kg (median, 353 mL; background infusion) in random order on 2 occasions. Spirometry was used to measure pulmonary function, the submaximal treadmill test to measure exercise capacity, and the Balance-Masher test to determine balance function. Patients were also weighed before and 0, 2, 4, 8, and 24 hours after the infusion was completed.

Results.—Spirometry showed that, after receiving the 40-mL/kg infusion, patients' forced vital capacity significantly declined over the first 0 to 8 hours, as did forced expiratory volume at 1 second at 0, 2, and 8 hours. The background infusion produced no such changes. A decrease in peak flow was present 0 and 2 hours after the 40-mL/kg infusion; peak flow was significantly decreased after fluid administrations 8 and 24 hours after the infusion was complete. A significant increase in oxygen saturation was found 0 hours after the infusion but at no other points. No difference was seen in subjects' exercise capacity regardless of the fluid volume. The median 24-hour weight gain was 0.85 kg with the 40-mL/kg infusion and 0 kg with the background infusion. A significantly greater urine output was measured throughout the first 24 hours with the 40-mL/kg infusion. The median cumulated urine output was 3413 mL for the 40-mL/kg infusion and 1888 mL for the background infusion. No differences in the occurrence of dizziness, headache, drowsiness, or general well-being were noted between the 2 fluid infusion volumes. Static balance function was similar for the 2 fluid infusions, but some aspects of dynamic balance improved slightly with the background fluid administration.

Conclusions.—Pulmonary function was inhibited for 8 hours by the 40-mL/kg infusion, and patients gained an average of 0.85 kg in 24 hours. Exercise capacity and balance function were essentially unaffected by either fluid administration. Further studies comparing the same fluid in differing amounts may help to determine the optimal amount of perioperative fluid to infuse.

▶ Controversy exists not only on the type of ideal IV fluid administered during the perioperative period, but also for the amount. We do not have adequate information on the effects of the fluid themselves, and regimens vary widely. This study showed that the effects on pulmonary function were greatest in the high-volume lactated Ringer's solution group, suggesting that high-volume fluid administration and low-volume administration should be investigated in formal randomized clinical trials.

M. Wood, MD, FRCA

Obesity in Adulthood and Its Consequences for Life Expectancy: A Life-Table Analysis
Peeters A, for NEDCOM, the Netherlands Epidemiology and Demography Compression of Morbidity Research Group (Erasmus MC, Rotterdam, The Netherlands; et al)
Ann Intern Med 138:24-32, 2003   9–4

Introduction.—Overweight and obesity in adulthood are associated with an increased risk of death and disease. It is challenging to estimate the public health impact of overweight and obesity caused by complex interactions with age, smoking, and obesity-associated risk factors, including diabetes, hypertension, and lipid disorders. Thus, the potential effect of overweight and obesity on life expectancy and premature death have yet to be determined. Reductions in life expectancy and increases in premature death correlated with overweight and obesity at age 40 years were examined in the Framingham Heart Study, a prospective cohort investigation with follow-up from 1948 through 1990.

Methods.—All 3457 Framingham Heart Study participants were 30 to 49 years old at baseline. Mortality rates specific for age and body mass index group (normal weight, overweight, or obese at baseline) were obtained from gender and smoking status strata. Life expectancy and the probability of death before age 70 were assessed via life tables.

Results.—Large reductions in life expectancy were linked with overweight and obesity. Female nonsmokers aged 40 lost 3.3 years of life expectancy and male nonsmokers aged 40 lost 3.1 because of being overweight. In obese participants, nonsmoking women aged 40 lost 7.1 years and nonsmoking men aged 40 lost 5.8 years. Obese female and male smokers lost 7.2 and 6.7 years of life expectancy, respectively, compared with normal-weight smokers. Obese female and male smokers lost 13.3 and 13.7 years, respectively, of life expectancy, compared with normal weight nonsmokers. Body mass index at ages 30 to 49 years predicted mortality after ages 50 to 69 years, even after adjusting for body mass index at ages 50 to 69.

Conclusion.—Obesity and overweight in adulthood is linked with large reductions in life expectancy and increases in early mortality. These reductions are similar to those observed with smoking. Obesity in adulthood is an important predictor of death at older ages. More efficient prevention and treatment of obesity should become high public health priorities.

▶ This article would seem strange in an anesthesia review, except for what it says about obesity and the prevalence of obesity in our patients. For general information, we should remember that a body mass index of less than 25 is considered normal weight; from 25 to 29.9, overweight; and greater than 30, obesity. For the average 5 ft 4 inch person, you don't get to a body mass index greater than 25 until you get over 147 pounds, and you don't get obese until your are greater than 175 pounds—almost 50 pounds more than the ideal weight of 128 pounds or so.

From a longevity standpoint, what these authors have shown is that obesity—regardless of high blood pressure, diabetes, and other traits—will shorten life expectancy by between 5.8 and 20 years, depending on whether you are a smoker or nonsmoker and whether you are Caucasian or African American. If one factors out diabetes and hypertension and the complications of obesity per se, there is much less effect, meaning the effect is between 3.3 and 10 years (very similar to what we calculated as the "real age" effect of obesity from other studies).

What do I take as the implications of this study for anesthesia? This study means that when you are dealing with obese patients who have nothing other than obesity (that is, they don't have high blood pressure, diabetes, sleep apnea, arthritis, etc.) they are still 3 to 10 years older than their thin counterparts. I guess this fits with another article that we are reviewing in this YEAR BOOK on patients taking advice much better from physicians who are thin and follow their own advice on diet, nutrition, physical activity, and other health behaviors (Abstract 9–5).

So the thin doctor has advantages in longer life expectancy and less disability and patients following the advice. It is your life and your patients' lives. I hope you use your ability to help yourself and influence your patients.

M. F. Roizen, MD

Does Physician Weight Affect Perception of Health Advice?
Hash RB, Munna RK, Vogel RL, et al (Mercer Univ, Macon, Ga; Altanta Med Ctr, Ga; Univ of Georgia, Athens)
Prev Med 36:41-44, 2003   9–5

Background.—Obesity has been recognized and well publicized as an important public health concern in the United States, yet the incidence of obesity continues to increase. Physicians are playing an increasingly important role in the identification of obesity and risk factors for obesity and in counseling patients on risk factor reduction and prevention. Counseling obese and overweight patients regarding lifestyle modifications is considered a most important component in the prevention and treatment of obesity. Unfortunately, many physicians are themselves overweight, which may compromise the effectiveness of overweight and obesity counseling. Whether there is a difference in the way in which patients perceive health care advice in general, and weight management advice in particular, when it is given by obese and nonobese physicians was investigated.

Methods.—A 43-item survey was administered to 226 patients in 5 physician offices. Two of the physicians were classified as obese according to body mass index calculations; the remaining 3 physicians were not obese. The 3 scales of this survey instrument were related to physician characteristics, health locus of control, and perceptions on receiving health advice from overweight physicians. Responses to the surveys were grouped into those from obese and nonobese physicians.

Results.—There were significant differences in patient receptiveness to counseling for treatment of illness and health advice, with the patients of nonobese physicians demonstrating greater confidence scores. The differences for weight and fitness counseling did not achieve statistical significance. Analysis showed that the patient's body mass index was not a significant covariate, nor were items related to physician characteristics in general or health locus of control.

Conclusion.—Patients who sought care from nonobese physicians responded that they had greater confidence in general health counseling and treatment of illness compared with patients seeing obese physicians. However, it is unknown whether these findings can be useful in increasing the success of obesity prevention and treatment.

▶ This study from a primary care practice, examines the practices of just 2 obese doctors and 3 thin doctors. It reports a trend that patients do what physicians do, not what physicians say to do. In this study, the general health advice and illness advice was taken considerably more seriously by those patients of thin doctors than by those patients of obese doctors. How pertinent is that to be in your practice, whether for pain therapy or preoperative therapy? We don't know, but this also confirms the data of Frank et al.[1]

Physician disclosure of healthy habits, whether by appearance in this case or by oral disclosure in the Frank et al study, shows ability to motivate patients toward healthier behaviors. So even if we don't do it for ourselves, we should do it for our patients, and choose healthy behaviors.

M. F. Roizen, MD

Reference

1. Frank E, Breyan J, Elon L: Physician disclosure of healthy personal behaviors improves credibility and ability to motivate. *Arch Fam Med* 9:287-290, 2000.

Hand-Cleansing During Postanesthesia Care
Pittet D, Stéphan F, Hugonnet S, et al (Univ of Geneva Hosps)
Anesthesiology 99:519-520, 2003   9–6

Introduction.—Most endemic infections that occur in ICUs result from the carriage of microorganisms on the hands of health care workers (HCWs). Thus, compliance with recommended hand-cleansing practices is the simplest and most effective preventive measure. The compliance of HCWs with hand cleansing and factors associated with poor compliance were examined in a postanesthesia care unit (PACU).

Methods.—The study was conducted during a 3-week period in a 12-bed PACU with 25 to 35 daily admissions and a nurse-to-patient ratio of 1:3. Three sinks, each with medicated soap, individual bottles of handrub solution, and paper towels, are available. Trained observers worked simultaneously to record hand-cleansing compliance by HCWs during weekday care sessions. Two periods were reported: immediately at PACU admission and at least 30 minutes after admission.

Results.—A total of 187 patients were cared for in the PACU during the observation period. The 3143 patient care activities recorded included 1091 opportunities for hand cleansing at high or medium risk for cross-transmission. With higher workloads, the number of indications for hand cleansing increased, and compliance with hand cleansing decreased. The average compliance at PACU admission was 19.6%; for patients already admitted, the average compliance was 12.5%. Factors associated with noncompliance included caring for patients older than 65 years (odds ratio, 2.23) and those recovering from clean/clean-contaminated surgery (odds ratio, 2.27), as well as a high intensity of patient care (odds ratio, 1.01). During both observation periods, handrub with alcohol was selected more often (approximately 80%) than washing with soap and water.

Conclusion.—There was a low rate of compliance with hand-cleansing requirements in the PACU, both at the time of patient admission and during the stay. Possible causes include a lack of awareness of cross-transmission risks on the part of HCWs, uneven distribution of the workload when several patients are admitted at once, and the open ward nature of the PACU. All staff members must be responsible for making hand cleansing an everyday part of the PACU routine.

▶ This is another example of an opportunity to reduce nosocomial infections. The accompanying editorial by Herwaldt says it as well as anyone can. The fact that in this non-US hospital there was only 19.6% compliance, means to me that maybe even less hand washing occurs at US facilities, and that we may be responsible for even more of such infections. Whether it be food-borne illness and washing of fruit and utensils, or whether it be our hands and going from patient to patient, water and use of more water should be our friend. Everybody should read this article and the accompanying editorial, as they are important for decreasing the risk of disease transmission in hospitals.

M. F. Roizen, MD

Anemia and Blood Tranfusion in Critically Ill Patients
Vincent JL, for the ABC Investigators (Erasme Univ, Brussels, Belgium; et al)
JAMA 288:1499-1507, 2002   9–7

Background.—Anemia is a common finding in critically ill patients admitted to the ICU. The adverse effects of anemia—which include increased risk of cardiac-related morbidity and mortality and a generalized decrease in oxygen-carrying capacity—may be compounded because critical illness often increases metabolic demands. Some of the most significant causes of anemia in critically ill patients are sepsis, overt or occult blood loss, decreased production of endogenous erythropoietin, and immune-associated functional iron deficiency. However, the consequences of anemia on morbidity and mortality in critically ill patients have not been clearly elucidated. The purpose of this study was to prospectively define the incidence of anemia and use of red blood cell transfusion in critically ill patients and to explore the potential benefits and risks associated with transfusion in the ICU.

Methods.—This prospective observational study was conducted in November 1999 and consisted of a blood sampling study and an anemia and blood transfusion study. A total of 1136 patients were enrolled in 145 western European ICUs for the blood sampling study, and 3534 patients from 146 western European ICUs were included in the blood transfusion study. Patients were followed up for 28 days or until hospital discharge, institutional transfer, or death. The main outcome measures were (1) frequency of blood drawing and associated volume of drawn blood, collected over a 24-hour period; and (2) hemoglobin, transfusion rate, organ dysfunction, and mortality, collected throughout a 2-week period.

Results.—The mean (standard deviation) volume per blood draw was 10.3 (6.6) mL, with an average total volume of 41.1 (39.7) mL over a 24-hour period. A positive correlation was observed between organ dysfunction and the number of blood draws and total volume drawn. The mean hemoglobin concentration at ICU admission was 11.3 (2.3) g/dL, with 29% having a concentration of less than 10 g/dL. The transfusion rate during the ICU period was 37%. Older patients and those with a longer length of stay in the ICU were more commonly transfused. Both ICU and overall mortality rates were significantly higher in patients who had a transfusion versus those who had not (ICU rates, 18.5% vs 10.1%, respectively; overall rates, 29% vs 14.9%, respectively). For similar degrees of organ dysfunction, patients who had a transfusion had a higher mortality rate. The 28-day mortality rate for matched patients in the propensity analysis was 22.7% among patients with transfusions and 17.1% among patients without transfusions, a difference that was confirmed by the Kaplan-Meier log-rank test.

Conclusion.—Anemia and the large use of blood transfusion are common in critically ill patients. In addition, the results of this study showed evidence for an association between transfusions and decreased organ function and between transfusions and mortality in these patients.

▶ A very nice study reporting on the demographics of anemia and transfusion practices from 15 different western European countries. It includes data from both academic and community facilities. Generic, medical, and surgical ICUs are represented. It was interesting that the average hemoglobin trigger in this study was 8.4 g/dL. The study was performed in 1999. Looks like a "restrictive" transfusion practice was nearly being adhered to. This study also brings to light the issue of transfusion reduction strategies, such as recombinant erythropoietin, which can be helpful in the critically ill patient.

J. D. Lang, Jr, MD

Use of Perflubron Emulsion to Decrease Allogeneic Blood Transfusion in High Blood Loss Non-Cardiac Surgery: Results of a European Phase 3 Study

Spahn DR, the European Perflubron Emulsion in Non-Cardiac Surgery Study Group (UniversitätsSpital Zürich, Switzerland; et al)

Anesthesiology 97:1338-1349, 2002   9–8

Background.—The limited availability of allogeneic erythrocyte transfusions and the public concern over the safety and availability of donor erythrocytes have prompted the development of artificial oxygen carriers. There are hemoglobin-based solutions and perfluorochemical-based solutions. The safety and efficacy of perflubron emulsion (PFC) given after preoperative acute normovolemic hemodilution were evaluated to see if this approach can decrease the need for allogeneic erythrocyte transfusions among patients having major noncardiac surgery with significant blood loss.

Methods.—The 492 individuals had hemoglobin concentrations between 12 and 15 g/dL. All were scheduled for noncardiac surgery with a 20 mL/kg or greater expected blood loss. The 251 control patients were transfused intraoperatively at a hemoglobin concentration less than 8.0 g/dL or at protocol-defined physiologic triggers. The 241 patients randomly assigned to the PFC group underwent acute normovolemic hemodilution to a hemoglobin level of 8.0 g/dL, then PFC at 1.8 g/kg. An added 0.9 g/kg dose was administered if the hemoglobin level fell to less than 6.5 g/dL. Transfusions were given to PFC patients at hemoglobin levels less than 5.5 g/dL or at predefined physiologic triggers. Postoperative hemoglobin levels were maintained at a minimum of 8.5 g/dL until discharge. Measures included the number of allogeneic and preoperative autologous donation units required and the percentage of patients who avoided transfusion.

Results.—Fewer transfusions were needed by the PFC group than the control subjects even though they had a higher estimated intraoperative blood loss. Transfusions were reduced by 26%. Approximately 21% more patients in the PFC group avoided allogeneic and preoperative autologous donation transfusions compared with control patients. When the estimated surgical blood loss was 10 mL/kg or greater, as noted in 86% of the subjects, transfusion was significantly reduced in patients receiving PFC compared with control subjects at all time points. Platelet counts were approximately 15% to 25% lower on the first through the third postoperative days in the group receiving PFC than in control subjects. By the seventh day, the platelet counts had recovered to normal screening levels in both groups, although those of the PFC group remained lower. The incidence of adverse events was similar between the 2 groups. However, more serious adverse events were noted in the PFC group than among control subjects, with 4 serious cases of ileus in the PFC group and none among control subjects. Mortality rate was 4% among the PFC group and 2% among control subjects, a difference that was not statistically significant.

Conclusions.—The efficacy of PFC was greatest when the estimated surgical blood loss was at least 20 mL/kg. However, the ability to avoid transfusion was significant among those receiving PFC compared with control patients even in procedures estimated to have a blood loss of 10 mL/kg or greater. The use of PFC as an IV oxygen therapeutic agent to augment autologous blood harvesting was a suggested benefit yet to be evaluated.

▶ Many physicians and patients would like to avoid or minimize the use of transfusions during major surgery. This phase 3 study demonstrated that transfusion requirements were decreased with PFC. The use of an artificial IV carrier has been attempted for almost as long as I have been an anesthesiologist; morbidity and adverse events have been an issue for these products, and they have not yet become a clinical reality in day-to-day anesthetic practice.

M. Wood, MD, FRCA

In Vitro Immunosuppressive Activity of Soluble HLA Class I and Fas Ligand Molecules: Do They Play a Role in Autologous Blood Transfusion?
Ghio M, Contini P, Mazzei C, et al (Univ of Genoa, Italy; Imperia Hosp, Italy)
Transfusion 41:988-996, 2001   9–9

Background.—Preoperative autologous blood donation is a common method for reducing exposure to allogeneic transfusion among patients undergoing elective surgery. The goal of this procedure is to limit the occurrence of viral infection transmission through blood components. The immunomodulatory effects of allogeneic blood transfusion may be contributing factors to a poor prognosis in patients with cancer who are undergoing surgery, and it has been postulated that these patients would benefit from autologous blood donation. The immunomodulatory effects of allogeneic blood transfusion have been associated with soluble molecules released from residual white blood cells during storage. The in vitro immunomodulatory activity of soluble molecules detected in supernatants from stored autologous blood was evaluated.

Methods.—Blood was obtained from 4 healthy volunteers. Packed white blood cell–reduced red blood cells (RBCs) were obtained and stored for 30 days, and supernatants were collected. Serum and fresh frozen plasma were also obtained. The concentration of soluble molecules was determined by immunoenzymatic assays, and the in vitro immunomodulatory activity of undiluted blood component supernatant was assessed with antigen-specific cytotoxic T-cell activity and mixed lymphocyte reactions in autologous combinations and by apoptosis induction in Fas+ cells.

Results.—The packed RBCs had higher concentrations of soluble Fas ligand and HLA class I molecules than the white blood cell–reduced RBCs, fresh frozen plasma, and serum. Undiluted supernatants of packed RBCs were observed to strongly inhibit functional assays and to induce apoptosis in Fas+ cells. The immunomodulatory effects were correlated with the amount of soluble Fas ligand and HLA class I molecules.

Conclusion.—These findings are compatible with findings previously reported in allogeneic blood components. It is apparent from these findings that undiluted supernatants of autologous blood components may have immunosuppressive effects in vitro.

▶ In transfusion therapy, we learned that renal transplant patients had fewer rejections if they had received a blood transfusion. In fact, for a period of time, all kidney transplant patients were getting blood transfusions to provide extra rejection proof. But obviously that therapy doesn't work when you want to have an immune system that is strong, such as in surgery for a patient with cancer or even warding off your own cancer cells or infections.

This study showed, interestingly, that the undiluted supernatants of fresh frozen plasma, and even white blood cell–reduced RBCs or radioactively treated red cells, probably have significant immunosuppressive compounds in them. This is another article and piece of data that say we should really be careful with transfusions, even platelet transfusions, and should develop, as soon as possible, artificial hemoglobin solutions. Until then, we might consider washing all RBCs and maybe all platelets prior to transfusion.

M. F. Roizen, MD

Blood Transfusions Correlate With Infections in Trauma Patients in a Dose-Dependent Manner
Claridge JA, Sawyer RG, Schulman AM, et al (Univ of Virginia, Charlottesville)
Am Surg 68:566-572, 2002   9–10

Background.—Because of the high morbidity and mortality rates associated with infections after trauma, it is important to identify risk factors for such infections. Evidence that transfusion of packed red blood cells (pRBCs) may predispose to an increased risk of infection has been reported. The relation between pRBC transfusion and infection in trauma patients was assessed.

Methods.—The analysis included trauma registry data on all 1593 adult patients admitted to a level 1 trauma center over a 3-year period. The mean age was 41 years, the average Injury Severity Score was 15.5, and the mean initial Glasgow Coma Scale score was 13.1. Transfusion of pRBCs during the first 48 hours was assessed and correlated with the infection rate.

Results.—The transfusion rate was 19.4% and the infection rate 12.6%. Patients receiving transfusions had an infection rate of 33.0% compared with 7.6% for those receiving no pRBC transfusions. As the number of transfusions increased from 0 to 15, the risk of infection increased exponentially. On multivariate analysis, pRBC transfusion was the strongest predictor of infection (odds ratio, 1.084).

Conclusions.—For trauma patients, pRBC transfusion is an independent and dose-dependent risk factor for infections. The results suggest that no more pRBC transfusions should be given than absolutely necessary. More research is needed to define their true risk-benefit ratio.

▶ It reports no new or novel information, but this study continues to add to the rapidly accruing literature reporting that transfusion can have detrimental consequences. Interest has focused on the negative immunomodulatory effects of transfusion. Stored blood may itself also be infected. In addition, novel agents that may assist in circumventing the need for pRBCs (synthetic hemoglobin solutions) should remain under evaluation. Lastly, don't buy in to the dogma, "if you transfuse 1 unit, you might as well give 2."

J. D. Lang, Jr, MD

The Forkhead Box m1b Transcription Factor Is Essential for Hepatocyte DNA Replication and Mitosis During Mouse Liver Regeneration

Wang X, Kiyokawa H, Dennewitz MB, et al (Univ of Illinois, Chicago)
Proc Natl Acad Sci U S A 99:16881-16886, 2002   9–11

Background.—The Forkhead Box (Fox) transcription factors are an extensive family of transcription factors, comprising over 50 mammalian proteins. The members of this family of transcription factors share homology in the winged helix DNA-binding domain and have essential roles in cellular proliferation, differentiation, transformation, longevity, and metabolic homeostasis. Previous studies of liver regeneration with transgenic mice have shown that the FoxM1B transcription factor regulates the onset of hepatocyte DNA replication and mitosis by the stimulation of expression of cell cycle genes. The hypothesis that FoxM1B controls the transcriptional network of genes that is essential for progression of the cell cycle was investigated..

Methods.—Mouse *FoxM1B* genomic DNA was isolated from mouse 129SvJ genomic library, and characterization of the intron and exon boundaries was determined. Partial hepatectomy was performed in 8-week-old Alb-Cre *Foxm1b* f1/f1 littermates to induce liver regeneration. Regenerating livers were harvested and divided into 3 portions for isolation of RNA and total protein extract and for paraffin embedding. Antibodies specific to FoxM1B or Cdc25B proteins were used for immunohistochemical detection of paraffin-embedded 5-μm sections of regenerating liver.

Results.—The albumin-promoter-driven Cre recombinase-mediated hepatocyte-specific deletion of the *Foxm1b* Floxed (fl) targeted allele resulted in significant reduction in hepatocyte DNA replication and inhibition of mitosis after partial hepatectomy. Reduced DNA replication in regenerating *Foxm1b*−'− hepatocytes was associated with sustained increase in nuclear staining of the cyclin-dependent kinase inhibitor p21[Cip1] (p21) protein from 24 to 40 hours after partial hepatectomy. In addition, increased levels of nuclear p21 and reduced expression of Cdc25A phosphatase coincided with decreases in cyclin-dependent kinase–2 activation and hepatocyte progression into S-phase.

Conclusion.—The findings of this study demonstrated that FoxM1B transcription factor is responsible for the regulation of the expression of cell cycle proteins that are essential for hepatocyte entry into DNA replication and mitosis.

▶ Clearly, with age, the body deteriorates, muscles atrophy, bones grow thin, the skin loses its elasticity, and wounds are slow to heal. Our tissues don't regenerate the way they did in youth. This article implies that one of the reasons why, is that the *FoxM1B* gene retires. This gene, found in human chromosome number 12, is critical for tissues to heal and replenish themselves. When this gene fails, there is a pileup of a protein called p21^{Cip1}. When this protein accumulates, it sets in motion a series of molecular events that prevent DNA from doubling, and it gives a green light to genes to produce proteins that are associated with old age, such as those proteins that produce the abnormalities found in Alzheimer's disease. Thus, keeping the *FoxM1B* gene healthy, or even finding it, may be important. This study is fun to read and may help all of us understand how genetic knowledge may, in fact, really transform the way we treat diseases and how protein, such as the p21^{Cip1} protein that may be found in some of the substances we eat, may make us older or younger, depending of how much of it we have.

M. F. Roizen, MD

Surgical Procedure Logging With Use of a Hand-Held Computer
Fischer S, Lapinsky SE, Weshler J, et al (Univ of Toronto)
Can J Surg 45:345-350, 2002   9–12

Background.—Medicine continues to trail most other information-rich industries in the adoption of computer technology. Some of the obstacles to computerization are lack of accessibility, costs, and user knowledge. Hand-held devices are becoming increasingly popular because they address many of these concerns. Clinical applications of hand-held computers include tracking of patient information, as a medical reference source, and for performing medical calculations. Hand-held computers are also being used in medical education, for documentation of procedural reports in a family medicine residency program, for procedure and resuscitation tracking in emergency medicine, and in obstetrics and gynecology and anesthesiology.

Despite the many advantages in documenting procedures on hand-held computers, the implementation of this technology is not widespread in medicine. This study evaluated the feasibility of incorporating hand-held computer technology into a surgical residency program by use of hand-held devices for surgical procedure logging linked through the Internet to a central database.

Methods.—This study was conducted at a university general surgery division in Toronto. The 69 residents enrolled in the general surgery training program were given hand-held computers with preinstalled medical programs and a program designed for surgical procedure logging. The procedural data were uploaded via the Internet to a central database. Survey data were collected on previous computer use and previous procedure logging methods. The main outcome measure was the use of this procedure logging system.

Results.—At the end of a 5-month pilot period, 38% of surgical residents were using the hand-held computer procedure-logging system successfully and with regularity. The use of the program was higher among more junior trainees. Analysis of the database provided valuable data on individual trainees, hospital programs, and supervising surgeons. These data would have been useful in program development.

Conclusion.—Hand-held devices can be implemented successfully in a large division of general surgery to provide a reference database and a procedure-logging platform. However, acceptance is not uniform among users of the technology, and ongoing training and support will be required to increased adoption.

▶ This was an interesting study. The authors provided the computers, provided the database, and then saw how many of the surgical host staff used the computers. It turned out that 38% did so for virtually every case. Use correlated with the age of the surgical residents, even though the difference in age wasn't much between the youngest and the oldest surgical resident. This program seems to report on an appropriate wave of the future that is here now.

M. F. Roizen, MD

10 Complications and Mishaps in Anesthesia

Excess Length of Stay, Charges, and Mortality Attributable to Medical Injuries During Hospitalization
Zhan C, Miller MR (Ctr for Quality Improvement and Patient Safety, Rockville, Md; Johns Hopkins Univ, Baltimore, Md)
JAMA 290:1868-1874, 2003   10–1

Introduction.—Medical injuries are a known and important hazard within the health care system, yet little is understood about their prevalence, adverse outcomes, or effective prevention. What is considered preventable is debatable. Medical injures may occur during all stages of care, vary widely in nature, and are relatively infrequent. Patient Safety Indicators (PSIs) were used to evaluate length of stay, charges, and deaths attributable to medical injuries during hospitalization.

Methods.—The Agency for Healthcare Research and Quality (AHRQ) PSIs were used to ascertain medical injuries in 7.45 million hospital discharge abstracts from 994 acute care hospitals across 28 states in 2000 in the AHRQ Healthcare Cost and Utilization Project Nationwide Inpatient Sample database. The primary outcome measures were length of stay, charges, and mortality that were documented in hospital discharge abstracts and were attributable to medical injuries according to 18 PSIs.

Results.—Excess length of stay due to medical injuries ranged from 0 days for injury to a neonate to 10.89 days for postoperative sepsis. Excess charges ranged from $0 for obstetric trauma (without vaginal instrumentation) to $57,727 for postoperative sepsis. The rate of excess mortality ranged from 0% for obstetric trauma to 21.96% for postoperative sepsis ($P < .001$). After postoperative sepsis, the second most serious event was postoperative wound dehiscence (9.42 extra days in the hospital, $40,323 in excess charges, and 9.63% in attributable mortality). Infection resulting from medical care was linked with 9.58 extra days, $38,656 in excess charges, and 4.31% in attributable mortality.

Conclusion.—Medical injuries in hospitals pose a substantial risk to patients and are associated with significant costs to society.

▶ Excess length of stay for hospital patients is monitored on a daily basis not only by academic health centers but also community hospitals. The process of

163

patient care is more and more a team approach, and patient safety requires protocols that reduce the number of adverse events and injury. Strategies to reduce adverse patient events need to be developed. These studies (tip of the iceberg) indicate the increased costs that result, but also the very real effect on patient morbidity and mortality.

M. Wood, MD, FRCA

Severe Bradycardia During Spinal and Epidural Anesthesia Recorded by an Anesthesia Information Management System
Lesser JB, Sanborn KV, Valskys R, et al (Columbia Univ, New York; Northwestern Univ, Chicago)
Anesthesiology 99:859-866, 2003   10–2

Background.—Bradycardia and asystole may occur unexpectedly in healthy patients who are receiving neuraxial anesthesia. Among the risk factors for bradycardia and asystole in these patients are low baseline heart rate (BHR), first-degree heart block, American Society of Anesthesiologists (ASA) physical status 1, β-blockers, male sex, and high sensory level. Anesthesia information management systems automatically record a large number of physiologic variables, which are then combined with data from the anesthesiologist to produce the anesthesia record. Large databases such as these can be scanned for episodes of bradycardia. Whether younger age, male sex, β-blockers, ASA 1 or 2 physical status, or low preinduction BHR increase the risk for bradycardia during neuraxial anesthesia was investigated.

Methods.—A total of 57,240 automated anesthesia records were scanned to identify spinal and epidural anesthetics that did not also involve general anesthesia. The search excluded obstetric patients and patients younger than 12 years. The selected records where then scanned for episodes of moderate (heart rate, < 50 but ≥ 40 beats/min) or severe (<40 beats/min) bradycardia.

Results.—A total of 6663 cases (11.6%) were identified. Of the 677 cases with bradycardia (10.2%), 46 cases (0.7%) were severe. Final multivariate logistic regression analysis showed that a BHR of less than 60 beats/min and male sex were significant risk factors for the risk of severe bradycardia (Table 2). Multivariate logistic regression analysis of the 631 episodes of moderate bradycardia found that a BHR of less than 60 beats/min, age younger than 37 years, male sex, and case duration were significant risk factors (Fig 1). The time of occurrence of bradycardia was widely distributed across the entire duration of a case.

Conclusions.—It seems that a risk of bradycardia and asystole may occur at any time during neuraxial anesthesia in otherwise healthy patients, regardless of the type of anesthesia used. The risk of bradycardia is increased in patients with a low BHR.

TABLE 2.—Risk of Severe Bradycardia (<40 beats/min) in Patients Undergoing Neuraxial Anesthesia: Steps in Multivariate Analysis

	Patient Characteristics		Patient Characteristics + Medical History		Patient Characteristics + Medical History + Chronic Medications		Patient Characteristics + Medical History + Chronic Medications + Case Duration	
	OR (Risk)	95% CI	OR (Risk)	95% CI	OR (Risk)	95% CI	OR (Risk)	95% CI
Baseline heart rate < 60 bpm	14.2	7.0-28.9	14.2	7.0-29.0	14.0	6.8-28.8	14.1	6.9-28.0
Age < 37 yr	NS		NS		NS		NS	
Male gender	2.0*	1.0-4.0	2.0*	1.0-4.0	2.0	1.0-4.1	2.1	1.0-4.3
Nonemergency	NS		NS		NS		NS	
ASA physical status 1-2	NS		NS		NS		NS	
Body mass index < 30	NS		NS		NS		NS	
Hypertension			NS		NS		NS	
Absence of diabetes			NS		NS		NS	
β-blockers					NS		NS	
α$_1$-blockers					NS		NS	
Case duration (min)							NS	

Note: Values are expressed as odds ratios (OR) with $P < .05$ with their 95% CIs.
*$P < .06$.
Abbreviations: ASA, American Society of Anesthesiologists; *NS*, not significant, $P > .05$.
(Courtesy of Lesser JB, Sanborn KV, Valskys R, et al: Severe bradycardia during spinal and epidural anesthesia recorded by an anesthesia information management system. *Anesthesiology* 99:859-866, 2003. Copyright American Society of Anesthesiologists, Inc. Used with permission of Lippincott-Raven Publishers.)

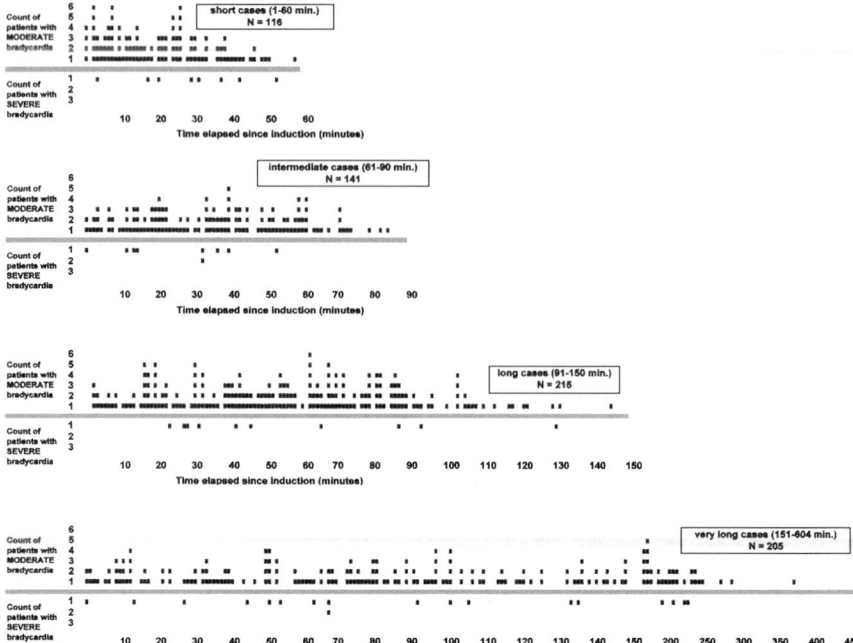

FIGURE 1.—Relationship between case duration and timing of episode of bradycardia. Each point corresponds to an episode of bradycardia. The points are plotted at the time elapsed since induction of neuraxial anesthesia when the episode of bradycardia occurred. The purpose of separating short, intermediate, long, and very long cases is to illustrate that episodes of bradycardia occur throughout the period of the anesthetic, regardless of case duration. (Courtesy of Lesser JB, Sanborn KV, Valskys R, et al: Severe bradycardia during spinal and epidural anesthesia recorded by an anesthesia information management system. *Anesthesiology* 99:859-866, 2003. Copyright American Society of Anesthesiologists, Inc. Used with permission of Lippincott-Raven Publishers.)

▶ This large retrospective study confirms the previously reported incidence of bradycardia after neuraxial blockade of approximately 10%. They found a statistically different but clinically similar incidence in epidural (9.1%) and spinal (10.6%) anesthetics. They also found different risk factors for severe bradycardia (<40 beats/min) and moderate bradycardia. Interestingly, a low BHR and male gender were the only risk factors for severe bradycardia; however, the use of β-blockers, young age, elective surgery, and the absence of diabetes were also risk factors for moderate bradycardia. In both groups, a low BHR was, by far, the most important predictor for development of bradycardia. There are 2 important clinical points evident from this study: patients with baseline bradycardia are at risk of developing moderate to severe bradycardia and it can occur at any point in the anesthetic—not just in the first half hour or so after performance of the block, when our vigilance tends to be greater.

S. Black, MD

Recovery Room Incidents: A Review of 419 Reports From the Anaesthetic Incident Monitoring Study (AIMS)
Kluger MT, Bullock MFM (North Shore Hosp, Auckland, New Zealand; Australian Patient Safety Foundation, Adelaide, Australia)
Anaesthesia 57:1060-1066, 2002   10–3

Background.—The recovery area is no longer a place for passive observation but serves as an important determinant of the rapidity of recovery and patient discharge. The problems that occur in the recovery area, their appearance, and how to deal with them most effectively were reviewed. In addition, factors that can be improved were identified.

Methods.—The Anaesthetic Incident Monitoring Study (AIMS) database supplied the information on 419 incidents occurring in the recovery room.

Results.—Ninety-two percent of the incidents reported involved persons older than 14 years, with 24 (6%) involving children younger than 14 years and 7 (2%) infants younger than 1 year. Ninety percent took place during daytime hours, with 4% at night and 6% having no time recorded. Most patients had undergone general surgical or orthopedic procedures and had mild or moderate coexisting disease. Cardiovascular, respiratory, airway-related, or drug error problems were involved in the majority of cases. Pulmonary edema developed in response to airway obstruction in 3% of cases, fluid overload in 2%, ischemic heart disease in 1%, drugs in 1%, sepsis in 0.2%, and no discernible cause in 0.2%. Drugs, anesthetic techniques, allergy, bleeding, sepsis, and myocardial ischemia produced hypotension. Twenty patients had cardiac arrest, 7 of whom were orthopedic patients and 17 of whom had ASA grades between 1 and 3. Respiratory failure resulted from inadequate reversal of neuromuscular blockade in 7% of cases. Two percent of patients were sick and debilitated, 2% had lung collapse or consolidation, 1% had opioid overdose, 1% had obesity-related factors, and 3% had inadequate reversal of neuromuscular blockade of unknown cause. Of the 9 patients who died, 2 had emergency surgery and 7 had elective surgery; 7 died of cardiovascular causes and 1 of respiratory complications. Factors that contributed to the incident ranged from error of judgment (18% of cases) to unfamiliar equipment (0.2% of cases). The top 5 factors after error of judgment were communication (14%), fault of the technique (7%), inadequate patient assessment (7%), a sick patient (3%), and inattention (3%). Factors found to minimize the seriousness of the incident included previous experience or training (23%), detection by a monitoring device (17%), skilled assistance (13%), supervision (4%), a healthy patient (3%), a relief anesthetist (2%), improved communication (0.2%), and quality assurance activity (0.2%).

Conclusions.—Improved care and avoidance of recovery room incidents rely on ensuring that the area can deal with a wide cross-section of procedures, that adequate staff numbers and competencies are represented, that an automated drug delivery system with feedback is used, and that the area is realistically viewed as a medium-term recovery unit. Ongoing education and quality assurance programs are needed to prepare recovery room personnel to handle the current and future demands of this area.

▶ There is a good reason for the existence of recovery rooms; 419 reports were reviewed and important incidents documented. It is from such an analysis that we can develop quality assurance and improvement programs to reduce such adverse events. It is of interest that many adverse events occurred in ASA I patients.

M. Wood, MD, FRCA

Residual Paralysis in the PACU After a Single Intubating Dose of Nondepolarizing Muscle Relaxant With an Intermediate Duration of Action
Debaene B, Plaud B, Dilly M-P, et al (Hôpital Jean Bernard, Poitiers, France; Fondation Adolphe de Rothschild, Paris; Hôpital Beaujon, Clichy, France)
Anesthesiology 98:1042-1048, 2003   10–4

Background.—Even short surgical procedures can produce residual neuromuscular blockade in the postanesthesia care unit (PACU). Residual neuromuscular blockade was initially defined as a train-of-four (TOF) ratio at the adductor pollicis less than 0.7 or 0.75 but recently has been revised to 0.9. The incidence of residual paralysis after receiving a single intubating dose of nondepolarizing muscle relaxant with an intermediate duration of action was determined and then correlated with the duration of surgery. The incidence was also compared between having residual paralysis defined by a TOF ratio less than 0.7 and having one less than 0.9.

Methods.—Of the 526 patients, 76% received rocuronium, 15% atracurium, and 9% vecuronium at initial doses of 0.58, 0.55, and 0.09 mg/kg, respectively. No other relaxant was administered, and neuromuscular blockade was not reversed at the procedure's end. Patients' TOF ratio was determined by acceleromyography at the adductor pollicis on arrival at the PACU. Other tests included head lift, tongue depressor test, and manual assessment of TOF and double-burst stimulation (DBS) fade. Computerized anesthetic records were used to calculate the time delay between the injection of the muscle relaxant and quantitative measurement of neuromuscular blockade.

Results.—Sixteen percent of patients had a TOF ratio less than 0.7 and 45% had one less than 0.9 when they arrived at the PACU. Partial paralysis was noted in 15.9% of patients receiving rocuronium, 16.9% of those receiving atracurium, and 17.0% of those receiving vecuronium at a ratio of 0.7. The incidences with a ratio of 0.9 were 45.0%, 41.6%, and 46.8%, respectively. When 238 patients were assessed over a 2-hour period after receiving the relaxant, residual blockade was found in 10% at a TOF ratio of 0.7 and 37% at a TOF of 0.9, which was a significant difference. With a TOF ratio of 0.7, the rate of residual paralysis began to diminish 90 minutes after receiving the relaxant. More than 120 minutes passed before the rate of residual paralysis declined with a TOF ratio of 0.9. The head lift test and tongue depressor test could not be assessed in 37% and 41% of patients, respectively, primarily because of residual effects of the anesthetic agents. Both TOF ratios and the DBS fade were easily performed in all cases. All tests had poor sensitivity, especially with the 0.9 TOF ratio cutoff point, and good specificity, especially the tactile TOF and DBS assessments.

Conclusions.—Residual paralysis was noted in the PACU more than 2 hours after patients received a dose of muscle relaxant. The sensitivity of all the tests performed to detect neuromuscular blockade was insufficient to recommend them for clinical use. The TOF ratio threshold allowing complete recovery is closer to 0.9 than to 0.7. Quantitative assessment of TOF ratio should be mandatory at the end of the surgical procedure to assess for the presence of residual paralysis, and it should be performed in the operating room to permit reversal of the block if needed before extubation. Because none of the quantitative measures of neuromuscular recovery was sufficient in itself, reversal agents may be safer even if more than 2 hours has passed since the muscle relaxant was administered.

▶ Residual paralysis remains a problem in the PACU, even after the use of an intermediate duration muscle relaxant. Manual tests such as head lift are a poor way to assess the degree of neuromuscular blockade, and routine use of the train-of-four ration is mandatory.

M. Wood, MD, FRCA

Medicolegal Claims in Vascular Surgery
Campbell WB, for the Research and Audit Committee of the Vascular Surgical Society of Great Britain and Ireland (Royal College of Surgeons of England, London; et al)
Ann R Coll Surg Engl 84:181-184, 2002   10–5

Background.—There has been a significant increase in recent years in the number of medicolegal claims in the United States as well as in the United Kingdom (UK). This has resulted in an increasing emphasis on counseling of patients, particularly in terms of risks of procedures, the provision of written information, and improved record keeping, all of which address the 3 most common themes in claims for negligence. This increasing medicolegal pressure has also resulted in the rise of defensive medicine, which is usually associated with medical practice in the United States.

The number of lawsuits in the United States continues to exceed the number in the UK. Good risk management is an essential component of the limiting of litigation, and this requires knowledge of the areas of highest risk. However, detailed information about claims for clinical negligence has been difficult to obtain. The first comprehensive collated data regarding vascular surgical practice in the UK was presented.

Methods.—Data were obtained from the UK's National Health Service Litigation Authority from its inception to 1995 and from the Medical Defence Union from 1990 to 1999. Details of claims posted to these services were analyzed.

Results.—A total of 424 claims were identified, including 176 from surgeons who described themselves as "vascular" and 248 from "general surgeons." The most common condition was varicose veins (244 claims); nerve damage was the most frequent complaint (79 claims) followed by incorrect or unsatisfactory surgery (35 claims) and damage to the femoral vein (16 claims) or arteries (13 claims). Arterial claims against vascular surgeons comprised 88% of claims in the National Health Service but only 39% in private practice, including 45 claims related to aortic grafting, 28 to other bypass grafts, and 36 related to alleged failure to recognize or treat ischemia.

Conclusion.—It is evident from these findings that the most probable cause of many of the medicolegal claims against vascular surgical practices involved failure to advise patients about potential risks and expected benefits. Future claims may be limited by recognition of the areas of highest risk, with improvements in communication and record keeping.

▶ I wonder what the total number of claims against vascular surgeons in the United States is compared to this number. Obviously, I think the incidences of suing in the United States are greater than in Great Britain. Clearly, in 5 or 10 years of claims, 424 claims for vascular surgery seems relatively low. I do not know the denominator of vascular operations in Great Britain, nor how often poor results result in suits. Nevertheless, the authors come to the conclusion that these adverse suits are directed because many of the surgeons did not advise the patients about the possibility of adverse outcomes. I guess what it comes down to is what patients want is information, appropriate expectations, and respect. Good results cannot hurt either.

M. F. Roizen, MD

Complications of Tracheobronchial Airway Stents
Zakaluzny SA, Lane JD, Mair EA (Walter Reed Army Med Ctr, Washington, DC)
Otolaryngol Head Neck Surg 128:478-488, 2003   10–6

Background.—Used in the management of difficult tracheobronchial obstruction, elegantly simple, and easy to apply, airway stents carry the potential for significant complications. The most common stent complications, how to avoid them, and how to manage the complications should they occur were outlined.

Methods.—Twenty-eight airway stents were placed for benign tracheobronchial diseases in 15 patients and for malignant diseases in 13 patients. Signs of complications were sought in each case.

Results.—Nine complications occurred, with 8 of them involving underlying benign airway pathology. Included were stent migration, breakage, excessive granulation, poor patient tolerance because of ongoing dysphagia and chest pain, and a technical inability to seat the stent optimally. The 1 complication linked to a malignant disease was migration into a tumor-laden right main bronchus. Endoscopic removal was undertaken in 7 cases, with 2 undergoing endoscopic stent manipulation. Metal stents became epithelialized in the airway within a month of placement, making removal endoscopically difficult. Plastic stents had more instances of migration but were easier to remove. One patient died as a result of ventilation failure linked to granulation occluding the lumen after laser treatment and pulmonary artery hemorrhage.

Conclusion.—Among the patients evaluated, stent complications occurred more frequently in the long-term treatment of benign conditions than with malignant disorders. The most common complications were migration, granulation, diminished mucociliary clearance, and patient intolerance. Endoscopic removal of the stent was successful, although metal stents proved to be more challenging than plastic stents because the former become epithelialized within 1 month of placement. Overall, tracheobronchial stents provided minimally invasive therapy for significant airway obstruction and led to improvement in many patients.

▶ These types of cases are increasing at a dramatic frequency. They require an intimate relationship to exist between anesthesiolgist, surgeon, and intensivist. This series demonstrated a 33% complication rate requiring some form of stent manipulation. One case resulted in a postoperative airway emergency but, unfortunately, that patient died. Within each institution, knowledge about the types of devices being used and the potential problems with insertion and deployment should be discussed. Other issues that merit discussion are interventions to prevent, or at least minimize, bleeding, edema formation, and excessive granulation tissue formation. In addition, house staff in particular should be aware that most problems that arise are going to be in the mid to distal trachea, so communication with otolaryngology and/or thoracic surgery is of paramount importance to appropriately address the problem.

J. D. Lang, Jr, MD

Small Risk of Serious Neurologic Complications Related to Lumbar Epidural Catheter Placement in Anesthetized Patients
Horlocker TT, Abel MD, Messick JM, et al (Mayo Clinic, Rochester, Minn)
Anesth Analg 96:1547-1552, 2003   10–7

Background.—When regional blockade is performed in an anesthetized or heavily sedated patient, nerve injury caused by needle or catheter placement or local anesthetic injection may go unrecognized because the patient cannot respond to painful stimuli. The incidence of this type of injury has not been established for adult patients. The frequency of neurologic complications after lumbar epidural catheter placement was assessed in anesthetized adult patients.

Methods.—A total of 4298 patients were undergoing lumber epidural catheter placement under general anesthesia for thoracic surgery. Catheter placement was performed immediately after induction and tracheal intubation or after completing the surgical procedure and before emergence. More than 98% of the catheters were used solely for postoperative analgesia; 1.8% were used for intraoperative anesthesia. Most patients received an opioid only, with 1.3% receiving a local anesthetic or combination local anesthetic and opioid epidurally.

Results.—A total of 1207 (28.1%) reported side effects. These included sedation (10.6%), nausea or emesis (7.6%), pruritus (2.7%), and respiratory depression (7.2%). Reintubation to address respiratory failure was performed in 34 patients; only 1 case of respiratory failure was attributed to the sedation or respiratory depression produced by the epidural agent. No neurologic complications or long-term sequelae developed in any of the patients. Six patients had new neurologic symptoms or worsening of previous neurologic symptoms after surgery, but epidural catheterization was not found to have caused these deficits.

Conclusions.—Neurologic complications were shown to occur rarely after epidural catheter placement in anesthetized patients. However, these findings should not be expanded to apply with either thoracic epidural block or the administration of epidural local anesthetic solution because these were not evaluated. Performing regional blockade in a heavily sedated or anesthetized patient must still be approached with caution.

▶ Many anesthesiologists are loathe to place an epidural catheter in an anesthetized patient and prefer an awake patient who can give guidance to the operator. This study evaluating data from a large number of patients at the Mayo Clinic concludes that the risk is small.

M. Wood, MD, FRCA

Epidural Hematoma Associated With Dextran Infusion
Muir JJ, Church EJ, Weinmeister KP (Mayo Clinic, Scottsdale, Ariz)
South Med J 96:811-814, 2003   10–8

Background.—Epidural hematoma is a rare complication of epidural anesthesia. Patients who are scheduled for anticoagulation therapy are usually not considered as candidates for epidural anesthesia. However, it has generally been considered safe to administer low-dose subcutaneous or IV standard (unfractionated) heparin if the needle puncture is performed 1 hour before heparin administration and the epidural catheter is removed when bleeding study results are normal. Dextran was commonly used for volume resuscitation, but it is no longer used because of adverse reactions associated with large-volume infusion of the drug. However, some vascular surgeons make use of the antithrombotic character of dextran to promote graft patency by low-dose infusions after peripheral vascularization. Presented is the first description of epidural hematoma in association with dextran infusion.

Case Report.—A 79-year-old woman with known peripheral vascular disease and a long-standing history of right lower extremity claudication presented for right femoral-popliteal bypass grafting. The patient had a history of coronary artery disease, hypertension, and asymptomatic chronic lymphocytic leukemia. The patient also had an unspecified hyperlipidemia. The patient was legally blind after an occipital cerebrovascular accident 2 years earlier. Her past surgical history included right cataract extraction and placement of a left vertebral artery stent. The patient denied a history of anesthetic complications. She had a 35-pack/year smoking history but had quit smoking 1 year preoperatively. Medications included atorvastatin and 325 mg aspirin daily. The patient reported using alcohol only occasionally. The results of a preoperative anesthetic examination were satisfactory, and a combined general-regional anesthestic technique was chosen. A lumbar epidural catheter was included for intraoperative anesthesia and analgesia. General anesthesia was accomplished with a laryngeal mask airway. After induction of epidural and general anesthesia, IV heparin 4000 U was administered. After surgery, infusion of 50 µg/hr of fentanyl was initiated and the patient was transferred to the immediate care ward, where a dextran 40 infusion of 30 mL/hr was started for maintenance of graft patency. Standard procedure at this institution was to continue dextran infusion for 24 hours. Overnight the patient complained of mid- to low back pain. The epidural infusion was increased and the patient repositioned, but pain persisted. MRI showed an epidural hematoma extending from T8 to T12, with displacement and mild compression of the lower thoracic spinal cord. Emergency decompressive laminectomy and evacuation of the epidural hematoma were performed, and the patient made a complete recovery.

Conclusions.—A case of epidural hematoma in association with a dextran infusion and epidural anesthesia and analgesia is presented. It is recommended that patients who receive epidural anesthesia and analgesia and dextran infusions be carefully monitored for potential complications.

► This review from Muir et al is typical of the excellent reports that Muir has shared with us in the past. I feel a loss because Jesse has largely left academic medicine; his articles were so good. The discussion in this paper is worthy of all this reading.

M. F. Roizen, MD

Postoperative Sudden Sensorineural Hearing Loss After Posterior Lumbar Decompression: A Case Report

Mak PHK, Tumber PS (Univ of Toronto)
Can J Anesth 50:519-521, 2003   10–9

Background.—Postoperative hearing loss is a rare occurrence after general anesthesia (5-20:100,000). It has been reported in patients after cardiopulmonary bypass. In patients undergoing subarachnoid anesthesia or intradural surgery, loss of CSF and the resulting drop in intracranial pressure can lead to hearing loss and cranial nerve palsy. In this report, a patient sustained a dural tear during spinal surgery under general anesthesia, complicated by a severe and persistent unilateral sensorineural hearing loss.

> *Case Report.*—A 51-year-old man underwent a posterior lumbar decompression procedure in the prone position under general anesthesia. The patient had no history of preoperative otologic disease or symptoms of auditory dysfunction. The patient also had no history of taking medications that can make an individual susceptible to hearing impairment, such as aminoglycosides or diuretics. A small dural tear was discovered intraoperatively and was repaired with sutures. The surgery lasted for 8 hours, and the patient lost more than 3 L of blood. Recovery from anesthesia was otherwise uneventful. A unilateral right-sided sensorineural hearing loss was discovered soon after surgery. The hearing loss was associated with mild tinnitus but no vertigo. The patient experienced no aural fullness, pain, headache, or postural difficulties. The symptoms failed to improve 18 months after surgery despite extensive investigation, treatment, and follow-up by an otorhinolaryngologist.

Conclusions.—The amount of blood loss and resulting fluid replacement has been correlated with low frequency hearing loss. Severe changes in blood volume, intracranial pressure, and osmolarity are thought to be triggering factors. A persistent CSF leak is also a possibility in this case, but no evidence exists to support this hypothesis. Preventive approaches to postoperative sudden sensorineural hearing loss (SSNHL) may include avoidance of nitrous oxide and the Valsalva maneuver in patients with a history of auditory dysfunction, dysequilibrium, or vertigo. The management of postoperative SSNHL is inconclusive. However, a recent study reported a higher incidence of success with the use of a cervicothoracic epidural compared with a stellate ganglion block. The mechanism of improvement in SSNHL with cervicothoracic epidural may be a higher blood flow to the cochlear region. Better understanding of postoperative SSNHL is needed to improve the safety profile.

▶ This case report presents a troubling complication after prone spine surgery. It reminds us that unanticipated complications continue to occur. Complications such as this one, which is rare but devastating, are particularly worrisome because the etiology and risk factors are unknown. The clinical scenario resembles some of the early case reports of posterior ischemic optic neuropathy: prone spine surgery of long duration with large intraoperative blood loss.

S. Black, MD

Operating on Patients Wearing Personal Identity Devices: A Report of Two Cases
Hart WJ, White SH (Royal Shrewsbury Hosp, England)
Ann R Coll Surg Engl 85:279-280, 2003   10–10

Background.—It is increasingly common for those convicted of minor crimes to be monitored through electronic personal identity devices. Two patients who presented to the Royal Shrewsbury Hospital while wearing these devices and the dilemmas they posed are described.

Case Reports.—Man, 25, admitted with contaminated lacerations that required surgical debridement and suturing. The device management company was called to determine whether it was safe to leave the device in place during surgery. Because no information was available, it was recommended that the device be removed and a replacement scheduled postoperatively. In a second case, a man, 32, was admitted unconscious after motor vehicle accident. He could not give informed consent to contact the device management company. After contacting the company, it was also decided to remove the device before treatment.

Discussion.—Personal identity devices such as these present a confidentiality dilemma for the physician, particularly in cases where the patient is not able to give informed consent for contact with the management company. There is no legal obligation for the physician to disclose the patient's private information to the management company. It is recommended that the device be removed before surgery.

▶ These devices were for people under electronic surveillance because of a prior crime record. Other personal identity devices can involve those worn for multiple other purposes, including medical risks. This is an interesting brief article that you are advised to read if you have an interest in this field.

M. F. Roizen, MD

11 Obstetric Anesthesia

Analgesia for Labor

Regional Anesthesia and Analgesia for Labor and Delivery
Eltzschig HK, Lieberman ES, Camann WR (Harvard Med School, Boston)
N Engl J Med 348:319-332, 2003   11–1

Background.—The maternal and fetal effects of analgesia during labor have been subjects of discussion and controversy for more than 150 years—since a Scottish obstetrician, James Simpson, first administered analgesia to a woman during labor. Numerous randomized trials have addressed the effects of different analgesic strategies on maternal and fetal outcomes. However, it has become increasingly clear that potentially unwanted effects of analgesia for women in labor and their children cannot be easily determined. Among the remaining controversial topics are the effects of regional anesthesia on the progress and outcome of labor and its effects on the neonate. Advances in the administration of epidural, spinal, or combined spinal–epidural analgesia during labor are discussed.

Overview.—Approximately 60% of women annually choose epidural or combined spinal–epidural analgesia for pain relief during labor. The use of epidural analgesia is associated with better pain relief than are systemic opioids. Many observational studies of epidural analgesia have compared women who selected epidural analgesia with those who did not, and these studies have shown an association between the use of epidural analgesia and a higher rate of cesarean delivery. However, women who select epidural analgesia are different from those who do not in that they are more frequently nulliparous, come to the hospital earlier in the course of labor, have slower cervical dilation, deliver larger babies, and have smaller pelvic outlets. Studies that control for these factors have found differences in outcomes between women who receive epidural analgesia and those who do not. Prospective, randomized trials studying the association between epidural analgesia and cesarean delivery have shown variable results. In terms of other reported complications of regional analgesia, current data do not support an association between a new onset of back pain and the use of epidural analgesia during labor. Inadvertent puncturing of the subarachnoid space during placement of an epidural catheter occurs in about 3% of women in labor, and a severe headache occurs in up to 70% of women with such a puncture. Data on other complications, including effects on the neonate, are inadequate and do not allow definitive conclusions to be drawn.

Conclusions.—According to a joint statement in 2002 from the American College of Obstetricians and Gynecologists and the American Society of Anesthesiologists, a woman's request for pain relief is sufficient medical indication for its use. The opinion presented in this article is that epidural analgesia is a safe, widely used, effective method of pain relief during labor and cesarean delivery. However, many questions remain to be answered, and the side effects of pharmacologic pain relief during labor are subjects of ongoing concern.

▶ This is a landmark review article. Two of the authors have been on opposite sides of the debate regarding the assessment of risks and benefits after the administration of regional analgesia in laboring women. This review represents a remarkable collaboration. I recommend that every anesthesiologist who provides obstetric anesthesia services read this article in its entirety.

D. H. Chestnut, MD

Comparison of Povidone Iodine and DuraPrep, an Iodophor-in-Isopropyl Alcohol Solution, for Skin Disinfection Prior to Epidural Catheter Insertion in Parturients

Birnbach DJ, Meadows W, Stein DJ, et al (Univ of Miami, Fla; Beth Israel Med Ctr, New York; Columbia Univ, New York)
Anesthesiology 98:164-169, 2003   11–2

Background.—Neuraxial techniques have become increasingly popular for analgesia and anesthesia during labor. Infectious sequelae of epidural analgesia are rare but can occur. These complications can be devastating and may result in paralysis or death. Bacteria can be introduced into the puncture

TABLE 1.—Positive Skin and Distal Catheter Tip Cultures Obtained From Parturients Who Requested Epidural Analgesia for Labor and Whose Backs Were Disinfected With DuraPrep or Povidone Iodine

Positive Cultures	DuraPrep n (%)	Povidone Iodine n (%)	P*
Skin			
Before disinfection	27 (90)	27 (90)	NS
After disinfection	1 (3)	9 (30)	0.01
At catheter removal	15 (50)	29 (97)	0.0001
Catheter tip			
All positives	2 (7)	13 (43)	0.002
Roll plate technique	0	6 (20)	0.02

Note: Data are expressed as the number of parturients (percent values are in parentheses).
*Fisher exact test.
Abbreviation: NS, Not significant.
(Courtesy of Birnbach DJ, Meadows W, Stein DJ, et al: Comparison of povidone iodine and DuraPrep, an iodophor-in-isopropyl alcohol solution, for skin disinfection prior to epidural catheter insertion in parturients. *Anesthesiology* 98:164-169, 2003. Copyright American Society of Anesthesiologists, Inc. Used with permission of Lippincott-Raven Publishers.)

TABLE 2.—Comparison of Bacterial Yield From Skin Cultures Obtained From Parturients Before and After Disinfection With DuraPrep or Povidone Iodine and at Catheter Removal

| | Log CFU* | | |
	DuraPrep	Povidone Iodine	*P*
Before disinfection	3.23 ± 0.36	2.85 ± 0.36	NS
After disinfection	0.35 ± 0.14	0.74 ± 0.22	NS
At catheter removal	0.90 ± 0.23	1.93 ± 0.40	0.03

*Values shown are mean ± SEM.
Abbreviations: CFU, Colony forming unit; *NS*, not significant.
(Courtesy of Birnbach DJ, Meadows W, Stein DJ, et al: Comparison of povidone iodine and DuraPrep, an iodophor-in-isopropyl alcohol solution, for skin disinfection prior to epidural catheter insertion in parturients. *Anesthesiology* 98:164-169, 2003. Copyright American Society of Anesthesiologists, Inc. Used with permission of Lippincott-Raven Publishers.)

site from the bloodstream, in association with contaminants, by spread to the epidural catheter from other sites, such as the vaginal tract, or during breaches in sterile technique by the anesthesiologist. DuraPrep is a recently marketed solution that contains an iodophor in isopropyl alcohol. This solution may provide longer lasting and enhanced antimicrobial activity; thus, it may be of value in the obstetric setting. The antisepsis provided by DuraPrep was evaluated in comparison with that provided by povidone iodine (PI).

Methods.—The study group included 60 women in active labor who requested epidural analgesia. The women were randomly assigned to receive skin preparation with either PI or the DuraPrep solution. Three cultures were obtained from each patient: the first just before skin disinfection, the second immediately after antisepsis, and the third just before removal of the catheter. A culture from the distal tip of the catheter was also obtained.

Results.—The 2 groups were similar in their clinical characteristics and the risk factors for infection. Significantly more patients had positive skin cultures immediately after skin disinfection in the PI group (30%) compared with the DuraPrep group (3%) (Table 1). In addition, the number of patients with any positive skin cultures at the time of catheter removal was greater in the PI group than in the DuraPrep group (97% vs 50%, respectively), as was the number of organisms cultured from skin (Table 2). Six catheters, all from the PI group, yielded positive cultures by the roll-plate technique.

Conclusions.—In this comparison with PI, the DuraPrep solution provided a greater decrease in the number of positive skin cultures immediately after disinfection. DuraPrep was also superior to PI in retarding bacterial regrowth and colonization of the epidural catheters.

▶ Bacterial meningitis and epidural abscess are rare complications of regional anesthesia in obstetric patients. However, these complications do occur and can be devastating. This study suggests that the addition of alcohol to an iodinated disinfectant offers advantages over the use of PI solution alone in performing skin disinfection before placement of an epidural catheter. The authors suggested that "antisepsis that eliminates bacteria at the time of insertion and that minimizes bacterial regrowth may be particularly important for indwelling labor epidural catheters that remain in situ for extended periods of time or in immunocompromised patients."

D. H. Chestnut, MD

Injecting Saline Through the Epidural Needle Decreases the IV Epidural Catheter Placement Rate During Combined Spinal-Epidural Labour Analgesia
Gadalla F, Lee S-HR, Choi KC, et al (Cornell Univ, New York; Women and Infants' Hosp, Providence, RI)
Can J Anesth 50:382-385, 2003   11–3

Background.—The problem of IV epidural catheter placement during needle-through-needle combined spinal–epidural (CSE) anesthesia during labor has not received sufficient attention in the literature. Injection of a sufficiently large volume of epidural fluid before catheter threading decreases the incidence of accidental venous catheter placement during epidural anesthesia. The rate of accidental IV epidural catheter placement is significantly decreased after injection of 10 mL of 0.5% bupivacaine (9% vs 3%) or saline (16% vs 0%) through the epidural needle but not after injection of 3 mL saline. Whether injection of 10 mL of saline before epidural catheter threading (ie, precannulation epidural fluid injection) can decrease the incidence of IV epidural catheter placement during CSE labor analgesia was determined.

Methods.—A total of 100 healthy women who requested CSE labor analgesia with either 20 µg fentanyl or 10 µg sufentanil were randomly assigned to receive either no epidural injection (dry group) or 10-mL epidural saline injection (saline group) before epidural catheter placement. A nylon multiport catheter was then threaded 3 to 5 cm into the epidural space, and the needle was removed. IV catheter placement was diagnosed if blood was freely aspirated, if the mother became tachycardic after injection of 15 µg epinephrine, or if intracardiac air was heard on US after injection of 1.5 mL air.

Results.—IV epidural catheter placement occurred in 1 of 50 patients in the saline group and in 10 of 50 patients in the dry group. No complications resulted from excessive cephalad intrathecal opioid spreading.

Conclusions.—The injection of 10 mL of saline through the epidural needle after intrathecal opioid injection and before threading the catheter significantly decreased the incidence of accidental venous catheter placement. No increase in complications seemed to occur from excessive cephalad intrathecal opioid spreading.

▶ For many years, I have injected approximately 10 mL of saline through the epidural needle into the epidural space before placement of an epidural catheter in obstetric patients. Other studies have suggested that this practice reduces the incidence of unintentional IV cannulation of the epidural catheter. To my knowledge, this is the first study that has demonstrated the efficacy of epidural injection of saline before insertion of the epidural catheter during administration of CSE analgesia. The authors observed no evidence of excessive cephalad spreading of the intrathecal opioid. However, given the small sample size and the low baseline incidence of this complication, the authors acknowledged that their study does not establish the safety of this technique. It would seem intuitive that epidural administration of 10 mL of saline (immediately after intrathecal opioid injection) might result in higher cephalad spreading of the intrathecal opioid. For that reason, additional studies of safety are needed.

D. H. Chestnut, MD

A Multicenter, Randomized, Controlled Trial Comparing Bupivacaine With Ropivacaine for Labor Analgesia

Halpern SH, Breen TW, Campbell DC, et al (Univ of Toronto; Duke Univ, Durham, NC; Univ of Saskatchewan, Saskatoon, Canada; et al)
Anesthesiology 98:1431-1435, 2003   11–4

Background.—Ropivacaine is a newer local anesthetic that was developed to reduce cardiovascular and CNS toxic effects. Ropivacaine may offer other advantages when compared with bupivacaine, such as reduced lower extremity motor block in women in labor and better neonatal outcomes. A meta-analysis of studies comparing high doses of bupivacaine with ropivacaine for labor pain found a higher incidence of forceps deliveries and motor block and poorer neonatal outcomes with bupivacaine. Whether these outcomes differ between patients receiving a low concentration of patient-controlled epidural bupivacaine combined with fentanyl and patients receiving a combination of ropivacaine and fentanyl was determined.

Methods.—This multicenter, randomized, controlled trial included term nulliparous women undergoing induction of labor. Patients were randomly assigned to receive either 15 mL bupivacaine 0.1% (276 patients) or 15 mL ropivacaine 0.1% (279 patients), each with 5 µg/mL fentanyl. The main outcome measure was the incidence of operative delivery. Obstetric, neonatal, and analgesic outcomes were also evaluated.

TABLE 2.—Obstetric Outcomes

Outcome	Bupivacaine No. (%) of Patients	Ropivacaine No. (%) of Patients	*P*
			0.175
Spontaneous vaginal delivery	128 (46)	144 (51)	
Instrumental vaginal delivery	80 (29)	84 (30)	
Cesarean delivery	68 (25)	51 (18)	
Total	276	279	
Operative delivery (instrumental plus cesarean delivery)	148 (54)	135 (48)	0.25
Episiotomy/total no. (%)	70/202 (35)	74/220 (34)	0.84

(Courtesy of Halpern SH, Breen TW, Campbell DC, et al: A multicenter, randomized, controlled trial comparing bupivacaine with ropivacaine for labor analgesia. *Anesthesiology* 98:1431-1435, 2003. Copyright American Society of Anesthesiologists, Inc. Used with permission of Lippincott-Raven Publishers.)

Results.—No significant difference was found between the 2 groups in the incidence of operative delivery (148 of 276 bupivacaine recipients vs 135 of 279 ropivacaine recipients). However, the incidence of motor block was significantly increased in the bupivacaine group compared with the ropivacaine group at 6 hours and at 10 hours after injection (Table 2). Satisfaction with mobility was higher with ropivacaine than with bupivacaine; however, satisfaction with analgesia at delivery was higher with bupivacaine than with ropivacaine.

Conclusions.—This study found no difference in the incidence of operative delivery or neonatal outcomes among nulliparous patients who received low concentrations of bupivacaine or ropivacaine for labor analgesia.

Epidural Ropivacaine Versus Bupivacaine for Labor: A Meta-Analysis
Halpern SH, Walsh V (Univ of Toronto)
Anesth Analg 96:1473-1479, 2003   11–5

Background.—Epidural bupivacaine has been used for many years for analgesia during labor. Bupivacaine provides excellent sensory analgesia, but some patients have experienced unacceptable motor block when large concentrations (0.25% or greater) were used. Accidental IV injection of large doses of bupivacaine have been associated with cardiac and CNS toxic effects. Ropivacaine was developed to reduce these side effects and was released for clinical use in 1996. Numerous studies have been performed since that time to determine whether ropivacaine is suitable for labor analgesia and to determine whether it is superior to bupivacaine. A meta-analysis of 6 selected clinical trials comparing epidural ropivacaine with bupivacaine found that an increased incidence of spontaneous vaginal delivery was associated with ropivacaine, primarily resulting from a reduction in the rate of forceps delivery. This meta-analysis also reported a less frequent incidence of maternal motor block and better neuroadaptive capacity scores in the neonate. In the present meta-analysis, all previous studies of these 2 drugs were reviewed in an effort to determine whether the incidence of motor block differs.

Methods.—This meta-analysis systematically reviewed and combined the results of randomized controlled trials comparing ropivacaine with bupivacaine to determine whether outcomes for the 2 drugs differ. Electronic databases and journals were searched for randomized controlled trials comprising women in labor. The primary outcome measure was the incidence of spontaneous vaginal delivery. Other obstetric, neonatal, and analgesic outcomes were also examined and combined when possible with the use of meta-analysis techniques and random effects modeling.

Results.—A total of 23 randomized trials were identified, composed of 1043 patients who received ropivacaine and 1031 who received bupivacaine. No significant difference was observed in the incidence of spontaneous vaginal delivery (Fig 1) or in any of the other outcomes. More studies

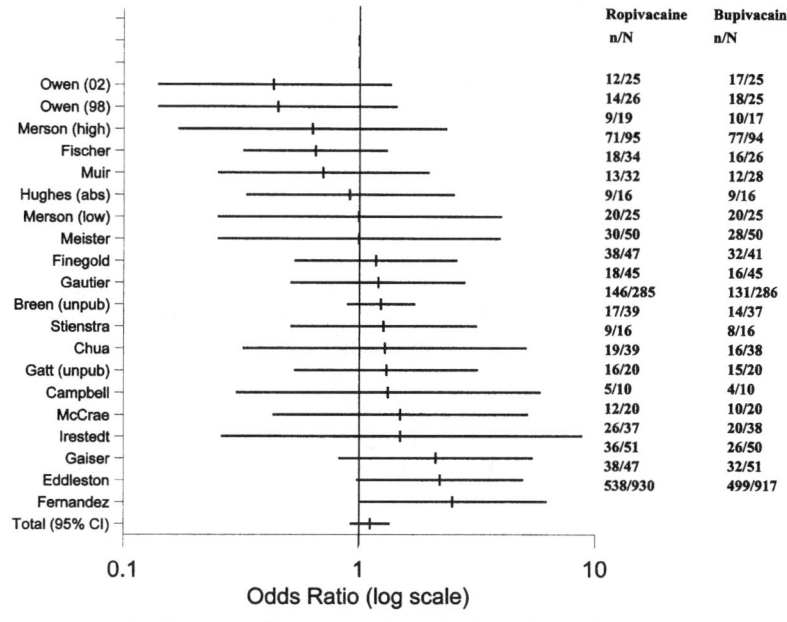

	Ropivacaine n/N	Bupivacaine n/N
Owen (02)	12/25	17/25
Owen (98)	14/26	18/25
Merson (high)	9/19	10/17
Fischer	71/95	77/94
Muir	18/34	16/26
Hughes (abs)	13/32	12/28
Merson (low)	9/16	9/16
Meister	20/25	20/25
Finegold	30/50	28/50
Gautier	38/47	32/41
Breen (unpub)	18/45	16/45
Stienstra	146/285	131/286
Chua	17/39	14/37
Gatt (unpub)	9/16	8/16
Campbell	19/39	16/38
McCrae	16/20	15/20
Irestedt	5/10	4/10
Gaiser	12/20	10/20
Eddleston	26/37	20/38
Fernandez	36/51	26/50
Total (95% CI)	38/47	32/51
	538/930	499/917

Odds Ratio (log scale)

FIGURE 1.—The odds ratios and 95% CIs are shown for the incidence of spontaneous vaginal delivery for each study. The number of patients in each study who had a vaginal delivery (n) and the total number of patients in the study (N) are shown in the table. The pooled odds ratio is also shown. Odds ratios less than 1.0 favor bupivacaine, and odds ratios more than 1.0 favor ropivacaine. (Courtesy of Halpern SH, Walsh V: Epidural ropivacaine versus bupivacaine for labor: A meta-analysis. *Anesth Analg* 96(5):1473-1479, 2003.)

reported a higher incidence of motor block with bupivacaine, but the results were heterogeneous and, therefore, were not combined.

Conclusions.—The findings of this meta-analysis indicate that no statistically significant difference occurs between bupivacaine and ropivacaine in the incidence of any obstetric or neonatal outcome. Additional studies with clinically appropriate concentrations are needed to determine whether these 2 drugs differ in the incidence of motor block.

▶ Both the multicenter, randomized controlled trial (see Abstract 11–4) and this meta-analysis (Abstract 11–5) suggest that there was no significant difference in obstetric outcome (eg, method of delivery) or neonatal outcome among parturients who received either epidural ropivacaine or bupivacaine for intrapartum analgesia. The randomized controlled trial suggests that administration of ropivacaine is associated with decreased motor block. However, earlier studies of motor block have reported conflicting results, so that additional studies are needed to resolve this issue.

D. H. Chestnut, MD

Relative Analgesic Potencies of Levobupivacaine and Ropivacaine for Epidural Analgesia in Labor

Polley LS, Columb MO, Naughton NN, et al (Univ of Michigan, Ann Arbor)
Anesthesiology 99:1354-1358, 2003   11–6

Background.—Although epidural bupivacaine is widely used for obstetric analgesia, it may be associated with cardiovascular toxicity. Two other agents, levobupivacaine and ropivacaine, which are structurally similar to bupivacaine, have been introduced. Minimum local analgesic concentration was used to directly compare their relative potencies in obstetric patients.

Study Design.—The study group consisted of 70 parturients in active labor who requested epidural anesthesia. They were randomly allocated to either levobupivacaine or ropivacaine by using an up-down sequential allocation technique. Efficacy was evaluated by a 100-mm visual analog pain scale at 10-minute intervals for the first 30 minutes after bolus injection. Sensory level, degree of motor blockade, and fetal hemodynamics were also evaluated.

Findings.—There were no significant demographic, obstetric, or hemodynamic characteristics between the 2 treatment groups. The minimum local analgesic concentration of levobupivacaine was 0.087% wt/vol and 0.089% wt/vol for ropivacaine. The ropivacaine/bupivacaine potency ratio was 0.98. There were no significant differences in motor effects between the 2 groups.

Conclusions.—This study found that levobupivacaine and ropivacaine were of similar potency for epidural analgesia during the first stage of labor.

A Randomized Sequential Allocation Study to Determine the Minimum Effective Analgesic Concentration of Levobupivacaine and Ropivacaine in Patients Receiving Epidural Analgesia for Labor

Benhamou D, Ghosh C, Mercier FJ (Hôpital Antoine Béclere, Clamart, France)
Anesthesiology 99:1383-1386, 2003   11–7

Background.—The advantages of bupivacaine over other local anesthetic agents is its sustained duration of action and its beneficial ratio of sensory to motor blockade. These characteristics have made bupivacaine a useful agent in obstetric epidural analgesia. Bupivacaine is available as a racemate or as a 50:50 mixture of levobupivacaine and dextrobupivacaine. Clinical studies have shown that levobupivacaine retains local anesthetic properties and potency similar to racemate bupivacaine, and that ropivacaine is less potent than racemic bupivacaine in terms of their minimum local anesthetic concentrations (MLACs). The MLACs of levobupivacaine and ropivacaine, when used in epidural obstetric analgesia, were compared.

Methods.—Healthy women who required epidural analgesia for labor pain were recruited for this double-blind study. The women were randomly assigned to receive either ropivacaine (47 patients) or levobupivacaine (47 patients) as a 20-mL epidural bolus. The concentration of both drugs was

0.11% at the initial administration and was increased or decreased at intervals of 0.01%, depending on the response of the previous patient, using up-down sequential allocation. MLACs were calculated by using the Dixon and Massey formula. Efficacy was assessed with visual analogue pain scores and motor and sensory block assessments. Safety was assessed by recording maternal and fetal/neonate vital signs and adverse events.

Results.—The MLACs for levobupivacaine (mean, 0.077%) were lower than those for ropivacaine (mean, 0.092%), but the difference was not statistically significant. There were no significant differences between the treatment groups in the proportion of patients reporting drug-related adverse events.

Conclusions.—The use of the MLAC method in women in labor demonstrated that levobupivacaine was 19.3% more potent than ropivacaine (a difference that was not statistically significant) and provided similar degrees of safety.

▶ Together, these 2 studies (Abstracts 11–6 and 11–7) suggest that there is little, if any, significant difference in the analgesic potency of levobupivacaine and ropivacaine when given to provide epidural analgesia in laboring women. These findings are puzzling, given that other studies have suggested that ropivacaine is less potent than racemic bupivacaine, and that levobupivacaine and racemic bupivacaine have similar potency. A single study of all 3 drugs would help provide clarification.

D. H. Chestnut, MD

The Relative Motor Blocking Potencies of Bupivacaine and Levobupivacaine in Labor
Lacassie HJ, Columb MO (Pontificia Universidad Católica de Chile, Santiago, Chile; South Manchester Univ, Wythenshawe, England)
Anesth Analg 97:1509-1513, 2003   11–8

Background.—Epidural administration of local anesthetic produces analgesia, anesthesia, and motor block during labor. The minimum motor block local analgesic concentration was compared for racemic bupivacaine and levobupivacaine during first-stage labor, and the relative potency ratio was determined.

Methods.—This study was double blind, randomized, and prospective and used an up-down sequential allocation technique. The study group consisted of 60 patients who requested epidural analgesia during first-stage induced labor. A baseline assessment of pain and muscle strength was made with a 100-mm visual analog pain score; 30 minutes after bolus injection, patients from each treatment group were re-evaluated.

Findings.—Demographic and obstetric data were similar for the 2 treatment groups. The minimum motor block local analgesic concentration for bupivacaine was 0.27% wt/vol and was 0.31% wt/vol for levobupivacaine, for a levobupivacaine/bupivacaine potency ratio of 0.87.

Conclusions.—This study demonstrated that levobupivacaine induces a less potent motor blockade than its racemate bupivacaine after epidural administration during early-stage labor.

▶ This study suggests that the S-enantiomer levobupivacaine has a motor-blocking potency that is approximately 13% less than that of the racemate when administered to provide epidural analgesia during labor. The clinical significance is unclear, given that most parturients have little motor block when receiving the dilute solutions of bupivacaine used in contemporary obstetric anesthesia practice.

D. H. Chestnut, MD

The Site of Action of Epidural Fentanyl Infusions in the Presence of Local Anesthetics: A Minimum Local Analgesic Concentration Infusion Study in Nulliparous Labor
Ginosar Y, Columb MO, Cohen SE, et al (Hadassah Hebrew Univ, Jerusalem, Israel; South Manchester Univ Hosps, Wythenshawe, England; Stanford Univ, Calif)
Anesth Analg 97:1439-1445, 2003   11–9

Background.—Although continuous epidural infusions of fentanyl induce analgesia by a systemic mechanism, it is not known whether this is true in the presence of local anesthetics. Whether epidural fentanyl induces analgesia by a predominantly spinal mechanism in the presence of local anesthetics was analyzed in a prospective, randomized, double-blind study.

Study Design.—The study group consisted of 48 adult, nulliparous women in active labor who requested epidural anesthesia. All women received an epidural infusion of bupivacaine at a concentration that was determined by the response of the previous woman in the same group. All were randomized to either an epidural infusion of bupivacaine with or without fentanyl and an IV infusion of either fentanyl or saline. The patients and all medical personnel were blinded regarding treatment group. By an up-down sequential analysis, the 3 possible outcomes were success (no supplemental analgesia required until 8 mm cervical dilation), failure (supplemental analgesia requested before 8 mm dilation), or reject (don't include in analysis). Analgesia was assessed during labor with a 100-mm visual analog pain score. Demographic and anesthetic/obstetric outcomes were compared between these 2 treatment groups.

Findings.—This study measured the minimum local analgesic concentration for maintenance of analgesia through the first stage of labor. There were 8 rejects out of 48 patients, who were not counted in the analysis. The infusion of epidural bupivacaine was 0.063% in the IV fentanyl group and 0.019% in the epidural fentanyl group (Fig 1). Continuous infusion of fentanyl was more than 3 times more potent when administered by the epidural rather than the IV route.

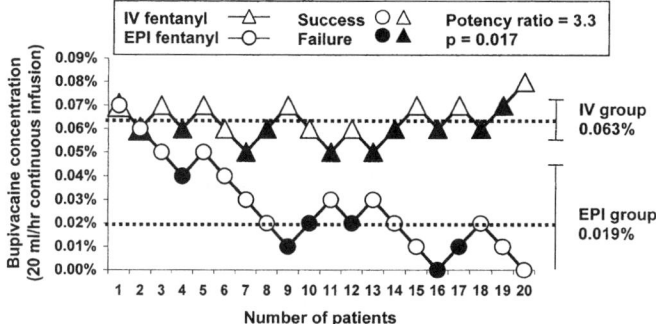

FIGURE 1.—Minimum local analgesic concentration for epidural bupivacaine with coadministration of either IV or epidural infusions of fentanyl. Minimum local analgesic concentration for a 20 mL/h continuous infusion of bupivacaine ($MLAC_{infusion}$) in 2 groups of patients, those receiving 30 μg/h fentanyl IV infusions (*triangles*, n = 20) and those receiving 30 μg/h fentanyl infusions (*circles*, n = 20). *Solid symbols* depict treatment failure and *open symbols* depict treatment success. Based on up-down sequential analysis, the $MLAC_{infusion}$ for bupivacaine in the IV group is 0.063 (95% confidence interval, 0.058-0.068) and 0.019 in the EPI group (95% confidence interval, 0.000-0.038). *Error bars* represent 95% confidence intervals. (Courtesy of Ginosar Y, Columb MO, Cohen SE, et al: The site of action of epidural fentanyl infusions in the presence of local anesthetics: A minimum local analgesic concentration infusion study in nulliparous labor. *Anesth Analg* 97:1439-1445, 2003.)

Conclusions.—These findings show that when coadministered with local anesthetics, a continuous infusion of epidural fentanyl is more potent than IV fentanyl, suggesting that epidural fentanyl induces analgesia predominantly by a spinal mechanism in these circumstances. This also suggests a synergy between epidural opioids and epidural local anesthetics. These data support the use of epidural fentanyl in labor when coadministered with local anesthetic to reduce dosage while providing comfort.

▶ The authors speculated that the coadministration of epidural bupivacaine with epidural fentanyl would enhance "the otherwise clinically insignificant spinal analgesic effect of the epidural fentanyl." Thus, the authors suggested the "occurrence of synergy" between epidural bupivacaine and epidural fentanyl. Coadministration of epidural fentanyl with an epidural local anesthetic results in administration of a smaller total dose of local anesthetic and less intense motor block.

D. H. Chestnut, MD

Minimum Analgesic Doses of Fentanyl and Sufentanil for Epidural Analgesia in the First Stage of Labor

Capogna G, Camorcia M, Columb MO (Città di Roma Hosp, Rome; South Manchester Univ, England)
Anesth Analg 96:1178-1182, 2003   11–10

Background.—Studies have reported that epidural opioids may provide pain relief during the first stage of labor. A previous study reported that an epidural bolus of 100 μg of fentanyl or 20 μg of sufentanil produced comparable labor analgesia after administration of a lidocaine and epinephrine test dose. However, the lidocaine test dose may contribute to the analgesic effects of epidural opioids. Both epidural fentanyl and sufentanil are used in combination with various concentrations of local anesthetic solutions for labor analgesia. However, there is little information regarding the analgesic potency, which is important for determination of the best possible analgesia at the smallest dosage with the fewest possible maternal and fetal side effects. The median effective dose of fentanyl and sufentanil and the relative potency ratio of these opioids when used as the only epidural analgesic in the first stage of labor were investigated.

Methods.—A series of 66 nulliparous women in spontaneous labor at term gestation who requested epidural analgesia were enrolled in this prospective, double-blind, randomized study. Each women received fentanyl or sufentanil diluted with 0.9% wt/vol saline to a volume of 10 mL. The initial dose was arbitrarily selected to be 125 μg for fentanyl and 25 μg for sufentanil, with subsequent doses determined by the response of the previous patient. The analgesia was considered efficacious if the visual analogue score decreased to less than 10 mm on a 100-mm scale within 30 minutes.

Results.—The minimum analgesic dose or median effective dose was 21.1 μg for sufentanil and 124.2 μg for fentanyl. The sufentanil/fentanyl potency ratio was 5.9.

Conclusion.—This study has established the equivalent doses and relative potencies of fentanyl and sufentanil for provision of epidural analgesia in the first stage of labor.

▶ The authors' observations apply to circumstances when either fentanyl or sufentanil is administered epidurally as the sole analgesic drug during the first stage of labor. Anesthesiologists in the United States rarely give an opioid alone when providing epidural analgesia in laboring women. Further, it is not clear that the potency ratios observed in this study apply to circumstances when an opioid is combined with a local anesthetic. Thus, the authors' observations are of greater interest academically than clinically.

D. H. Chestnut, MD

PCEA Compared to Continuous Epidural Infusion in an Ultra-Low-Dose Regimen for Labor Pain Relief: A Randomized Study
Eriksson SL, Gentele C, Olofsson CH (Gävle-Sandviken County Hosp, Sweden; Söder Hosp, Stockholm; Karolinska Hosp, Stockholm)
Acta Anaesthesiol Scand 47:1085-1090, 2003   11–11

Background.—Drug consumption during labor appears to decrease when patient-controlled epidural analgesia (PCEA) is used rather than continuous epidural infusion (CEI). Whether an ultra–low-dose local anesthetic with an opioid regimen can be used throughout labor and still show a decrease in drug consumption with PCEA compared to CEI was explored. In addition,

TABLE 2.—Dosage Requirements

	CEI (n = 40)			PCEA (n = 40)			
Total consumption (ml)*	52 (19.6)			35 (18.0)			P<0.001
Hourly consumption (ml h⁻¹)*	6.9 (1.31)			5.2 (2.54)			P<0.001
	1st	2nd	3rd	1st	2nd	3rd	
Need for extra bolus dose (No)	14	2	2	9	3	1	

*Mean (standard deviation).
Abbreviations: CEI, continuous epidural infusion.; PCEA, patient-controlled epidural analgesia.
(Courtesy of Eriksson SL, Gentele C, Olofsson CH: PCEA compared to continuous epidural infusion in an ultra-low-dose regimen for labor pain relief: A randomized study. *Acta Anaesthesiol Scand* 47:1085-1090, 2003.)

the combination of ropivacaine, 1 mg/mL, with sufentanil was assessed in the ultra–low-dose protocol.

Methods.—Forty patients were randomly assigned to receive CEI with ropivacaine and sufentanil and 40 to receive PCEA with 4-mL demand doses with a 20-minute lockout. Eight milliliters of the study solution constituted the epidural start dose, with rescue bolus doses given as needed. The continuous infusion could be increased so that the 2 groups had the same maximum possible dose. Measures included pain intensity (documented using a visual analogue score), patient's opinion of the epidural efficacy, motor block, development of pruritus, and need for nitrous oxide.

Results.—Participants' assessments of pain relief were similar in the 2 groups. However, the PCEA group's total consumption was 33% lower and their hourly consumption 25% lower than those of the CEI group (Table 2). After delivery, the epidural was rated as achieving the pain relief promised by 82.5% of the PCEA group and 85% of the CEI group. Insufficient relief from pressure experienced in the second stage of labor was noted as the reason for any dissatisfaction in both groups. Among the women receiving PCEA, 97.5% believed it was safe and 92.5% approved of being in control of their own doses and would choose this method to relieve labor pain again.

The duration of labor after the epidural was slightly shorter for the PCEA than for the CEI patients. Fifty percent of each group reported pruritus that was mild to moderate in intensity. Motor ability was impaired sporadically in 4 women in the CEI group and 2 in the PCEA group, with 1 CEI parturient having affected motor ability throughout labor. Hypotension developed in 1 patient in the CEI group; she responded to treatment.

Conclusion.—The consumption of analgesic was lower with PCEA than with CEI, even with the ultra–low-dose regimen using ropivacaine and sufentanil. Most patients expressed satisfaction with the analgesia obtained, and the side effects were few and manageable.

▶ The preponderance of evidence suggests that PCEA—*without* a continuous "background" infusion—results in administration of a lower total dose of local anesthetic and opioid than CEI in laboring women.

D. H. Chestnut, MD

Hyperbaric Bupivacaine 2.5 mg Prolongs Analgesia Compared With Plain Bupivacaine When Added to Intrathecal Fentaynl 25 µg in Advanced Labor

Teoh WHL, Sia ATH (KK Women's & Children's Hosp, Singapore)
Anesth Analg 97:873-877, 2003   11–12

Background.—In the search to identify the optimal intrapartum analgesia, various combinations of intrathecal (IT) fentanyl and plain bupivacaine have been used. The visceral afferent nerves mediate the pain experienced early in the first labor stage, with perineal pain becoming more prominent as the descending fetus exerts pressure. The viability of using "dissociative" spinal analgesia using a sequential subarachnoid block with IT fentanyl, 25 µg, diluted in normal saline solution for the visceral component and IT hyperbaric bupivacaine, 2.5 mg, to achieve a sacral block was assessed. This sequential subarachnoid block was induced while the woman was seated upright. Use of the combined spinal/epidural (CSE) mode delivered in this way was designed to induce the hyperbaric bupivacaine, 2.5 mg, to pool to the dependent area and produce optimal analgesic effects on the sacral nerve roots and hopefully prolong the spinal analgesic effect.

Methods.—Participants included 37 nulliparous women whose cervical dilation was at least 5 cm. Nineteen were randomly assigned to receive IT fentanyl, 25 µg, plus plain bupivacaine (group P) and 18 were assigned to receive IT fentanyl, 25 µg, plus hyperbaric bupivacaine 2.5 mg (group H). Sequential administration was carried out for the 2 components; then patients were positioned with their torsos elevated at 30° for 30 minutes. Visual analogue scales were completed to obtain pain scores ranging from 0 to 100 before CSE analgesia and 5, 15, and 30 minutes after the block was administered.

Results.—A significantly longer duration of effective spinal analgesia was obtained by group H patients using the IT hyperbaric bupivacaine than by the group P patients. Values ranged from 80 to 210 minutes (mean, 122.5 minutes) for group H and from 75 to 125 minutes (mean, 95.0 minutes) for group P. Two patients in group H and 4 in group P delivered before they lost spinal analgesia. Group H patients had a more limited dermatomal spread than those in group P. Side effects were seen at equal rates in the 2 groups, and the reduction in visual analogue scale over 30 minutes after CSE administration did not differ significantly between the groups.

Conclusion.—Compared to the use of plain bupivacaine, the use of hyperbaric preparations given with the parturients in a head-up position during late labor prolonged the duration of analgesia with the use of the same amount of local anesthetic.

▶ In this study, administration of hyperbaric bupivacaine, 2.5 mg, immediately after administration of fentanyl, 25 µg, resulted in a lesser degree of dermatomal spread but a modest prolongation of analgesia when compared with administration of plain (marginally hypobaric) bupivacaine and fentanyl.

D. H. Chestnut, MD

Small Dose Bupivacaine-Fentanyl Spinal Analgesia Combined With Morphine for Labor

Hess PE, Vasudevan A, Snowman C, et al (Beth Israel Deaconess Med Ctr, Boston)
Anesth Analg 97:247-252, 2003   11–13

Background.—The combined spinal–epidural technique is a popular method for providing labor analgesia because it provides a rapid onset of pain relief achieved with the spinal injection and prolonged analgesia maintained via epidural infusion. A number of drugs have been used to initiate the spinal component of analgesia. Large doses of lipid-soluble opioids will produce rapid and profound analgesia but are associated with significant side effects. The synergistic effect of combining local anesthetics allows a significant reduction in the dose of opioids required to provide effective analgesia during labor, and some studies have shown that reducing the dose of spinal medications reduces the duration of analgesia without affecting the quality of pain relief. The duration of labor analgesia obtained from a small dose of spinal bupivacaine–fentanyl alone or in combination with a small dose of morphine was investigated.

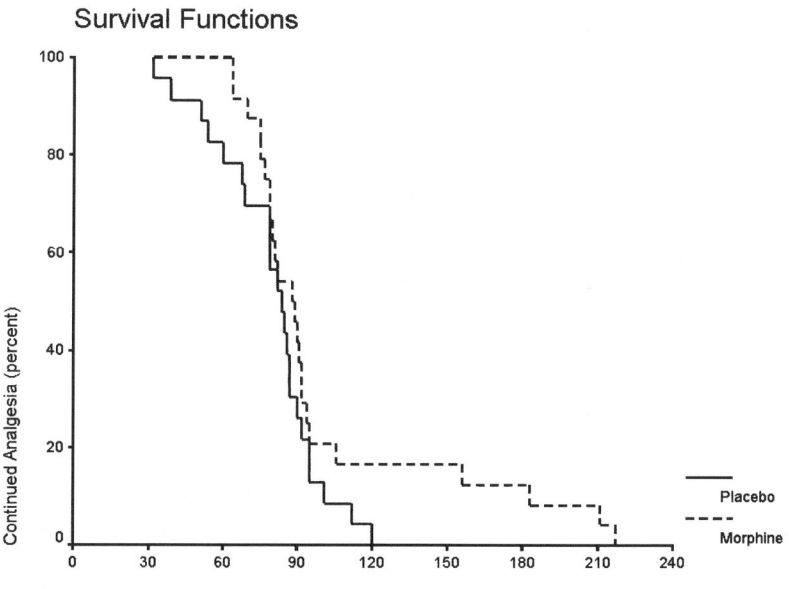

FIGURE 1.—Life table of duration of spinal analgesia. This figure illustrates the percentage of research subjects with continued analgesia after spinal injection. Both groups received 12.5 μg of fentanyl and 2 mg of bupivacaine. The morphine group received 125 μg of morphine in addition. Placebo indicates the bupivacaine–fentanyl group; morphine indicates the morphine/bupivacaine/fentanyl group. (Courtesy of Hess PE, Vasudevan A, Snowman C, et al: Small dose bupivacaine-fentanyl spinal analgesia combined with morphine for labor. *Anesth Analg* 97(1):247-252, 2003.)

Methods.—This placebo-controlled, double-blind, randomized study enrolled 60 women in labor. All the women received a spinal injection of 12.5 µg fentanyl with 2 mg of bupivacaine. The morphine group (MBF) also received 125 µg of morphine, but the placebo group (BF) received saline.

Results.—Pain scores were rated as less than 3 of 10 within 10 minutes of injection. The median duration of analgesia was similar between groups (89 minutes vs 84 minutes), and only 20% of the MBF group experienced prolonged analgesia (Fig 1). The MBF group had a significantly lower rate of breakthrough pain than did the BF group during subsequent epidural analgesia. In addition, the MBF group required significantly fewer medications (3.3 ± 3.7 doses) than did the BF group (4.7 ± 3.5 doses).

Conclusions.—Intrathecal administration of a small dose of bupivacaine–fentanyl produced a rapid onset of labor analgesia. Analgesia was not significantly prolonged by the addition of a small dose of morphine, but morphine did improve subsequent pain relief. The approach presented in this study may provide a useful method for improving intrapartum and postpartum pain relief.

► In this study, the addition of 0.125 mg morphine to 2 mg intrathecal bupivacaine with 12.5 µg fentanyl did not prolong the duration of intrathecal analgesia in laboring women. During subsequent administration of epidural analgesia, women in the morphine group had less breakthrough pain, and they also required fewer doses of analgesic drugs after delivery. It is unclear whether this modest benefit warrants the risks (eg, postpartum respiratory depression) associated with intrathecal administration of morphine during labor.

D. H. Chestnut, MD

Analgesia for Labor: Obstetric Outcome and Economic Issues

Physician Contribution to a Cesarean Delivery Risk Model
Luthy DA, Malmgren JA, Zingheim RW, et al (Swedish Med Ctr, Seattle; HealthStat Consulting Inc, Seattle)
Am J Obstet Gynecol 188:1579-1587, 2003   11–14

Introduction.—The percentage of births that are cesarean deliveries has increased in recent years, reaching nearly 23% in 2000. The impact of individual physician practice on the cesarean delivery rate remains unclear. The effects of physicians' labor management on the rate of cesarean delivery among women with singleton pregnancies and planned vaginal delivery were assessed.

Methods.—This 2-year, prospective study included 10,027 live births of babies with birth weights of at least 500 g. Of these births, 7940 were planned to be vaginal deliveries at the time the mother went into labor. Predictors of cesarean delivery were identified using a risk-adjusted logistic regression model. The effects of physician management on cesarean delivery risk were evaluated using data on 6563 babies delivered by physicians with at least 45 deliveries during the study period.

Results.—In the planned vaginal delivery sample, the rate of cesarean delivery was 11.3% in the first year of the study and 11.6% in the second year. For physicians with at least 45 deliveries, the cesarean delivery rate varied widely, from 3.7% to 21.2%. On multivariate analysis, the strongest predictors of cesarean delivery were abnormal fetal position, odds ratio (OR), 4.21, and nulliparity, OR, 6.13. Other contributing factors included birth weight more than 4000 g, meconium staining, amnionitis, and spontaneous labor. A forward stepwise regression model including these variables had a predictive ability of 43.8%. Adding physician management data to the model improved predictive ability to 50.2%.

Conclusions.—Physician management is a significant, independent factor affecting the likelihood of cesarean delivery in a population of women with planned vaginal delivery. Because the other predictors are nonmodifiable, including parity, birthweight, and fetal position, labor and delivery practices that affect the cesarean delivery rate should be identified and modified.

▶ For many years I have contended that maternal-fetal factors and obstetric management—not epidural analgesia—are the primary determinants of the cesarean section rate. This study provides further evidence of the importance of physician management as a significant independent factor that affects the rate of cesarean section.

D. H. Chestnut, MD

Local Anesthetic Requirements Are Greater in Dystocia Than in Normal Labor
Panni MK, Segal S (Duke Univ, Durham, NC; Harvard Med School, Boston)
Anesthesiology 98:957-963, 2003   11–15

Objective.—Many cesarean sections result from dystocia, or abnormal progression of labor. Some retrospective studies have suggested that epidural analgesia is a contributing factor to dystocia. However, these studies overlook the possibility that women opting for epidural analgesia may have more difficult labor and other risk factors for dystocia. The minimum local analgesic concentration (MLAC) approach was used to compare the bupivacaine requirements during early labor for women who went on to require cesarean section for dystocia versus the requirements for those who delivered vaginally.

Methods.—The analysis included 57 nulliparous women in labor who were assigned on alternate days into a spontaneous vaginal delivery group and a cesarean section for dystocia group. At the time of epidural catheter placement, they were also assigned to either receiving or not receiving IV oxytocin. Using an up-down sequential allocation technique, the investigators compared the MLAC of bupivacaine for patients who delivered by their assigned route (vaginal or cesarean section).

Results.—The final analysis included 40 women who delivered by cesarean section, 20 on oxytocin; and 17 who delivered vaginally, 9 on oxytocin and 8 not on oxytocin. In the cesarean section group, MLAC values were 0.102% wt/vol bupivacaine for women who received oxytocin and 1.06% wt/vol for those who did not. For women who delivered vaginally, MLAC values were 0.078% and 0.085% wt/vol bupivacaine for those who did and did not receive oxytocin, respectively. Thus, MLAC values were significantly less for women who went on to deliver vaginally: 25% lower for those who received oxytocin and 31% lower for those who did not.

Conclusions.—Women who require larger amounts of local anesthetic during epidural labor analgesia experience more intense pain, associated with the later development of dystocia. Among women in early, clinically normal labor, those who go on to have dystocia appear to experience more pain, and thus require more local anesthetic than those who proceed to vaginal delivery. The findings should inform the ongoing debate over the effects of labor analgesia on labor outcomes.

▶ For many years I have argued that women at increased risk for operative delivery are more likely to request and receive epidural analgesia during labor. Other studies have noted that severe pain during early labor predicts an increased risk of operative delivery. Indirectly, this study confirms those earlier observations. Specifically, these authors noted higher MLAC (ie, increased local anesthetic requirements) during administration of epidural analgesia in laboring women who subsequently required cesarean section for dystocia.

This study illustrates that retrospective studies of epidural analgesia and obstetric outcome are subject to selection bias. In recent years, most of the evidence from randomized controlled trials suggests that the contemporary administration of epidural analgesia does not increase the incidence of cesarean section in laboring women.

D. H. Chestnut, MD

Randomized Controlled Trial Comparing Traditional With Two "Mobile" Epidural Techniques: Anesthetic and Analgesic Efficacy
MacArthur C, for the Comparative Obstetric Mobile Epidural Trial (COMET) Study Group UK (Univ of Birmingham, England; et al)
Anesthesiology 97:1567-1575, 2002   11–16

Purpose.—The use of low-dose combinations of local anesthetics and opioids for "mobile" epidural analgesia during labor can reduce the effect of epidural analgesia on instrumental vaginal delivery, relative to a traditional technique. In the authors' previous study of this approach, postpartum estimates of labor pain after epidural catheter placement did not differ significantly for women undergoing mobile epidural analgesia compared with traditional techniques. The anesthetic and analgesic efficacy of mobile epidural analgesia during labor was evaluated.

Methods.—The randomized trial included 1054 nulliparous women who requested epidural analgesia during labor. Two mobile epidural approaches were evaluated, both using 0.1% bupivacaine with 2 µg/mL fentanyl: a combined spinal-epidural (CSE) technique and a low-dose infusion (LDI) technique. In addition to recording visual analogue scale pain scores during labor and delivery and at 24 hours' follow-up, data were collected on the course of epidural analgesia, medication use, and the need for anesthesiologist reattendance.

Results.—Five minutes after insertion, the median pain score was 20 in the CSE group versus 64 in the traditional analgesia group and 57 in the LDI group. The difference in pain scores with CSE was significant and persistent through 1 hour; pain scores in the LDI group were not significantly different than in the traditional group. The mean bupivacaine dose during labor was also significantly lower with CSE. The 2 mobile epidural techniques were associated with more frequent anesthesiologist reattendance.

Conclusions.—For women undergoing labor analgesia, the CSE mobile epidural technique provides a faster onset of analgesia and lower pain scores than traditional techniques. The LDI technique is equally effective as traditional epidural analgesia. Their good analgesic efficacy together with their beneficial effects on mode of delivery make these mobile epidural techniques the preferred approach to pain relief during labor.

Ambulatory Epidural Anesthesia and the Duration of Labor
Karraz MA (Hôpital Louise Michel, Evry, France)
Int J Gynaecol Obstet 80:117-122, 2003   11–17

Background.—Epidural analgesia is usually administered to patients in the supine position, preventing women in labor from walking around. Ambulatory epidural analgesia has become common at the Beauvais Central Hospital in France. The effect of ambulatory epidural analgesia on delivery mode, oxytocin dosage, and labor duration was evaluated.

Study Design.—The study group consisted of 221 women in labor at 36 to 42 weeks of gestation, with a singleton pregnancy and cephalic presentation. These women were randomly assigned to either ambulatory epidural analgesia or supine epidural analgesia. Use of oxytocin, amount of local anesthetic used, duration of labor, and mode of delivery were recorded. This study was conducted only for daytime deliveries, because women in labor at night are less inclined to walk.

Findings.—There were no significant differences between these 2 groups in mode of delivery or use of local anesthetic or oxytocin. There was a significant difference in labor duration.

Conclusion.—Ambulatory epidural analgesia shortens labor duration when compared with supine epidural analgesia but has no other effect on labor progress or outcome.

▶ The preponderance of evidence suggests that epidural administration of a dilute solution of local anesthetic results in a decreased risk of operative delivery, when compared with epidural administration of higher doses of local anesthetic. This relationship remains true, with or without the intrathecal in-

jection of analgesic drugs to initiate analgesia. Further, it is clear that most patients prefer the decreased motor block associated with the use of these low-
dose epidural techniques. The importance of ambulation during labor remains
unclear. The study by Karraz (Abstract 11–17) suggests that ambulation shortens labor but does not have any other effect on obstetric outcome in laboring
women receiving epidural analgesia.

D. H. Chestnut, MD

Postural Stability Following Ambulatory Regional Analgesia for Labor
Davies J, Fernando R, McLeod A, et al (Royal Free Hosp, London)
Anesthesiology 97:1576-1581, 2002   11–18

Background.—Ambulatory, or "mobile," epidural analgesia is an attrac-
tive alternative for pain relief for women in labor. Recent studies have shown
good balance function despite the presence of clinical sensory deficits, but
there is continued concern over the safety of allowing mobilization after
low-dose regional analgesia. A computerized balance function test was used
to assess postural stability in women in labor who have received low-dose
combined spinal-epidural analgesia.

Methods.—The study used the computerized Balance Master version 6.1,
which provides real-time analysis of balance function during ambulation.
This device was used to measure balance during various simple tasks, such as
walking and standing from a seated position, in 50 women in labor who had
received combined spinal-epidural analgesia with bupivacaine and fentanyl.
Two control groups were studied for comparison: 50 pregnant women who
were not in labor and 50 nonpregnant women.

Results.—Compared with both pregnant groups, the nonpregnant
women scored better on 6 of 13 balance function measures evaluated. Pregnancy was associated with impaired function in standing from a seated position, walking speed, step length, and stepping over a 20-cm obstacle. The
initial dose of spinal analgesia did not adversely affect balance function,
compared with that of the pregnant control group. Seventeen women in the
combined spinal-epidural group were retested after receiving supplemental
epidural analgesia after an initial spinal injection. These tests showed impairment of 4 balance function measures, compared with those of women
who received spinal injection only.

Conclusions.—Pregnant women at term have significantly reduced balance function, compared with that of women who are not pregnant. The
initial dose of spinal-epidural analgesia does not further impair balance,
compared with the effects of pregnancy alone. Women receiving additional
supplemental analgesia may show further detrimental effects on balance.
This issue requires further study, but the results support the safety of allowing parturients to ambulate after their initial dose of spinal-epidural
analgesia.

▶ This study confirms that pregnancy significantly affects balance function. This study provides some objective evidence that intrathecal administration of bupivacaine 2.5 mg with fentanyl 5 µg does not result in further impairment of maternal balance function. However, women who received supplemental epidural doses of local anesthetic showed evidence of impaired balance function when compared with women who received intrathecal analgesia alone.

Supervised ambulation seems safe for both the mother and the fetus, provided the mother retains adequate motor function, proprioception, and balance, and provided there is no evidence of postural hypotension. It seems wise for these patients to sit on the side of the bed for 1 or 2 minutes before standing up. In addition, they should not be allowed to walk unsupervised. Instead, these patients should ambulate only with assistance.

D. H. Chestnut, MD

A Randomized Clinical Trial Comparing the Effects of Delayed *Versus* Immediate Pushing With Epidural Analgesia on Mode of Delivery and Faecal Continence
Fitzpatrick M, Harkin R, McQuillan K, et al (Univ College Dublin; Mater Misericordiae Hosp, Dublin)
Br J Obstet Gynaecol 109:1359-1365, 2002   11–19

Background.—For women in labor receiving epidural analgesia, delayed active pushing has been proposed as 1 way of reducing the risk of instrumental delivery. Although this practice has been widely adopted, studies of its efficacy have yielded conflicting results. Also data are contradictory on the effects of epidural analgesia and delayed pushing on pelvic floor physiology and postpartum fecal continence. The effects of delayed pushing on mode of delivery, fecal continence, and other outcomes were evaluated in a randomized, controlled trial.

Methods.—The study included 178 nulliparous women who were receiving continuous epidural analgesia. The women were selected randomly and stratified into 2 groups when they reached full dilation, but before the fetal head reached the pelvic floor. One group was told to delay pushing for 1 hour, and the other group was told to push immediately. The mode of delivery was assessed, with all women undergoing postpartum evaluation of anal sphincter function, including manometry. Further evaluations included neurophysiologic studies in women undergoing normal delivery and endoanal US in those undergoing instrumental delivery.

Results.—Spontaneous delivery occurred in 52% of women assigned to delayed pushing and 56% of those assigned to immediate pushing. The mean duration of labor was 480 and 427 minutes for the 2 groups, respectively. Oxytocin was given to augment labor in 81% of patients in the delayed-pushing group, 31% in the second-stage only; and in 84% in the immediate-pushing group, 28% in the second stage (Fig 1).

Fetal outcomes were similar with delayed versus immediate pushing; episiotomy rates were 69% and 73%, respectively. After delivery, changes in

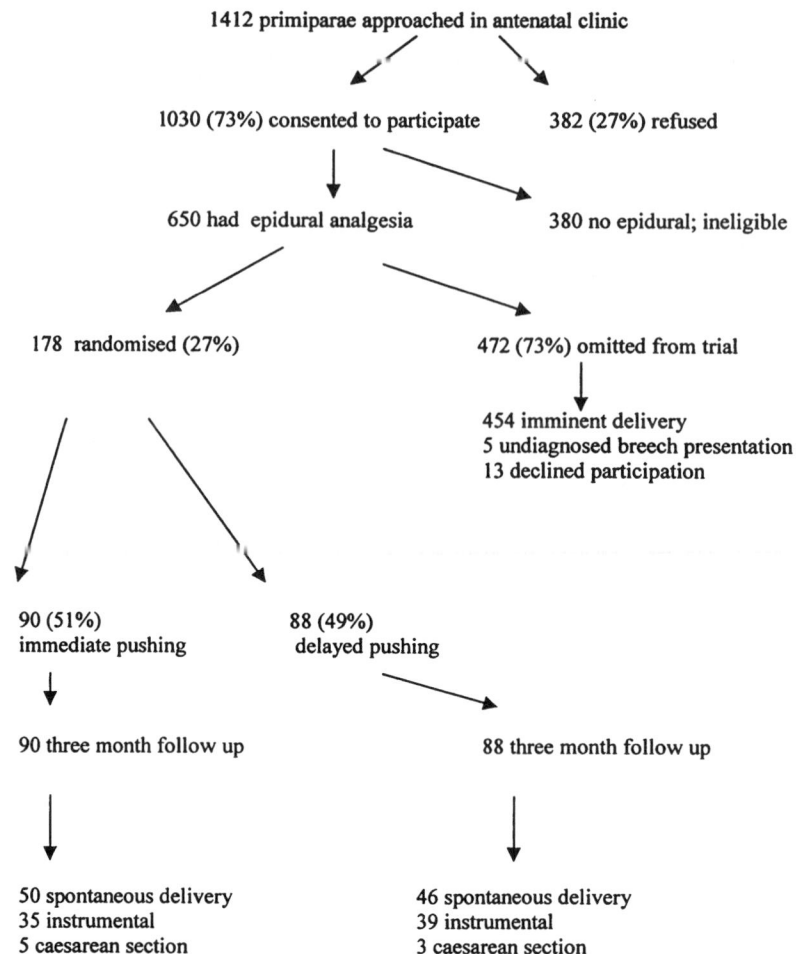

FIGURE 1.—Comparison of the effects of delayed versus immediate pushing with epidural analgesia on mode of delivery and fecal continence—flow chart. (Courtesy of Fitzpatrick M, Harkin R, McQuillan K, et al: A randomized clinical trial comparing the effects of delayed *versus* immediate pushing with epidural analgesia on mode of delivery and faecal continence. *Br J Obstet Gynaecol* 109:1359-1365, 2002. With permission from Elsevier Science.)

fecal continence were reported by 38% of women in the delayed-pushing group versus 26% of those in the immediate-pushing group; however, the difference was not significant. The findings of manometry, US, and neurophysiologic studies were similar between groups. Anal sphincter damage was observed on endosonography in 55% of women undergoing instrumental delivery, while neurophysiologic studies were abnormal in 36% of women undergoing spontaneous delivery.

Conclusions.—No difference was found in the risk of instrumental delivery in laboring women on epidural analgesia assigned to delayed versus immediate pushing. Delayed pushing is associated with a longer duration of labor, yet it does not lead to an increased risk of anal sphincter injury or changes in fecal continence. Other outcomes and postpartum evaluations are also similar between groups.

▶ The value of delayed pushing during the second stage of labor in women receiving epidural analgesia remains a matter of some dispute. It seems intuitive to allow the force of uterine contractions to promote fetal descent, until such time that pushing is likely to be effective. Some studies have suggested that delayed pushing is associated with an increased likelihood of spontaneous vaginal delivery. However, the authors of this study did not confirm any benefit as a result of delayed pushing. Instead, delayed pushing prolonged labor by approximately 1 hour, without resulting in an increased likelihood of spontaneous vaginal delivery. Of interest, the authors observed no difference between groups in the use of episiotomy, postpartum continence, or postpartum assessment of anal sphincter function.

D. H. Chestnut, MD

Fetal and Neonatal Considerations

Analgesia in Labour and Fetal Acid-Base Balance: A Meta-Analysis Comparing Epidural With Systemic Opioid Analgesia
Reynolds F, Sharma SK, Seed PT (St Thomas' Hosp, London; Univ of Texas, Dallas; King's College, London)
Br J Obstet Gynaecol 109:1344-1353, 2002   11–20

Objective.—Epidural analgesia during labor provides superior pain relief, compared with that of other approaches. However, there is ongoing concern over the potential for adverse effects on the fetus and newborn, because of the maternal and obstetric changes during labor. The effects of epidural labor analgesia on fetal acid-based balance were analyzed in a meta-analysis.

Methods.—The analysis included data on previous studies, published or unpublished, comparing epidural with systemic analgesia during labor. Data on babies born to 2102 women were included in the study. Fetal pH data were obtained from 12 studies, 8 of them randomized (epidural, 1098 mothers; systemic, 1004 mothers [control subjects]). Base excess data were obtained from 8 studies, 4 of them randomized (epidural, 856 mothers; systemic, 842 mothers). Random effects meta-analysis was done to compare the 2 forms of analgesia for their effects on funic acid-base status at birth.

Results.—The randomized trial data suggested higher mean pH in infants in the epidural group versus the control group, with a mean difference of 0.009 (95% confidence interval [CI], 0.002-0.015). The difference became nonsignificant when data from the observational studies were also included (Fig 1). Epidural analgesia was consistently associated with greater fetal base excess: the difference in the randomized trial data was 0.779 mEq/L (95% CI, 0.056 to 1.502); and in all data, 0.837 mEq/L (95% CI, 0.330-1.343).

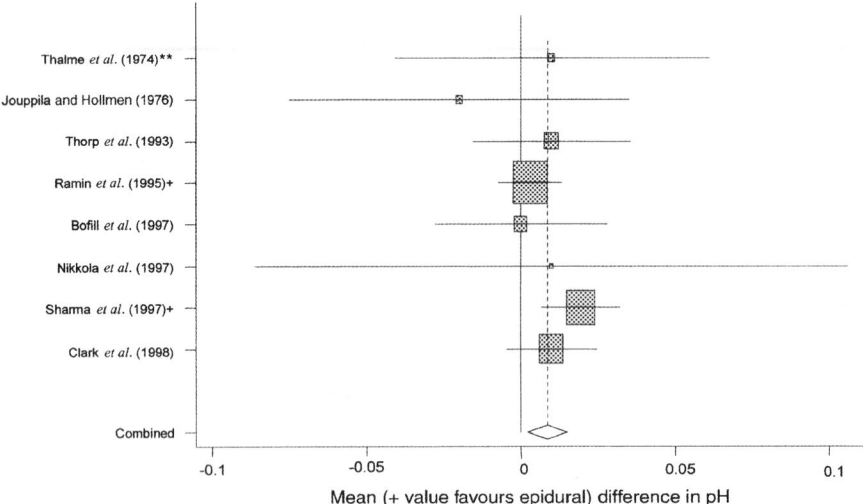

FIGURE 1.—Meta-analysis of difference (epidural minus control) between umbilical artery (**umbilical cord) pH values in eight randomized controlled trials of epidural versus systemic opioid analgesia. The *vertical line* represents unity, the size of the box gives an estimate of the weighting of the study, and the *horizontal lines* are the 95% confidence intervals. (Weighting is based on the amount of information provided by the study, defined as 1/the square of the standard error of the estimate.) There is a significant difference ($P = .007$) between the two treatment groups, favoring epidural analgesia. +Includes unpublished data. (Courtesy of Reynolds F, Sharma SK, Seed PT: Analgesia in labour and fetal acid-base balance: a meta-analysis comparing epidural with systemic opioid analgesia. *Br J Obstet Gynecol* 109:1344-1353, 2002. With permission from Elsevier Science.)

Conclusions.—For women in labor, epidural analgesia appears to lead to improvements in neonatal acid-base status. Thus, this form of analgesia appears to protect placental exchange while providing sympathetic blockade and effective pain control for the mother. The increased risk of adverse maternal or obstetric events with epidural analgesia, including a higher rate of instrumental vaginal deliveries may be outweighed by the beneficial effects on neonatal acid-base status. Because maternal hyperventilation affects umbilical artery pH, base excess may be a better indicator of metabolic acidosis after labor.

▶ Multiple studies have confirmed that epidural analgesia provides much better analgesia during labor than systemic opioids. Likewise, these studies have consistently noted that epidural analgesia is less likely to result in neonatal respiratory depression than systemic opioids. This meta-analysis also confirms that epidural analgesia is associated with improved neonatal acid-base status, suggesting that maternal sympathetic blockade and good analgesia help preserve placental gas exchange during labor. The authors concluded that epidural analgesia "does not exacerbate fetal acidosis, and if anything, may partially protect the fetus from fetal hypoxia."

D. H. Chestnut, MD

Spinal and Epidural Versus General Anesthesia for Elective Cesarean Section at Term: Effect on the Acid-Base Status of the Mother and Newborn

Petropoulos G, Siristatidis C, Salamalekis E, et al (Univ of Athens, Greece)
J Matern Fetal Neonatal Med 13:260-266, 2003   11–21

Background.—The use of regional anesthesia in cesarean deliveries is increasing. This has resulted in increased interest in the influence of choice of anesthetic modality on neonatal outcome. However, there is significant disagreement in the literature comparing the type of anesthesia and cord blood gas values, which has led to confusion regarding the type of anesthesia to be recommended. Both regional and general anesthesia have potential advantages. General, epidural, and combined spinal-epidural anesthesia were compared in regard to short-term outcome of newborns delivered by elective cesarean section by healthy women with normal pregnancies.

Methods.—A total of 238 pregnant women admitted to 1 institution between January 1998 and July 2002 and for whom elective cesarean section was planned after 38 weeks' gestation were grouped according to the kind of anesthesia used for the procedure. Several variables were analyzed, including maternal characteristics, birth weight, Apgar scores, and maternal and umbilical artery (UA) acid-base parameters.

Results.—The general anesthesia group had significantly lower maternal pH and significantly higher pCO_2 and pO_2 compared with the other 2 groups. The pH of the UA was higher in the general anesthesia group compared with the spinal-pidural group. The pO_2 and the O_2 saturation of the UA were higher when general anesthetic was administered, compared with the 2 regional modalities. UA O_2 saturation dropped to zero in some cases in the combined spinal-epidural group, with no apparent effect on fetal well-being. No fetal acidemia was noted in any group. The 3 groups were similar in neonatal outcomes.

Conclusion.—It appears that the type of anesthesia does not influence the short-term outcomes of infants born by elective cesarean section. However, differences in the acid-base status of the mother and particularly the newborn advocate the careful use of spinal anesthesia.

▶ These results are consistent with observations from earlier studies. The modest differences in acid-base status were not associated with clinically significant differences in neonatal outcome.

D. H. Chestnut, MD

Anesthesia for Cesarean Section

Aortocaval Compression in Pregnancy: The Effect of Changing the Degree and Direction of Lateral Tilt on Maternal Cardiac Output
Bamber JH, Dresner M (Leeds Gen Infirmary, England)
Anesth Analg 97:256-258, 2003   11–22

Background.—When a woman in late pregnancy lies supine, the gravid uterus will completely occlude the inferior vena cava and laterally displace the subrenal aorta. This aortocaval compression causes a reduction in maternal cardiac output, an event that is often concealed because only 10% of pregnant women will manifest supine hypotension syndrome. Some pregnant women will naturally avoid lying on their backs, but they are often positioned supine during their medical care. The consequent aortocaval compression is often alleviated by gravity by either placing a wedge under the woman's hip or by tilting the operating table.

There has been little study of what constitutes an adequate amount of lateral tilt and whether more tilt is better than less tilt. The hypothesis that increasing the amount and direction of lateral tilt has a significant effect on maternal cardiac output was tested.

Methods.—Thirty-two women were selected for study, as this sample size was calculated to be sufficient for detection of a 20% difference in cardiac output among each of 7 positions: supine on the left or right side and with varying degrees of lateral tilt. One woman was unable to complete the study. Each position was adopted for a total of 5 minutes, and measurements were obtained over the last 3 minutes of the position. Cardiac output, stroke volume, and heart rate were measured continuously with bioimpedance cardiography. Blood pressure was measured automatically over the left brachial artery.

Results.—Stroke volume and cardiac output were greatest when the women lay on the left side and least when they lay on the back with the table

TABLE 3.—Comparison of Measurements of Cardiac Output Between Left Lateral Position and the Tilt and Supine Positions

Comparison of Positions	Mean Difference (Mean % Change)	95% CI for Mean Difference	P Value
Cardiac output (L/min)			
Left lateral with:			
Left 12.5°	0.79 (8%)	−0.51-2.09	1.0
Left 5°	0.77 (8%)	−0.53-2.06	1.0
Supine	1.20 (13%)	−0.11-2.56	0.1
Right 5°	1.34 (15%)	0.04-2.64	0.04
Right 12.5°	1.46 (17%)	0.16-2.76	0.01

Note: A negative value represents a comparative increase in cardiac output. Statistical analysis was by analysis of variance with Bonferroni's correction.
Abbreviation: CI, Confidence interval.
(Courtesy of Bamber JH, Dresner M: Aortocaval compression in pregnancy: The effect of changing the degree and direction of lateral tilt on maternal cardiac output. *Anesth Analg* 97:256-258, 2003.)

tilted laterally to the right. There was a mean 17% reduction in cardiac output when women lying on their backs were tilted laterally to the right, compared with the cardiac output measured when they were lying on their left sides (Table 3). When the women were supine, increasing the amount of lateral table tilt to the left or right appeared to have no effect on cardiac output.

Conclusion.—This study found no significant effect on maternal cardiac output in healthy pregnant women when the amount and direction of lateral table tilt were increased. However, the significant reduction in maternal cardiac output when the maternal position was changed from lying on the left side to lying supine with lateral table tilt to the right may have greater importance for women with compromised cardiac output or ureteroplacental circulation.

▶ Readers should be aware that these measurements were performed in nonanesthetized, healthy pregnant women. Thus, it is not clear that the authors' conclusions can be applied to women subjected to sympathetic blockade during administration of either epidural or spinal anesthesia.

The authors concluded that "To avoid any detrimental effect on maternal cardiac output, the pregnant woman would ideally be kept in the full lateral tilt position, but this is often impractical." Of course, the parturient cannot remain in the full lateral position during cesarean section. However, there is one circumstance when it may be advantageous to keep the patient in the full lateral position during initial administration of regional anesthesia for cesarean section. Specifically, I have kept some patients with multiple gestation in the full lateral position during administration (ie, induction) of epidural anesthesia for cesarean section.

Patients with multiple gestation are at increased risk for aortocaval compression. Posture and gravity have little effect on the spread of a large "surgical" dose of local anesthetic in the epidural space. By maintaining the full lateral position during the onset of epidural anesthesia, the patient is able to compensate for the effect of sympathetic blockade, without the added stress of aortocaval compression. Once surgical anesthesia is achieved, the patient can be turned to the supine leftward tilt position, the abdomen can be prepped and draped, and surgery can begin immediately thereafter. In my experience, this regimen is associated with a reduced risk of significant hypotension during administration of epidural anesthesia for cesarean section in patients with multiple gestation.

D. H. Chestnut, MD

Efficacy of Augmentation of Epidural Analgesia for Caesarean Section
Tortosa JC, Parry NS, Mercier FJ, et al (Hôpital Antoine Béclère, Clamart Cedex, France; Hope Hosp, Manchester, England)
Br J Anaesth 91:532-535, 2003   11–23

Background.—Extension of a labor epidural for cesarean delivery, which obviates the need for general anesthesia, is believed to be successful in most patients. However, most research on the failure rate of pre-existing epidural catheters included small numbers of patients.

Methods.—Data on 194 consecutive extensions performed in a 1-year period were analyzed retrospectively to determine the failure rate of indwelling epidural catheters. The anesthetic team, led by a senior anesthetist specializing in obstetrics, was available at all times. Extension was done using lidocaine 2% with epinephrine. In most patients, it was combined with sufentanil and/or clonidine.

Findings.—General anesthesia was required in 2.6% of the patients. Another 13.9% needed sedation and/or IV analgesia. In 3 patients requiring general anesthesia, the interval between the decision to initiate such anesthesia and incision was less than 10 minutes. Correlates of failure could not be identified. Adding a lipophilic opioid or clonidine did not alter the efficacy of the block.

Conclusions.—The use of lidocaine 2% plus epinephrine to augment labor epidural for cesarean delivery appears to be reliable and effective. No variables could be associated with failure.

▶ This retrospective study demonstrates the utility of the epidural administration of 2% lidocaine with epinephrine for extension of preexisting epidural analgesia for cesarean section.

D. H. Chestnut, MD

Time Required for Surgical Readiness in Emergency Caesarean Section: Spinal Compared With General Anaesthesia
McCahon RA, Catling S (Singleton Hosp, Sketty Lane, Swansea, UK)
Int J Obstet Anesth 12:178-182, 2003   11–24

Background.—Findings of studies recently conducted in the United Kingdom have suggested that many cesarean section procedures performed in an emergent setting fall outside the auditable standard of 30 minutes between the decision to operate and the delivery of the fetus. Several factors have been cited as potentially contributing to the delay in delivery, including the transfer of the patient to the operating suite and the achievement of adequate anesthesia. The likelihood of delivery within 30 minutes has been shown to be greater if the patient arrives in the operating room within 10 minutes of the decision to operate. Safe and rapid provision of analgesia and anesthesia is not without risk in this situation. A concern for the potential for failed intubation in obstetric patients has prompted the increased use of regional anesthesia, which has implications for training in obstetric general anesthesia. The time required to be ready for emergency cesarean section when spinal anesthesia was used was compared with that required when general anesthesia was administered.

Methods.—The time for surgical readiness was defined as the interval from leaving the delivery room to the time of skin incision. This retrospective observational study was conducted in an obstetric tertiary referral hospital with more than 3000 obstetric patients per year.

Results.—Records were available for 137 women who had undergone emergency cesarean section with either spinal or general anesthesia from January 2000 through December 2000. The mean time for surgical readiness for general anesthesia was 15.4 minutes, with a range of 2 to 44 minutes; in comparison, the mean time for surgical readiness for spinal anesthesia was 27.6 minutes, with a range of 13 to 55 minutes. The proportion of patients in this study falling outside the 30-minute standard counting only surgical readiness was 31% for the spinal anesthesia group and 12% for the general anesthesia group.

Conclusions.—The 30-minute standard for surgical readiness in cesarean section is often unrealistic and unnecessary, and there appears to be little evidence to support the continued use of this standard. The few cases in which this standard is appropriate may be clarified by the new classification of clinical urgency of cesarean section endorsed by the Royal College of Obstetricians and Gynaecologists.

▶ Spinal anesthesia can be administered safely for many cases of emergency cesarean section. However, general anesthesia is usually more appropriate in cases of *stat* cesarean section, when delivery must be accomplished as soon as possible (eg, uterine rupture, placental abruption).

D. H. Chestnut, MD

Randomized, Double-blind Comparison of Different Inspired Oxygen Fractions During General Anaesthesia for Caesarean Section
Ngan Kee WD, Khaw KS, Ma KC, et al (Chinese Univ of Hong Kong, Shatin)
Br J Anaesth 89:556-561, 2002   11–25

Background.—Uncertainty exists regarding the optimum inspired oxygen fraction (FIO_2) for general anesthesia for cesarean section. Various articles have advocated FIO_2 values both smaller and greater than 0.5, combined with 50% nitrous oxide and a low concentration of a volatile agent. These different recommendations may be the result of differences in study design. Confounding factors that increase the difficulty of interpretation of earlier studies include a lack of lateral uterine displacement, inclusion of both laboring and nonlaboring patients, incomplete or undescribed methods of randomization, and inadequate compensation for changes in anesthetic depths when varying FIO_2. The effect of an FIO_2 value of 0.3, 0.5, and 1.0 on umbilical cord blood oxygen content was compared in patients having elective cesarean section under general anesthesia.

Methods.—Patients having elective cesarean section were randomly assigned to receive the following: 0.3 FIO_2, 0.7 FI_{N2O}, and 0.6% end-tidal sevoflurane (group 30, 20 patients); 0.5 FIO_2 and FI_{N2O}, 1.0% end-tidal sevoflurane (group 50, 20 patients); or 1.0 FIO_2 and 2.0% end-tidal sevoflurane (group 100, 20 patients) until delivery. Neonatal outcomes were compared biochemically and clinically.

Results.—At delivery, for umbilical venous blood, the mean PO_2 was greater in group 100 (7.6 kPa) than in either group 30 (4.0 kPa) or group 50 (4.7 kPa). The oxygen content was greater in group 100 (17.2 mL/dL) than in either group 30 (12.8 mL/dL) or group 50 (13.8 mL/dL). For umbilical arterial blood, PO_2 was greater in group 100 (3.2 kPa) than in group 30 (2.4 kPa) and greater in group 50 (2.9 kPa) than in group 30 (2.4 kPa). The oxygen content was greater in group 100 (10.8 mL/dL) than in group 30 (7.0 mL/dL). The groups had similar outcomes in terms of Apgar scores, neonatal neurologic and adaptive capacity scores, and maternal arterial plasma concentrations of epinephrine and norepinephrine before induction and at delivery. None of the patients reported intraoperative awareness.

Conclusions.—Although the findings of this study indicate that a high FIO_2 improved fetal oxygenation, the potential harmful effects should be considered. Fetal oxygenation improved in the group that received the highest FIO_2 (1.0), which suggests that this is not a significant concern in cases of elective cesarean section.

▶ The results of this study seem intuitive. However, this study does not address the observations from the authors' earlier study, namely that the use of a high FIO_2 during administration of regional anesthesia for cesarean section resulted in increased maternal and umbilical plasma concentrations of lipid peroxide markers of oxygen-free radical activity.[1] The clinical significance of those earlier findings is unclear. For now, the preponderance of evidence supports the administration of a high maternal FIO_2 during administration of either regional or general anesthesia for cesarean section, especially in patients with evidence of fetal stress (eg, a nonreassuring fetal heart rate tracing).

D. H. Chestnut, MD

Reference

1. Khaw KS, Wang CC, Ngan Kee WD, et al: High-inspired oxygen fraction during elective cesarean section under spinal anesthesia induces lipid-peroxidation in the mother and fetus. *Br J Anaesth* 88:18-23, 2002.

Fetal and Maternal Effects of Phenylephrine and Ephedrine During Spinal Anesthesia for Cesarean Delivery
Cooper DW, Carpenter M, Mowbray P, et al (James Cook Univ Hosp, Middlesbrough, Cleveland, England)
Anesthesiology 97:1582-1590, 2002   11–26

Purpose.—Previous studies have shown an increased rate of fetal acidosis after spinal anesthesia for elective cesarean delivery. Clinical experience suggests that this problem may be less frequent when phenylephrine is added to ephedrine as initial vasopressor therapy. This impression was tested in a randomized, double-blind trial.

Methods.—The study included 147 women undergoing elective cesarean section selected randomly to receive phenylephrine, 100 g/mL or ephedrine, 3 mg/mL; or a combination of phenylephrine 50 g/mL and ephedrine 1.5 mg/mL. All were given by infusion to maintain maternal systolic arterial pressure during spinal anesthesia. The rate of fetal acidosis, defined as an umbilical artery pH of less than 7.20, was compared among the 3 groups.

Results.—Fetal acidosis occurred at a rate of about 2% with phenylephrine, alone or in combination with ephedrine; compared with a rate of 21% with ephedrine alone. The 3 groups were similar in mean systolic arterial pressure, but mean heart rate was higher with ephedrine alone. Nausea occurred in 17% of women in the phenylephrine group versus nausea in 55% in the combination group and in 66% in the ephedrine group. Vomiting was also less frequent with phenylephrine.

Conclusions.—For women receiving spinal anesthesia for cesarean delivery, initial vasopressor therapy with phenylephrine alone or in combination with ephedrine reduces the rate of fetal acidosis. Phenylephrine also decreases the rate of maternal nausea and vomiting. The combination of phenylephrine and ephedrine provides no advantage; it increases nausea and vomiting with no further reduction in the risk of fetal acidosis.

▶ This study provides further confirmation of the safety of careful administration of small doses of phenylephrine for prevention or treatment of hypotension during administration of spinal anesthesia for cesarean section. The authors discussed the somewhat surprising increase in the incidence of fetal acidosis in the ephedrine group. This is puzzling, given the abundant evidence that ephedrine is superior to α-adrenergic agonists in restoring or protecting uteroplacental perfusion in pregnant animals and humans. Ephedrine crosses the placenta, and the authors speculated that "increased fetal metabolic rate, secondary to ephedrine-induced β-adrenergic stimulation, was the most likely mechanism for the increased incidence of fetal acidosis in the ephedrine group." The authors subsequently noted that "this does not necessarily mean that the use of α-adrenergic agonists is better for the fetus than ephedrine."

Anesthesiologists should remember that administration of ephedrine has the advantages of ease of use and a long history of safety in obstetric anesthesia practice. In my judgment, ephedrine remains the preferred first-line agent for treatment of most cases of hypotension during administration of regional anesthesia in obstetric patients. However, this study confirms that phenylephrine is also a safe vasopressor in obstetric patients.

Anesthesiologists might choose phenylephrine in patients with hypotension that is refractory to usual doses of ephedrine. Also, anesthesiologists might choose phenylephrine as a first-line agent in parturients who are tachycardic or in patients (eg, mitral stenosis) in whom tachycardia should be avoided.

D. H. Chestnut, MD

Should α-Agonists Be Used as First Line Management of Spinal Hypotension?

Vallejo MC, Ramanathan S (Univ of Pittsburgh, Pa)
Int J Obstet Anesth 12:243-245, 2003   11–27

Background.—The results of studies in the 1970s and 1990s led to a general misconception that α-agonists (particularly phenylephrine) were contraindicated in obstetric patients for the treatment of spinal hypotension because they would increase uterine vascular resistance and decrease uteroplacental perfusion and blood flow. Ephedrine is an indirect adrenergic agonist with mixed α- and β-agonist properties that increases both mean arterial pressure and cardiac output; thus, the use of ephedrine is not without maternal and fetal side effects. Recent studies of ephedrine administration in obstetric patients have provided mixed findings. The issues involved in selecting a vasopressor for the treatment of hypotension during administration of regional anesthesia in obstetric patients were reviewed.

Overview.—Prophylactic IM and IV infusions of vasopressors have been used for the prevention of hypotension for cesarean section under spinal anesthesia. However, a meta-analysis of controlled clinical trials found that prophylactic ephedrine, both IM and IV, did not improve neonatal outcome; thus, the routine use of prophylactic ephedrine could not be recommended. Numerous studies have shown that with the use of conservative measures (including volume preloading, left lateral uterine displacement, and Trendelenburg positioning), the use of α-agonists is safe and effective in the treatment of maternal hypotension. The clinical situation must determine which vasopressor is appropriate for the patient.

Conclusions.—Both ephedrine and phenylephrine can be used to maintain adequate maternal blood pressure and uteroplacental perfusion resulting from spinal anesthesia. It is proposed that a debate as to the optimal vasopressor for treatment of maternal hypotension is unnecessary. Provided the hypotension is transient, the choice of vasopressor should be determined by the clinical situation and consideration of not only the blood pressure, but also the heart rate.

▶ This editorial provides a nice review of the issues surrounding the choice of vasopressor for the treatment of hypotension during administration of regional anesthesia in obstetric patients. Laboratory studies suggest that ephedrine has a more favorable effect on uteroplacental perfusion than does phenylephrine. Further, ephedrine offers the advantages of familiarity, ease of administration, and a long history of safe use in obstetric patients. However, phenylephrine seems to be the preferred choice in parturients who are tachycardic or in whom tachycardia would be detrimental.

D. H. Chestnut, MD

Patients With Severe Preeclampsia Experience Less Hypotension During Spinal Anesthesia for Elective Cesarean Delivery Than Healthy Parturients: A Prospective Cohort Comparison
Aya AGM, Mangin R, Vialles N, et al (Univ Hosp, Nîmes, France)
Anesth Analg 97:867-872, 2003   11–28

Background.—Cesarean delivery under epidural anesthesia is usually performed when the patient is severely preeclamptic and there are no contraindications to the technique. Spinal anesthesia (SA) is avoided because of the risk of severe hypotension, but studies have indicated similar hemodynamic effects for spinal and epidural anesthesia. The hemodynamic effects of SA on patients with severe preeclampsia were compared with the effects on healthy women undergoing cesarean delivery.

Methods.—With the use of a prospective cohort design, the incidence and severity of SA-associated hypotension were evaluated in 30 severely preeclamptic and 30 healthy parturients who were having cesarean delivery. IV fluids were administered, then SA was performed using hyperbaric 0.5% bupivacaine, sufentanil, and morphine. Measurements of blood pressure (BP) were obtained before and every 2 minutes for 30 minutes after SA. The definition of a clinically significant hypotension was the need for ephedrine, which was prompted by systolic BP decline to less than 100 mm Hg in the healthy women or a 30% decline in the mean BP in either group of women.

Results.—The patients with severe preeclampsia tended to be nulliparous and to have pregnancies of younger gestational age than the healthy women. Effective anesthesia was achieved in both groups, permitting cesarean delivery. The preeclamptic group had higher baseline values of systolic and diastolic BP as well as mean BP, but all of the variables decreased significantly in both groups after the spinal block was accomplished. The incidence of clinically relevant hypotension was 16.6% among the preeclamptic group and 53.3% among the normotensive group; thus, the risk for development of hypotension was nearly 6 times less for patients with severe preeclampsia than for patients in the normotensive group. Treatment with ephedrine alleviated symptoms such as nausea, vomiting, and dizziness during the time of hypotension.

The mean BP tended to decline to a greater extent among the normotensive women and was somewhat restored by the use of ephedrine. Among the preeclamptic women, the mean BP declined at a slower pace and remained significantly lower than the baseline level. A significant decline in BP occurred 8 minutes after the injection of the spinal anesthetic. Women with preeclampsia had a time to the nadir of mean BP of 17.0 minutes, while the control group had a time of 13.3 minutes.

Conclusion.—Significant hypotension requiring ephedrine treatment occurred less often among the severely preeclamptic women who had SA for a cesarean delivery than among the normotensive women having the same procedure. The hypotension risk was nearly 6 times greater for the normotensive than for the preeclamptic patients. The severely preeclamptic group also had a smaller decrease in mean BP compared with the controls. The sample size limits the ability to draw conclusions about the safety of the preload and the technique in severely preeclamptic patients or to evaluate the effect of hypotensive treatments on the incidence of significant hypotension. However, it suggests that the incidence and severity of spinal hypotension may be less for preeclamptic patients than was previously thought.

Prospective, Randomized Trial Comparing General With Spinal Anesthesia for Cesarean Delivery in Preeclamptic Patients With a Nonreassuring Fetal Heart Trace

Dyer RA, Els I, Farbas J, et al (Univ of Cape Town, South Africa)
Anesthesiology 99:561-569, 2003   11–29

Background.—Understanding the cardiovascular pathophysiology of severe preeclampsia induces caution in using regional anesthesia in preeclamptic patients because of the possibility of development of hypotension, decreased cardiac output, and placental hypoperfusion. Use of spinal anesthesia (SA) for elective cesarean delivery has been linked to less favorable early markers of neonatal compromise compared with those for general anesthesia. To determine whether the mode of anesthesia influences markers of neonatal hypoxia, patients with preeclampsia and a nonreassuring fetal heart trace were given either spinal or general anesthesia for cesarean delivery and the results were compared.

Methods.—Thirty-five patients received general anesthesia with thiopentone, magnesium sulfate, and suxamethonium IV before intubation, then 50% nitrous oxide in oxygen, 0.75% to 1.5% isoflurane, and morphine after delivery; 35 received SA with 1.8 mL hyperbaric bupivacaine plus 10 µg fentanyl at the L3-L4 interspace. Measures included heart rate and blood pressure (BP); ephedrine was given for hypotension. At delivery, maternal arterial and neonatal umbilical arterial blood gas samples were obtained, and any need for resuscitation was documented.

Results.—One stillbirth and 1 case of sudden infant death syndrome occurred. Before anesthetic induction, the SA group received significantly more fluid. The time from induction to skin incision and that from induction to uterine incision was longer for the SA group. Patients receiving general anesthesia had significantly greater blood loss, but no transfusions were needed. The general anesthesia patients had arterial carbon dioxide tension values controlled at 32.4 mm Hg, while the SA group's value was 28.9 mm Hg.

A significantly higher mean base deficit was found in the SA than in the general anesthesia group (7.13 vs 4.68 mEq/L). Significantly lower median umbilical arterial pH and mean standard bicarbonate values were noted in the SA group (7.20 and 18.4 mEq/L, respectively) compared to the general anesthesia group (7.23 and 20.4 mEq/L, respectively). Although the median 1-minute Apgar scores were significantly lower for infants of mothers receiving general anesthesia, 5-minute Apgar scores did not differ significantly, nor was Apgar score linked to neonatal umbilical arterial base deficit values.

The SA group had significantly lower heart rate and systolic, diastolic, and mean BP values at various points, but no significant correlations were found between neonatal base deficit and duration of time at over 25% below baseline mean arterial BP or the absolute changes in mean arterial pressure. In addition, no significant between-group difference was found for duration of time spent at BPs 25% of baseline. Although women receiving SA required ephedrine more than those receiving general anesthesia, neither group showed a correlation between ephedrine use and neonatal base deficit.

Conclusion.—A significantly greater mean umbilical arterial base deficit and lower median umbilical arterial pH were found in the neonates of mothers given general anesthesia than those whose mothers received SA. General anesthesia was also associated with a lower 1-minute Apgar score. Both techniques produced similar and acceptable maternal hemodynamic profiles. The clinical significance of these findings remains unexplored.

▶ In the past, some obstetric anesthesiologists have argued that the presence of severe preeclampsia contraindicates the administration of SA, for 2 reasons: (1) SA results in an abrupt onset of sympathetic blockade, which may precipitate severe hypotension in preeclamptic women with a contracted intravascular volume; and (2) hypotension is not well tolerated in patients with preexisting uteroplacental insufficiency. During the last decade, several investigators have reevaluated the historical proscription against the use of SA in women with severe preeclampsia. However, published studies have been small and have excluded women with nonreassuring fetal heart rate tracings.

These 2 studies provide important new information regarding the administration of SA in preeclamptic women. In a prospective cohort study, Aya et al (Abstract 11–28) observed that the risk of hypotension was almost 6 times less in severely preeclamptic women than in healthy parturients receiving spinal anesthesia for elective cesarean section.

Dyer et al (Abstract 11–29) performed the first prospective, randomized study of spinal versus general anesthesia for cesarean section in preeclamptic women with a nonreassuring fetal heart rate tracing. Almost half of the study subjects had mild preeclampsia; the mean preinduction diastolic BP was 97 mm Hg in the SA group. The mean umbilical arterial blood base deficit was greater (7.13 vs 4.68 mEq/L) and the mean umbilical arterial blood pH was lower (7.20 vs 7.23) after SA than after general anesthesia. These modest differences are similar to the differences observed in healthy patients receiving either spinal or general anesthesia for cesarean section.

Further, there was no difference between groups in the number of infants with Apgar scores less than 7 or umbilical arterial blood pH less than 7.20. However, in a post hoc analysis of study subjects with severe preeclampsia (ie, diastolic BP greater than 110 mm Hg), the authors observed a significantly higher base deficit among neonates whose mothers received SA than among those exposed to general anesthesia.

When time allows, it seems intuitive that incremental administration of epidural anesthesia may be preferable to single-shot SA in women with severe preeclampsia. However, SA may be a better choice in cases of urgent—but not stat—cesarean section. In this circumstance, SA offers the advantages of rapid onset, reliability, and the ability to avoid general anesthesia, with its attendant risk of airway complications.

D. H. Chestnut, MD

Low Complication Rate Associated With Cesarean Section Under Spinal Anesthesia for HIV-1–Infected Women on Antiretroviral Therapy
Avidan MS, Groves P, Blott M, et al (Washington Univ, St Louis; King's College, London; Chelsea and Westminster Hosp NHS Trust, London)
Anesthesiology 97:320-324, 2002   11–30

Background.—An estimated 36 million individuals throughout the world are infected with HIV, which is thought to have killed approximately 20 million individuals thus far. The HIV infection is still spreading, and the most rapid increases are occurring in southern and central Africa and in South Asia. Heterosexual sex is the predominant mode of HIV transmission, and women represent a high proportion of new infections, including those in developed countries. The likelihood of vertical HIV transmission is reduced by elective cesarean section. Whether cesarean section performed with spinal anesthesia on HIV-1–infected pregnant women taking antiretroviral therapy is associated with intraoperative hemodynamic instability, postoperative complications, or changes in immune functioning or HIV-1 viral loads was determined.

Methods.—This 3-year case–control study was conducted in a London academic hospital. The study population included a group of 44 women infected with HIV-1 and a control group of 45 HIV-negative women undergoing cesarean section. The main outcome measures were intraoperative blood pressure, heart rate, blood loss, and ephedrine requirements and postoperative infective complications, blood transfusions, changes in blood HIV-1 viral loads and lymphocyte subsets, and time to hospital discharge.

Results.—No differences were found between the 2 groups in hemodynamic stability and postoperative complications. An acute postoperative increase in the CD4 T-lymphocyte count was found, but no changes in the CD4 T-cell:CD8 T-cell ratio and viral load occurred.

Conclusions.—These findings indicate that elective cesarean section under spinal anesthesia can be safely performed in women taking antiretroviral medication for HIV-1 infection. In this study, this procedure was not associated with intraoperative or postoperative complications.

▶ CNS involvement occurs early in the course of HIV infection. This study suggests that the administration of spinal anesthesia for elective cesarean section is safe in HIV-infected women who are taking antiretroviral therapy, provided that there are no contraindications to the administration of regional anesthesia.

D. H. Chestnut, MD

A Randomized, Controlled Trial to Compare Ketorolac Tromethamine Versus Placebo After Cesarean Section to Reduce Pain and Narcotic Usage
Lowder JL, Shackelford DP, Holbert D, et al (East Carolina Univ, Greenville, NC)
Am J Obstet Gynecol 189:1559-1562, 2003   11–31

Background.—Nonsteroidal anti-inflammatory drugs are usually given orally or rectally and so cannot be used in the immediate postoperative period for pain relief. Ketorolac tromethamine is a nonsteroidal anti-inflammatory that acts by inhibiting prostaglandin synthetase and can be administered IV, intramuscularly, or orally. This randomized, double-blind, placebo-controlled trial examined the efficacy of postcesarean administration of ketorolac tromethamine.

Methods.—The study group consisted of 44 patients undergoing cesarean section who were randomly assigned to either ketorolac or placebo immediately after the procedure. All patients received opioid patient-controlled analgesia. Pain control was evaluated hourly for the first 4 hours and then at 6, 12, and 24 hours by visual analog scales. Outcomes included visual analog scale scores, patient-controlled analgesia, time to discharge, and hematocrit levels.

Findings.—There were no demographic differences between these 2 treatment groups. The use of postoperative analgesics was significantly reduced at 2, 3, 4, 6, 12, and 24 hours in the ketorolac group. Despite using less narcotics, pain scores were also reduced in the ketorolac group compared with the placebo group.

Conclusions.—Postoperative ketorolac significantly reduces pain and narcotic use in patients after cesarean section.

▶ The manufacturer of ketorolac has stated that ketorolac is contraindicated in nursing mothers because of the possible adverse effects of prostaglandin synthetase inhibitors in neonates. In contrast, the American Academy of Pediatrics considers the use of ketorolac to be compatible with breastfeeding.[1]

D. H. Chestnut, MD

Reference

1. American Academy of Pediatrics Committee on Drugs: The transfer of drugs and other chemicals into human milk. *Pediatrics* 108:776-789, 2001.

Special Situations in Obstetric Anesthesia

Management of a Parturient With a History of Local Anesthetic Allergy
Balestrieri PJ, Ferguson JE II (Univ of Virginia, Charlottesville)
Anesth Analg 96:1489-1490, 2003   11–32

Introduction.—Adverse reactions to local anesthetics are rare, and most cases involve sensitivity to paraben or sulfite preservatives. The case reported here illustrates some of the problems encountered when a parturient has an allergy to local anesthetics. Recommendations on the optimal timing and nature of provocative testing are presented.

> *Case Report.*—Woman, 35, gravida 3, was seen for evaluation at 36 weeks of gestation. Important medical history items included mitral valve prolapse, pericarditis, deep vein thrombosis, and reported allergy to local anesthetics. During her first pregnancy, the patient reported poor labor pain relief after receiving a combined spinal epidural with 15 μg of intrathecal sufentanil and boluses of epidural fentanyl 50 to 100 μg. Provocative challenge with preservative-free (PF) bupivacaine was conducted when the patient returned to labor and delivery at 38 weeks' gestation. An obstetric team was on standby if emergency cesarean delivery was required. Subcutaneous injections of PF 0.25% bupivacaine were administered beginning with 0.1 mL and followed by 0.5, 1.0, and 2.0 mL doses. When no clinical signs were observed 15 minutes after each injection, labor was induced and PF bupivacaine was included as a local anesthetic. The patient had excellent pain relief.

Discussion.—The patient reported here had an unsatisfactory experience with neuraxial opioids alone for labor and a history of local anesthetic hypersensitivity. Because the safety and utility of provocative challenge testing is well established, a decision was made to test bupivacaine. The timing selected, at labor and delivery, allows emergent cesarean delivery to be performed if a serious reaction occurs.

▶ Allergy to local anesthetic agents—especially the amide agents typically used in clinical practice—is rare. Further, anaphylactic and anaphylactoid reactions may be the result of exposure to additives such as methylparaben or metabisulfite. This case report outlines one approach to the parturient with a history of local anesthetic allergy.

D. H. Chestnut, MD

Subarachnoid Small-Dose Bupivacaine Versus Lidocaine for Cervical Cerclage

Beilin Y, Zahn J, Abramovitz S, et al (New York Univ; Cornell Univ, New York)
Anesth Analg 97:56-61, 2003   11–33

Introduction.—Cervical cerclage is a brief ambulatory surgical procedure often performed under a subarachnoid anesthetic. Lidocaine is frequently used as the local anesthetic, yet its association with transient neurologic symptoms (TNS) has led alternative agents to be considered. In a randomized double-blind study, lidocaine and bupivacaine were compared for efficacy and safety in cervical cerclage.

TABLE 2.—Outcome Variables and Complications

Variable	Bupivacaine Group	Lidocaine Group	P Value
n	30	29	
Complete analgesia at start of surgery	29/30 (97%)	29/29 (100%)	NS
Highest sensory dermatome level (R)	T7 (T1 to T12)	T6 (T2 to T11)	0.31
Highest sensory dermatome level (L)	T7 (T1 to T10)	T6 (T2 to T11)	0.19
Time until peak level (min)	9 (3-21)	6 (3-30)	0.15
Duration of procedure (min)	15 (5-130)	17.5 (8-71)	NS
Time until Bromage score of 0 (min)	56 (15-150)	75 (30-150)	0.04
Time until T12 regression (min)	90 (45-150)	90 (30-120)	0.51
Time until ambulation (min)	117 (45-225)	117 (45-203)	0.72
Time until micturition (min)	164 (45-327)	133 (45-203)	0.12
Nausea	3/27 (3 mild)	5/26 (3 mild, 2 severe)	NS
Vomiting	1	1	NS
Pruritus	15/27 (56%)	16/26 (62%)	NS
Mild	12/15	14/16	
Moderate	2/15	2/16	
Severe	1/15	0/16	
Hypotension	3/30 (10%)	2/29 (7%)	NS
Ephedrine	1/30 (3%)	0/29	NS
Symptoms of TNS	0/29	2/29 (7%)	NS
Headache	0/27	1/23 (4%)	NS

All data are median and range or % if indicated.
Abbreviations: NS, Not significant; *R*, right; *L*, left.
(Courtesy of Beilin Y, Zahn J, Abramovitz S, et al: Subarachnoid small-dose bupivacaine versus lidocaine for cervical cerclage. *Anesth Analg* 97:56-61, 2003).

Methods.—The 59 women who participated in the study were scheduled to undergo elective cervical cerclage during the first or second trimester of pregnancy. Women received either 2 mL of lidocaine 1.5% (30 mg) with fentanyl 20 µg and 0.6 mL of 0.9% saline or 0.7 mL of bupivacaine 0.75% (5.25 mg) in dextrose 8.25% with fentanyl 20 µg and 1.9 mL of 0.9% saline. Outcomes recorded included the onset and highest dermatomal level of sensory block; quality of anesthesia; hypotension; and times until T12 regression, return of lower extremity motor function, ambulation, and micturition. Patients were telephoned 24 hours after surgery for reports of TNS.

Results.—Women in the 2 groups were similar in demographic data. All had at least a T12 dermatomal level of sensory anesthesia before onset of the procedure. Only 1 patient (in the bupivacaine group) rated analgesia as incomplete at this time, and another woman in this group required additional epidural medication during the procedure. The only difference in recovery times was a longer duration until the return of lower extremity motor strength in the lidocaine group. Two women in the lidocaine group reported symptoms consistent with TNS, but these symptoms resolved spontaneously with 48 hours. Other side effects were similar (Table 2) in the 2 groups.

Conclusion.—A small dose of subarachnoid bupivacaine with fentanyl provides reliable anesthesia for patients undergoing cervical cerclage. The pharmacodynamic profiles of bupivacaine and lidocaine are similar, and bupivacaine reduces the concerns about TNS associated with lidocaine.

▶ Most anesthesiologists consider spinal anesthesia to be the anesthetic technique of choice in patients undergoing elective cervical cerclage. In the past, lidocaine was the preferred local anesthetic agent because of its short duration of action. However, many anesthesiologists are now reluctant to give spinal lidocaine because of its association with TNS. In this study, spinal administration of bupivacaine 5.25 mg with fentanyl 20 μg was not associated with a significant delay in recovery from anesthesia when compared with spinal lidocaine 30 mg with fentanyl 20 μg. Thus, small-dose spinal bupivacaine seems to be a reasonable alternative to spinal lidocaine in patients undergoing elective cervical cerclage.

D. H. Chestnut, MD

The Direct Depressant Effects of Desflurane and Sevoflurane on Spontaneous Contractions of Isolated Gravid Rat Myometrium
Dogru K, Dalgic H, Yildiz K, et al (Erciyes Univ, Kayseri, Turkey)
Int J Obstet Anesth 12:74-78, 2003   11–34

Introduction.—Both desflurane and sevoflurane are used for obstetric anesthesia, and desflurane has been administered safely for analgesia during vaginal delivery. Experimental studies indicate that these agents can inhibit myometrial contractions. The direct depressant effects of desflurane and sevoflurane on spontaneous contractions of isolated gravid rat myometrium were investigated.

Methods.—Sixty myometrial strips were obtained from 10 gravid, albino Wistar rats killed before the onset of labor. The strips were subjected to a resting tension of 1 g (found to be optimal in previous studies) throughout all experiments. Baseline spontaneous contractions were recorded for 45 minutes, then the strips were washed with bath solution and exposed to 0.5, 1, or 2 minimum alveolar concentrations (MAC) of desflurane or sevoflurane for 15 minutes. Effects of the anesthetic agents were expressed as means ± SD and percent change in duration, amplitude, and frequency of myometrial contractions.

Results.—Desflurane 0.5 MAC had no effect on the duration or amplitude of spontaneous contractions, but their frequency significantly decreased. All 3 measures were significantly decreased by both desflurane 1 and 2 MAC. Sevoflurane at 0.5 MAC had no effect, but 1 MAC significantly decreased amplitude and frequency and 2 MAC significantly decreased all 3 measures. The frequency of contractions was decreased to a greater extent with 1 MAC desflurane (21.2%) than with 1 MAC sevoflurane (17.1%). At 2 MAC, the amplitude and frequency of contractions were decreased 48.2% and 48.7%, respectively, with desflurane, and 58.9% and 49.3%, respectively, with sevoflurane.

Conclusion.—Both 1 and 2 MAC of desflurane and sevoflurane decrease, to a similar degree, spontaneous contractions of isolated rat myometrium. Both agents have been used in patients undergoing cesarean section, and both could be useful in nonobstetric surgery during pregnancy because of their tocolytic activity.

The In-Vitro Effects of Sevoflurane and Desflurane on the Contractility of Pregnant Human Uterine Muscle
Turner RJ, Lambros M, Kenway L, et al (Prince of Wales Hosp, Randwick, NSW, Australia)
Int J Obstet Anesth 11:246-251, 2002   11–35

Introduction.—Sevoflurane and desflurane are widely used in obstetric practice, yet the influence of these agents on pregnant human uterine muscle contractility has not been established. Strips of human myometrium obtained at elective cesarean section were examined to determine the effect of sevoflurane and desflurane on the contractility of the uterine muscle.

Methods.—Uterine muscle biopsies were obtained from 12 nonlaboring term parturients undergoing routine elective cesarean section. Small strips of muscle were prepared and suspended in an organ bath containing oxygenated physiologic saline. Myometrial strips were exposed to varying concentrations of either sevoflurane or desflurane in concentrations corresponding to 0.5, 1.0, or 1.5 minimum alveolar concentration (MAC). An isometric tension transducer was used to record force of contraction continuously.

Results.—Baseline measurements were obtained after the onset of regular spontaneous contractions. Exposure to both sevoflurane and desflurane depressed contractility of the myometrial strips in a dose-dependent manner, effects that were statistically significant compared with control. Sevoflurane depressed contractility to a mean of 72% of control at 0.5 MAC, 37% at 1.0 MAC, and 27% at 1.5 MAC. Corresponding values for desflurane were 65%, 43%, and 22%. At all concentrations, the degree of depression of uterine muscle contractility produced by both sevoflurane and desflurane was significantly different from control.

Conclusion.—Both desflurane and sevoflurane were found to depress the contractility of gravid human myometrium, particularly at concentrations of 1.0 MAC or greater. The effects on contractility were similar for both agents, and both may be appropriate choices if rapid uterine relaxation is required.

▶ In some cases of obstetric emergency, the anesthesiologist is asked to facilitate uterine relaxation. Those situations include cases of fetal head entrapment, delivery of a second twin, uterine inversion, and retained placenta. Also, uterine relaxation is needed during intrauterine fetal surgery. Some anesthesiologists advocate the administration of nitroglycerin for this purpose. However, nitroglycerin does not provide anesthesia, and controversy exists regarding the efficacy of nitroglycerin as a tocolytic agent. Thus, in some patients it is necessary for the anesthesiologist to perform a rapid-sequence induction of general anesthesia, secure the airway, and administer a volatile halogenated agent. These 2 studies (Abstracts 11–34 and 11–35) suggest that administration of either sevoflurane or desflurane results in uterine smooth muscle relaxation similar to that observed after administration of the older volatile halogenated agents (eg, halothane, enflurane, isoflurane).

D. H. Chestnut, MD

Nitroglycerin for Fetal Surgery: Fetoscopy and Ex Utero Intrapartum Treatment Procedure With Malignant Hyperthermia Precautions

Rosen MA, Andreae MH, Cameron AG (Univ of California, San Francisco)
Anesth Analg 96:698-700, 2003   11–36

Introduction.—Anesthesia for hysterotomy and fetal intervention presents unique challenges related to providing care and monitoring both mother and fetus and avoiding intraoperative or postoperative preterm labor. In the case reported, a patient with a family history of malignant hyperthermia (MH) was managed successfully with IV nitroglycerin to avoid the use of volatile anesthetics.

Case Report.—Woman, 21, was referred at 25 weeks' gestation because the fetus had severe left congenital diaphragmatic hernia with liver herniation into the hemithorax. No other anomalies were present, and the fetus had a normal karyotype. The patient was considered potentially at risk for MH, but susceptibility testing could not be performed in time for surgery. Anesthetic gases, as triggering drugs for MH, were contraindicated. Laparotomy for fetoscopy and fetal tracheal occlusion was performed under epidural anesthesia. Continued postoperative tocolysis was provided by IV magnesium sulfate and terbutaline. Cesarean delivery and a fetal ex utero intrapartum treatment were performed under general anesthesia after 31 weeks and 3 days of gestation. Large-dose nitroglycerin was able to achieve adequate uterine relaxation. The mother's recovery was uneventful. After surgical repair of the diaphragmatic hernia with a trigger-free anesthetic, the infant was discharged home with a normal neurologic examination at age 2 months.

Discussion.—Volatile anesthetics, the most potent for intraoperative uterine relaxation, may trigger MH. In this patient, a regional technique without volatile gases was thus chosen for the fetoscopy and tracheal balloon placement. If increased uterine tone occurred during fetoscopy, IV boluses of nitroglycerin would have provided adequate tocolysis. And large-dose nitroglycerin, with the advantage of a short duration of action, achieved satisfactory uterine relaxation during the procedure, also performed without volatile anesthetics.

▶ This case report suggests that the anesthesiologist may give nitroglycerin rather than a volatile halogenated agent to facilitate uterine relaxation during intrauterine fetal surgery.

D. H. Chestnut, MD

Sublingual Nitroglycerin Versus Placebo as a Tocolytic for External Cephalic Version: A Randomized Controlled Trial in Parous Women

Bujold E, Boucher M, Rinfret D, et al (Univ of Montreal; Wayne State Univ, Detroit; Children's and Women's Health Centre of British Columbia)
Am J Obstet Gynecol 189:1070-1073, 2003   11–37

Introduction.—External cephalic version (ECV) is a safe and effective approach for reducing the rate of cesarean deliveries performed for breech presentation at term. Due to its ease of administration and rapid onset of action (2-4 minutes), sublingual nitroglycerin has been proposed as a tocolytic agent in ECV. The efficacy of sublingual nitroglycerin as a tocolytic agent for ECV was assessed in parous women in a double-blind, randomized investigation.

Methods.—Included were patients with parity of 1 or greater and at 36 to 40 weeks' gestation who were eligible for ECV between April 1999 and August 2002. Patients were randomly assigned to treatment with a sublingual spray of either 400 μg of nitroglycerin or 2 sprays of a placebo 3 minutes before the trial of ECV. Success rates of ECV and side effects were compared.

Results.—Of 99 patients evaluated, 50 received sublingual nitroglycerin, and 49 received placebo. There were no between-group differences in maternal age, estimated fetal weight, amniotic fluid index, or placental location between the 2 groups. Successful ECV was possible in 48% of the nitroglycerin group and 63% of the placebo group ($P = .13$). The nitroglycerin group had a higher rate of headache (42% vs 4%; $P < .001$).

Conclusion.—Sublingual nitroglycerin was linked to a higher incidence of headache and did not improve the success rate of ECV.

▶ This study suggests that sublingual nitroglycerin does not improve the rate of successful ECV.

D. H. Chestnut, MD

Epidural Anesthesia in Three Parturients With Lumbar Tattoos: A Review of Possible Implications

Douglas MJ, Swenerton JE (BC Women's Hosp, Vancouver, British Columbia, Canada)
Can J Anesth 49:1057-1060, 2002   11–38

Background.—Tattooing and body piercing are increasingly popular among youths. In the past, women tended to get their tattoos in areas remote from their backs, but this is no longer the case. The lumbar midline area has become a popular location for tattoos among young women. However, tattooing in this area can create problems if these young women later request epidural anesthesia for labor. In this report, 3 women requested epidural anesthesia for labor and were found to have tattoos on their lower backs. The possible implications of epidural anesthesia in women with lumbar tattoos are discussed.

Case Report.—The first woman was seen with a tattoo that covered the midline from approximately T12 to S1 and extended to either side of the midline for approximately 1 to 2 cm. Fortunately, a pigment-free area was located underneath 1 area of the tattoo at the level of L2-3. The epidural was inserted successfully at that location with the use of a paramedian approach. She then received a second epidural for labor, which avoided the tattoo. The second woman was seen with a tattoo that completely covered her back, extending to the midaxillary line bilaterally. No pigment-free area could be found. The epidural was placed through the tattoo because labor was painful and prolonged. This patient ultimately required a cesarean section. The third patient had a butterfly tattoo that was midline and extended 2 cm to each side. Fortunately, this was located over the L4-5 interspace, which left the L2-3 and L3-4 interspaces available. The epidural was successfully inserted at L2-3.

Discussion.—A search of the literature on tattoos and on coring with neuraxial anesthesia found that coring is a complication of neuraxial anesthesia that may result in epidermoid tumors in the subarachnoid space. In theory, a pigment-containing tissue core from a tattoo could be deposited into the epidural, subdural, or subarachnoid space, which could result in neurologic complications in the future.

Conclusions.—The possible implications of needle insertion for neuraxial anesthesia in women with lumbar tattoos are discussed. To date, there have been no reports in the literature of possible risks in this setting.

▶ The epidural needle was inserted through a tattoo in only 1 of these 3 patients. The authors implied that no complications occurred. This report neither establishes the safety nor confirms the hazards of regional anesthesia in patients with tattoos. However, the authors have nicely reviewed the possible risks associated with regional anesthesia in women with tattoos.

D. H. Chestnut, MD

Complications in Obstetrics and Obstetrics Anesthesia

Anaphylactoid Reaction to Hydroxyethylstarch During Cesarean Delivery in a Patient With HELLP Syndrome
Vercauteren MP, Coppejans HC, Sermeus L (Univ Hosp Antwerp, Edegem, Belgium)
Anesth Analg 96:859-861, 2003   11–39

Introduction.—Colloids are reported to be potentially superior to crystalloids for hydration before spinal anesthesia for cesarean delivery. Colloids increase the circulating blood volume while preserving the oncotic pressure, but some patients may have allergic reactions. In the case reported here, pentastarch caused an allergic reaction during cesarean delivery.

Case Report.—Nulliparous woman, 28, was admitted with worsening preeclampsia at 28 weeks' gestation. When several days of treatment failed to lower the patient's blood pressure, a semiurgent cesarean delivery was scheduled. Within the first minute after administration of less than 20 mL of a 6% pentastarch infusion, the patient had moderate bronchospasm, erythema, perifascial edema, and hypotension. Blood pressure gradually decreased to 100/77 mm Hg and oxygen saturation to 90%. Treatment included oxygen 5 L/min by face mask, ephedrine (total dose, 40 mg), ranitidine, transexaminic acid, promethazine, and aminophylline. Because the fetal condition was stable, a decision was made to delay surgery. The patient's condition improved, with liver function tests and platelet count better than before the attempted surgery. Cesarean delivery was performed successfully the next day, and both mother and infant recovered uneventfully.

Discussion.—Anaphylaxis can occur in a parturient receiving colloids at the time of cesarean delivery. Such an event presents the anesthesiologist with a serious dilemma. In this case, surgical delivery could be postponed because the fetus was stable.

▶ Most anesthesiologists typically give a bolus of crystalloid (eg, 1000 mL of Ringer's lactate) to increase intravascular volume and decrease the likelihood of maternal hypotension during administration of regional anesthesia for cesarean section. Recent studies have suggested that prophylactic crystalloid results in only a modest decrease in the incidence of maternal hypotension. Some anesthesiologists have suggested the use of colloid rather than crystalloid. This case report illustrates one disadvantage of colloid, namely, the risk of anaphylaxis. Other disadvantages of colloid include its increased cost as well as the risk of postpartum pulmonary edema in high-risk parturients (eg, women with severe preeclampsia or heart disease). In my judgment, prophylactic crystalloid remains preferable to prophylactic colloid in obstetric anesthesia practice.

D. H. Chestnut, MD

Intrathecal Morphine Overdose During Combined Spinal–Epidural Block for Caesarean Delivery
Cannesson M, Nargues N, Bryssine B, et al (Hôpital de l'Hôtel-Dieu, Lyon, France)
Br J Anaesth 89:925-927, 2002   11–40

Background.—The combined spinal–epidural block has gained popularity since its introduction in 1981 as a regional technique for cesarean delivery. Opioids associated with hyperbaric 0.5% bupivacaine (2.5 mL or 12.5 mg) are commonly selected for subarachnoid administration because they provide rapid and profound analgesia. In addition, the epidural block is used to extend spinal analgesia and to treat postoperative pain. Intrathecal morphine overdoses have occasionally been reported; however, most of them were reported in patients who were exposed to these drugs on a long-term basis and for whom tolerance levels were well known. A few reports have described the perioperative course of an intrathecal opioid overdose in patients undergoing orthopedic surgery and in whom CSF removal or mechanical ventilation or both were performed. A woman was successfully treated for an intrathecal 25-mg morphine overdose that did not require these invasive procedures during a combined spinal–epidural block for a cesarean delivery.

> *Case Report.*—A healthy 31-year-old gravida 7, para 4 woman was seen at 39 weeks' gestation (156 cm and 75 kg) with a singleton pregnancy. The woman's prenatal course was uncomplicated, and she was scheduled for an elective cesarean delivery because of a contracted pelvis. She had previously undergone 4 cesarean sections under spinal anesthesia. The anesthetist injected 30 μg fentanyl and 2.5 mL of what was thought to be sterile hyperbaric 0.5% bupivacaine through the spinal needle. However, the solution was identified as 10 mg/mL morphine immediately after the injection. Thus, the patient received 25 mg morphine intrathecally instead of bupivacaine. At 15 minutes, the patient reported no change in temperature sensation and had no motor block. The epidural block was performed, and the patient was immediately placed in the supine position. Her respiratory rate was 12 to 14 breaths per minute and she was hemodynamically stable. An IV naloxone infusion at 80 μg/h was initiated after a loading dose of 0.4 mg. A healthy 3800-g boy with Apgar scores of 9 and 10 at 1 and 5 minutes, respectively, was delivered. The plasma morphine level was measured in the baby immediately after delivery and in the mother at 15 minutes after the injection and 4, 8, 12, 16, 20, and 24 hours after the event. The patient was admitted to intensive care 6 hours after the cesarean procedure. Naloxone was discontinued at 24 hours after its introduction. She received a total of 5.24 mg IV naloxone over the 24-hour period.

Conclusions.—Accidental massive overdose of opioids have been reported in a variety of settings. In this case, naloxone infusion was begun before the patient became symptomatic and almost immediately after the morphine injection. However, in massive intrathecal morphine overdoses (250 mg or greater), it is important to consider more invasive treatments.

▶ The typical dose of intrathecal morphine (administered for postcesarean analgesia) is 0.1 to 0.2 mg. Incredibly, this patient received a more than 100-fold overdose of intrathecal morphine.

D. H. Chestnut, MD

Epidural Blood Patch Placed in the Presence of an Unknown Cervical Epidural Hematoma

Castillo D, Tsen LC (Harvard Med School, Boston)
Anesth Analg 97:885-887, 2003   11–41

Background.—Among the differential diagnoses for postdural puncture headaches (PDPH) is cervical epidural hematoma (CEH), for which urgent decompression may be needed. PDPH is generally treated with an epidural blood patch (EBP), which achieves compression of the dural sac. A case of PDPH treated with an EBP is reported in a patient found to have a preexisting CEH.

Case Report.—Woman, 31, with an uncomplicated term singleton first gestation was admitted to the hospital for labor and delivery. Mild hypertension, migraines, and chronic neck and upper back discomfort were being treated by a chiropractor with the diagnosis of cervical misalignment. As active labor commenced, the patient had an epidural catheter placed while she was in the sitting position. The epidural needle was initially placed incorrectly, as demonstrated by aspiration of blood once an epidural catheter was threaded. Successful placement at L4-L5 was finally confirmed, with the catheter located 5 cm into the epidural space.

The patient was administered 12 mL of bupivacaine, 0.25%, in divided doses through the epidural catheter to achieve analgesia, then given an infusion of bupivacaine, 0.125%, and fentanyl, 2 µg/mL at a rate of 10 mL/h. She had an uncomplicated and comfortable vaginal delivery. After delivery, she noted occipital cephalgia and neck pain but believed these symptoms resulted from accentuated head flexion during delivery. The following day the patient sought relief for increased neck discomfort, which was diagnosed as musculoskeletal and treated with ibuprofen 600 mg q 4-6 h prn and a soft collar.

Neck pain grew worse and was accompanied by severe postural frontal and occipital headache as well as mild right arm paresthesias when the patient was in the upright position. A cervical spine MRI showed no obvious pathologic conditions, and the patient was presumptively diagnosed with PDPH, for which an EBP was attempted. The first attempt found the L5-S1 epidural space. The 40 mL of autologous blood given was based on the appearance of back pressure, primarily in the cervical area.

The patient reported significant improvement in the headache and absence of the arm paresthesias when placed upright. Final cervical MRI results identified an epidural collection from C2–4 levels without cord compression. The nonsteroidal antiinflammatory drugs were discontinued, coagulation studies performed, and a neurosurgery consultation obtained. The patient was closely observed for 2 days, then discharged with baseline neck symptoms only. No change in these symptoms occurred over the succeeding 6 months.

Conclusion.—The EBP treatment successfully dealt with the problems of this patient in the presence of a CEH. The case supports the importance of using a spinal needle for epidural space confirmation and of waiting for final consultation and radiologic imaging results before proceeding, when possible.

▶ This patient apparently had a spontaneous CEH, without neurologic compromise. One of my colleagues recently provided care for a pregnant woman with a spontaneous thoracic epidural hematoma. The diagnosis was made after the abrupt onset of lower extremity paralysis before the onset of labor. This latter patient had not received either spinal or epidural anesthesia.

D. H. Chestnut, MD

Sodium Bisulfite: Scapegoat for Chloroprocaine Neurotoxicity?
Taniguchi M, Bollen AW, Drasner K (San Francisco Gen Hosp)
Anesthesiology 100:85-91, 2004   11–42

Background.—Chloroprocaine is an ester anesthetic that was used for epidural anesthesia. In the early 1980s, however, it was almost abandoned after reports of neurologic injury associated with use of Nesacaine-CE, a chloroprocaine solution containing sodium bisulfite. A rat model of intrathecal neurotoxicity was used to assess whether the chloroprocaine or the bisulfite was responsible for the neurotoxicity.

Methods.—In the first experiment male rats received either chloroprocaine with or without bisulfite or saline intrathecally. In the second experiment they received freshly prepared solutions of chloroprocaine, chloroprocaine plus sodium bisulfite, and sodium bisulfite and saline. Sensory impairment was evaluated by the tail flick test after 7 days. Histologic specimens were used to quantify nerve injury.

Results.—In the first experiment, tail flick latencies and nerve injury scores were significantly greater after administration of chloroprocaine than saline and were significantly greater in rats that received chloroprocaine alone than in those that also received bisulfite. In the second experiment, rats that received fresh chloroprocaine had the highest levels of neurotoxicity of all 4 groups. Tail flick scores of mice injected with bisulfite were similar to those injected with saline.

Conclusions.—In a rat model of intrathecal neurotoxicity, intrathecal administration of chloroprocaine induced significant neurotoxicity whereas administration of bisulfite did not. In fact, inclusion of bisulfite with chloroprocaine appeared to reduce neurotoxicity. This suggests that neurotoxicity after inadvertent intrathecal injection of Nesacaine-CE was caused by the anesthetic, not the preservative.

▶ This laboratory study suggests that neurologic deficits that have followed the apparent unintentional intrathecal injection of epidural doses of 2-chloroprocaine resulted from a direct effect of the local anesthetic and not the sodium bisulfite.

D. H. Chestnut, MD

Incidence, Treatment and Outcome of Peripartum Sepsis
Kankuri E, Kurki T, Carlson P, et al (Helsinki Univ)
Acta Obstet Gynecol Scand 82:730-735, 2003   11–43

Introduction.—Maternal sepsis is an important clinical problem responsible for up to 8% of maternal deaths and 15% of admissions to ICUs. Only limited data are available concerning the clinical outcome and causative microbes in peripartum sepsis. Maternal outcome and the clinical, microbiological, and laboratory findings in peripartum sepsis (7 days before to 7 days after delivery) were examined retrospectively to determine possible risk factors, optimal treatment, and outcome.

Methods.—The electronic database of the only tertiary referral center for the most complicated pregnancies in Helsinki, Finland was searched for delivery data from May 1990 to October 1998 for blood culture reports and ICD-9 and ICD-10 coded diagnoses of all obstetric infections. All blood culture results, hospital records, and records of ICD-9 and ICD-10 diagnoses of infection were reviewed. Of 43,483 deliveries between 1990 and 1998, laboratory-confirmed bacteremia was identified in 41 (5.1%) of 798 clinically suspected septic infections.

Results.—Preterm deliveries were linked with a crude 2.7-fold risk for peripartum sepsis compared with that of term deliveries. Antepartum sepsis was linked with a crude 2.6-fold risk for cesarean section. Postpartum sepsis was 3.2-fold more likely to occur after cesarean section versus vaginal delivery. Therapy involved a combination of cefuroxime and metronidazole in 80% (33/41) of patients. All mothers had a good recovery. One patient experienced septic shock. Forty-two bacterial strains involving 18 different bacterial species were isolated from blood cultures; 37 strains (88%) were aerobic and 5 (12%) were anaerobic. The most common species identified were betahemolytic streptococci, *Escherichia coli*, and *Staphylococcus aureus*. Most microbes were susceptible to first- or second-generation cephalosporins.

Conclusion.—Peripartum sepsis is linked with preterm pregnancies and cesarean sections. Treatment with second-generation cephalosporin is often effective and provides a good outcome.

▶ It is seemingly a rare occurrence, but when the septic parturient arrives at the ICU, tensions are high. Obstetricians and family members have a way of ratcheting up the anxiety level under these circumstances. Therefore, the intensivist should have some perspective regarding the occurrence, consequences, likely causes, and treatment approaches. This study went far to further define this. In the study, sepsis was associated with preterm labor and cesarean section. This study was conducted in Finland, and their preferences of antibiotics were cefuroxime and metronidazole for empirical antibiotic therapy. In the United States, that would probably differ, with ampicillin and gentamicin being the preferred empirical choice.

J. D. Lang, Jr, MD

12 Pain Management

Acute Pain Management

Effects of Preemptive Analgesia on Pain and Cytokine Production in the Postoperative Period

Beilin B, Bessler H, Mayburd E, et al (Tel-Aviv Univ, Israel; Hebrew Univ, Jerusalem)

Anesthesiology 98:151-155, 2003
12–1

Introduction.—Previous research by authors of the present study found patient-controlled epidural analgesia (PCEA) to be more effective than intermittent administration of systemic opiates or patient-controlled analgesia in the management of postoperative pain. Extending these findings, they examined the effects of preemptive PCEA on the production of proinflammatory cytokines and pain in the postoperative period.

Methods.—Study participants were 41 healthy women scheduled for transabdominal hysterectomy and randomly assigned to 1 of 2 perioperative pain management techniques. Twenty received PCEA in the postoperative period and 21 received preemptive epidural analgesia (PA) followed by PCEA (PA + PCEA). All patients underwent general anesthesia in a standardized manner and received bupivacaine plus fentanyl on demand, via the PCEA pump postoperatively. But 20 to 25 minutes before incision, PA + PCEA patients received an epidural mixture of 12 mL bupivacaine (0.5%) plus fentanyl (50-100 µg). Patients reported pain intensity by means of a visual analogue scale at 4, 8, 12, 24, 48, and 72 hours after surgery.

Results.—The 2 groups were similar in age, body weight, and duration of surgery, but differed significantly for visual analogue scale at rest or during coughing. Throughout the entire postoperative observation period, patients in the PA + PCEA group experienced less severe postoperative pain. The production of interleukin (IL)-1β, IL-6, IL-1ra, and IL10 was significantly less elevated and production of IL-2 significantly less suppressed in patients receiving preemptive analgesia.

Conclusion.—The production of inflammatory cytokines, known to amplify pain intensity, is increased in the postoperative period. When PA was administered in addition to postoperative PCEA, patients undergoing transabdominal hysterectomy exhibited reduced inflammatory cytokine production and experienced less postoperative pain than patients treated with post-operative PCEA only.

▶ There is increasing interest in and understanding of the role of pro-inflammatory cytokines in the generation of both acute and chronic pain. Hyperalgesia is mediated by the increased production and release of these substances following tissue or nerve injury and inflammation. This occurs in the periphery in mononuclear cells and in the CNS in microglia and astrocytes. This study is important in that it demonstrates a preemptive effect of regional anesthesia on both postoperative pain perception and levels of proinflammatory cytokines. A cause and effect relationship cannot be established but is likely. These data help explain the disappointing benefits of preemptive N-methyl-D-aspartate antagonists, which would block spinal sensitization induced through neuronal mechanisms but not through glial or peripheral activation of cytokines.

S. E. Abram, MD

A Single Infusion of Intravenous Ketamine Improves Pain Relief in Patients With Critical Limb Ischaemia: Results of a Double Blind Randomised Controlled Trial
Mitchell AC, Fallon MT (Western Infirmary, Glasgow, Scotland; Western Gen Hosp, Edinburgh, Scotland)
Pain 97:275-281, 2002   12–2

Background.—This study determined whether a combination of regular opioid analgesia and a single IV ketamine infusion could improve ischemia rest pain in patients with allodynia, hyperalgesia, and hyperpathia caused by critical limb ischemia.

Methods.—Thirty-five patients completed the double-blind randomized study. Seventeen patients received regular opioids plus placebo, and 18 received regular opioids plus an infusion of 0.6 mg/kg IV ketamine. The Brief Pain Inventory was used to assess levels of pain.

Findings.—The proportion of pain relief attributed to medication in the opioids plus ketamine group improved significantly from 50% immediately before infusion to 65% 24 hours after infusion and 69% 5 days after infusion. During the same period, pain relief in the placebo group decreased from 58% preinfusion to 56% at 24 hours after infusion, then declined to 50% 5 days later. Between-group differences were statistically significant. The group receiving ketamine infusion also had a significant improvement 24 hours after infusion in the effect of pain on general activity and enjoyment of life.

Conclusion.—The addition of a single infusion of low-dose ketamine to regular opioid analgesia can significantly improve pain relief in patients with allodynia, hyperalgesia, and hyperpathia caused by critical limb ischemia. Such treatment should improve patients' quality of life.

▶ The persistence of an antinociceptive effect 5 days postinfusion is encouraging. This suggests that there may be additive effects if the procedure is repeated. Ketamine is effective orally (first-pass metabolism is to the active metabolite nor-ketamine) and administration of subdissociative doses can be continued indefinitely.

Ischemic pain is often resistant of opioid therapy, possibly because it has a neuropathic component. Antihyperalgesic regimens, including *N*-methyl-D-aspartate antagonists and discontinuation of opioids, should be considered in selected patients. One promising area of investigation is the development of drugs that block hyperalgesia induced by glial activation and subsequent release of proinflammatory cytokines. Pentoxyfilline is a drug that has been shown in multiple experimental pain modes to block the development of hyperalgesia and allodynia. It would seem to be a logical choice for patients with ischemic pain.

S. E. Abram, MD

Modulation of Remifentanil-Induced Analgesia, Hyperalgesia, and Tolerance by Small-Dose Ketamine in Humans

Luginbñl M, Gerber A, Schnider TW, et al (Univ Hosp of Bern, Switzerland; Kantonsspital St Gallen, Switzerland; Univ of Aalborg, Denmark)
Anesth Analg 96:726-732, 2003   12–3

Background.—Animal studies have demonstrated that *N*-methyl-D-aspartic acid (NMDA) receptor antagonists inhibit central sensitization and prevent acute tolerance to opioids or opioid-induced hyperalgesia. The genesis of acute tolerance and opioid-induced hyperalgesia, and their prevention by NMDA receptor antagonists in humans are controversial. Some studies on postoperative pain have detected acute tolerance to opioids, whereas others have not. There is some evidence that the addition of a small dose of ketamine to opioids may increase the analgesic effect and prevent opioid-induced hyperalgesia and acute tolerance to opioids. The following 2 hypotheses were tested: (1) opioid-induced hyperalgesia and acute opioid tolerance, and their prevention by ketamine, occur with some but not all types of painful stimuli; and (2) ketamine enhances opioid analgesia and modifies its side effect profile.

Methods.—This randomized, double-blind, placebo-controlled crossover study investigated the effect of remifentanil combined with small concentrations of ketamine on different experimental pain models. Pain detection thresholds to single and repeated IM electrical stimulation and to repeated transcutaneous electrical stimulation, pressure pain tolerance threshold, and sedative, respiratory, and cardiovascular side effects were evaluated in 14 healthy volunteers. In 4 study sessions, saline, remifentanil alone, and remifentanil combined with ketamine at target plasma concentrations of 50 or 100 ng/mL were administered. Ketamine infusion was initiated after baseline testing at a constant target concentration. Remifentanil infusion was initiated after testing with ketamine alone at an initial target concentration of 1 ng/mL and then increased to 2 ng/mL before decreasing to 1 ng/mL. The last test series were begun 10 minutes after discontinuation of remifentanil.

Results.—Acute remifentanil-induced hyperalgesia and tolerance were only detected with the pressure pain test; they were not suppressed by ketamine infusion. A significant degree of analgesia was induced by remifentanil alone in all pain tests. Ketamine increased the effect of remifentanil only on IM electrical pain. The infusion of remifentanil at a target concentration of 2 ng/mL induced a slight respiratory depression that was antagonized by ketamine.

Conclusions.—The effects of ketamine on opioid analgesia are specific to the type of pain.

▶ Opioid tolerance and opioid-induced hyperalgesia are important phenomena clinically for patients with both acute and chronic pain. NMDA antagonists have been shown to be highly effective in animal models of pain and tolerance, and to be very effective at preventing and reversing both tolerance and hyperalgesia. The results in humans with acute and chronic pain have been less impressive. This study of experimental pain in humans does not show a very robust effect of ketamine in blocking the development of acute tolerance and hyperalgesia after a single dose of remifentanil.

Neuronally mediated mechanisms involving NMDA receptors are not the only sources of opioid-induced hyperalgesia. Glial cell–mediated mechanisms have recently been identified. These involve release of proinflammatory cytokines, nitric oxide, and glutamate and can be modified by a number of experimental agents as well as by some existing drugs.

S. E. Abram, MD

A Single Small Dose of Postoperative Ketamine Provides Rapid and Sustained Improvement in Morphine Analgesia in the Presence of Morphine-Resistant Pain
Weinbroum AA (Tel Aviv Univ, Israel)
Anesth Analg 96:789-795, 2003   12–4

Background.—Despite postoperative administration of IV morphine, many surgical patients experience pain. Ketamine, a noncompetitive N-methyl-D-aspartate (NMDA) receptor antagonist, can enhance opioid-induced antinociception. The effect of adding ketamine to morphine to reduce pain perception in patients after surgery was examined.

Study Design.—This randomized, double-blinded study enrolled 245 patients who were scheduled for elective surgery from January to March 2002. While recovering from surgery, patients were administered IV morphine. If after receiving 100 µg/kg of morphine within a 30-minute period, patients still complained of pain (≥6 on a visual analogue scale [VAS] of 10) and were alert, they were randomly assigned to receive injections of either 30 µg/kg of morphine plus saline (MS group), or 15 µg/kg of morphine plus 250 µg/kg of

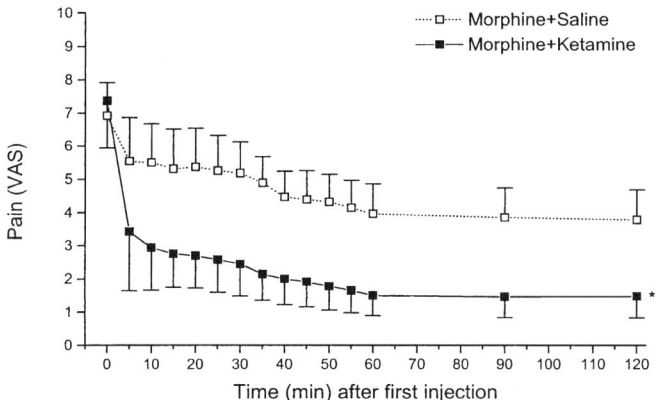

FIGURE 1.—Self-rated levels (by a 0-10 visual analog scale [*VAS*]) of pain intensity (mean ± SD). *Asterisk*, *P* < .001 between the groups (by analysis of variance). (Courtesy of Weinbroum AA: A single small dose of postoperative ketamine provides rapid and sustained improvement in morphine analgesia in the presence of morphine-resistant pain. *Anesth Analg* 96:789-795, 2003.)

ketamine (MK group). Up to 3 of these injections could be given until the pain VAS was 4 or less or 10 minutes had passed. VAS was reassessed every 5 minutes for the first hour and then every 15 minutes. Blood pressure, ECG, respiratory rate, fingertip pulse-derived oxygen saturation (SpO_2), alertness, and adverse effects were also compared between the 2 groups.

Findings.—The MK group had significantly lower VAS scores at 10 and 120 minutes (Fig 1). The level of alertness was significantly better in the MK group at 10 minutes (Fig 2). SpO_2 decreased in the MS group, but increased in the MK group (Fig 3). More MS patients experienced nausea or vomiting. Nine of the MK patients felt light-headed, and 1 had a weird dream.

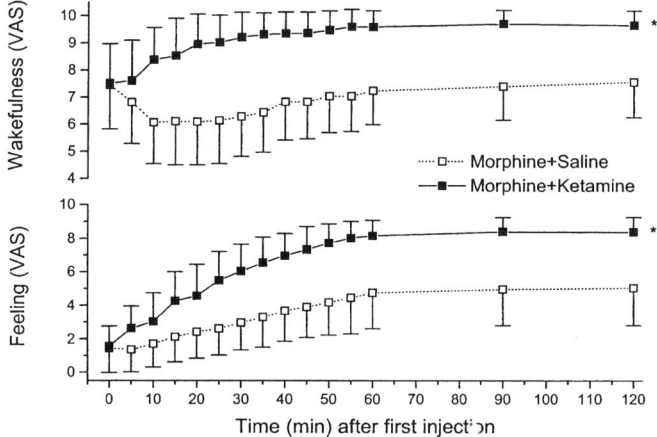

FIGURE 2.—Self-rated levels (by a 0-10 visual analog scale [*VAS*]) of awakening (**top**) and feelings of well-being (**bottom**) (mean ± SD). *Asterisk*, *P* < .001 between the groups (by analysis of variance). (Courtesy of Weinbroum AA: A single small dose of postoperative ketamine provides rapid and sustained improvement in morphine analgesia in the presence of morphine-resistant pain. *Anesth Analg* 96:789-795, 2003.)

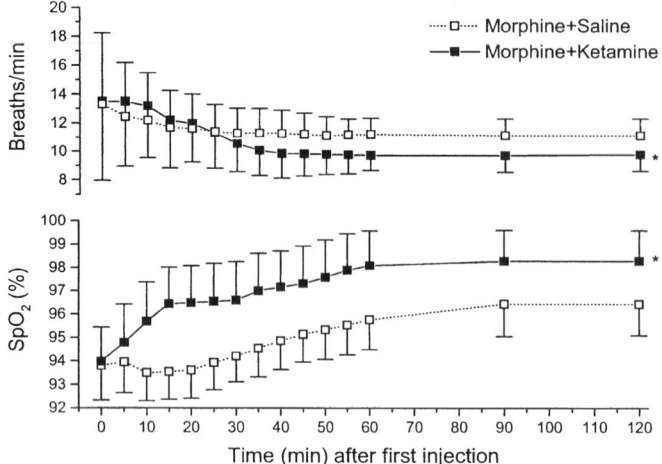

FIGURE 3.—Nurse assessed respiratory rate (**top**) and fingertip-derived arterial blood saturation on air (Sp_{O_2}) (**bottom**) (mean ± SD). *Asterisk*, $P < .001$ between the groups (by analysis of variance). (Courtesy of Weinbroum AA: A single small dose of postoperative ketamine provides rapid and sustained improvement in morphine analgesia in the presence of morphine-resistant pain. *Anesth Analg* 96:789-795, 2003.)

Conclusions.—Postoperative administration of small doses of morphine with ketamine provided rapid and sustained pain control that was better than that achieved with morphine alone. Side effects were minimized, blood SpO₂ was improved, and alertness was increased compared with morphine alone. Larger trials should be performed to confirm these promising results.

▶ In this study, patients who failed to respond adequately to usual doses of IV morphine were shown to benefit from a small rescue dose of ketamine in terms of better analgesia, lower further morphine requirements, and sedation. Most previous reports of postoperative ketamine use have been in chronic or cancer pain patients previously on high-dose opioids. Those patients typically experience transient relief, and ketamine administration must usually be continued for several days. It is possible that a single dose of ketamine in opioid-naive patients may provide lasting benefit by reversing spinally mediated hyperalgesia induced by surgical trauma. Unfortunately, the patients in this study were not followed up long enough to determine whether there was a lasting effect.

Another issue raised by this study is the possibility that the patients selected for this study (ie, those with unexpectedly high opioid requirements) were individuals susceptible to acute opioid tolerance and hyperalgesia. It has been shown in animal models that a single opioid dose can produce a period of hyperalgesia that can be blocked by pretreatment with ketamine.

S. E. Abram, MD

Influence of Thoracic Epidural Analgesia on Cardiovascular Autonomic Control After Thoracic Surgery

Licker M, Spiliopoulos A, Tschopp JM (Univ Hosp, Geneva; Centre Valaisan de Pneumologie, Montana, Switzerland)
Br J Anaesth 91:525-531, 2003   12–5

Background.—Thoracic epidural analgesia (TEA) effectively alleviates pain after major thoracoabdominal surgery. It may also decrease postoperative mortality and morbidity rates. Cardiovascular autonomic control and its modulation by continuous TEA were investigated in patients undergoing elective thoracic surgery.

Methods.—By random assignment, 38 patients received patient-controlled analgesia (PCA group) or TEA with bupivacaine, 0.25% intraoperatively and 0.125% postoperatively, and fentanyl, 2 μg ml^{-1}. Assessment included heart rate variability (HRV), baroreflex function, and pressure response to nitroglycerin and phenylephrine before surgery, 4 hours after surgery (POD 0) and on postoperative days 1 and 2 (POD 1 and 2).

Findings.—In the early postoperative period, both groups had markedly reduced HRV and baroreflex sensitivities. Total HRV and its high-frequency components (HF) increased toward preoperative values in the TEA group on POD 1 and 2. However, the ratio of low to high frequencies was significantly decreased, associated with blunting of the postoperative increase in heart rate and blood pressure. In the PCA group, the low-frequency/high-frequency ratio was unchanged, and HRV decrements persisted until POD 2. Baroreflex sensitivities and pressure responses returned to their preoperative values by POD 2 in both groups.

Conclusions.—Compared with PCA management, TEA with low bupivacaine and fentanyl concentrations blunted cardiac sympathetic neural drive. This resulted in vagal predominance. Postoperatively, HRV variables were restored.

▶ This is one of the few published randomized studies of TEA placed to provide pain after major thoracic surgery. The findings are important.

M. Wood, MD, FRCA

The Effect of Spinal Bupivacaine in Combination With Either Epidural Clonidine and/or 0.5% Bupivacaine Administered at the Incision Site on Postoperative Outcome in Patients Undergoing Lumbar Laminectomy

Jellish WS, Abodeely A, Fluder EM, et al (Loyola Univ, Maywood, Ill)
Anesth Analg 96:874-880, 2003   12–6

Background.—The advantages of spinal anesthesia for lumbar spine surgery are well-recognized. However, no studies have demonstrated a prolonged effect on intermediate postoperative pain relief (4-24 hours later) in comparison with general anesthesia. The addition of narcotics to spinal anesthesia is effective in prolonging the analgesic effect but has also been asso-

TABLE 2.—Intraoperative Data Comparing Groups Receiving Varying Combinations of Epidural and Subcutaneous Local Anesthetics Undergoing Lumbar Laminectomy

	Group 1 Spinal: Bupivacaine Epidural: Clonidine Local: Bupivacaine	Group 2 Spinal: Bupivacaine Epidural: Clonidine Local: Saline	Group 3 Spinal: Bupivacaine Epidural: Saline Local: Bupivacaine	Group 4 Spinal: Bupivacaine Epidural: Saline Local: Saline
Total anesthesia time, min	101.3 ± 4.6	96.2 ± 3.6	97.0 ± 5.0	102.5 ± 5.1
Total surgical time, min	66.3 ± 5.3	63.0 ± 3.8	67.2 ± 4.6	70.7 ± 5.1
Level of spinal achieved, T level	7.6 ± 0.4	7.8 ± 0.4	7.8 ± 0.4	8.2 ± 0.4*
Amount of SQ local anesthetic injected, mL	11 ± 1	13 ± 1	14 ± 2	13 ± 1
No. requiring additional SQ local anesthetic (%)	3 (10.0)	4 (13.3)	7 (23.3)	7 (24.1)
Intraoperative pain, n (%)	0 (0)	0 (0)	2 (6.7)	1 (3.4)
Hypotension, %	46.7	46.7	40.0	58.7
Bradycardia, %	13.3	3.4	13.3	17.2
Nausea, %	6.7	6.7	20.0	10.3
Total IV fluid intake, mL	1480 ± 128	1222 ± 67	1133 ± 71*	1200 ± 80
Calculated blood loss, mL	180 ± 54	204 ± 70	228 ± 50	198 ± 38

Note: Values are mean ± SEM. Bradycardia and hypotension defined as greater than 20% decrease from baseline values of mean arterial blood pressure and * P < .05 when compared with Group 1. (Courtesy of Jellish WS, Abodeely A, Fluder EM, et al: The effect of spinal bupivacaine in combination with either epidural clonidine and/or 0.5% bupivacaine administered at the incision site on postoperative outcome in patients undergoing lumbar laminectomy. Anesth Analg 96(3):874-880, 2003.)

TABLE 3.—Short-term Postanesthesia Care Unit Hemodynamic Outcomes

	Group 1 Spinal: Bupivacaine Epidural: Clonidine Local: Bupivacaine	Group 2 Spinal: Bupivacaine Epidural: Clonidine Local: Saline	Group 3 Spinal: Bupivacaine Epidural: Saline Local: Bupivacaine	Group 4 Spinal: Bupivacaine Epidural: Saline Local: Saline
Mean arterial blood pressure, mm Hg				
Admit	76 ± 2	75 ± 2	88 ± 2*†	87 ± 2*†
10 min	75 ± 2	75 ± 2	84 ± 2*†	85 ± 2*†
20 min	74 ± 2	76 ± 2	85 ± 2*†	86 ± 2*†
30 min	76 ± 2	76 ± 2	87 ± 2*†	89 ± 2*†
40 min	74 ± 2	75 ± 2	89 ± 2*†	87 ± 2*†
50 min	77 ± 2	74 ± 2	90 ± 3*†	89 ± 2*†
60 min	74 ± 3	74 ± 2	90 ± 4*†	92 ± 2*†
Heart rate, bpm				
Admit	68 ± 2	70 ± 2	74 ± 2	73 ± 2
10 min	66 ± 2	68 ± 2	72 ± 2	70 ± 2
20 min	66 ± 2	68 ± 2	71 ± 1	70 ± 2
30 min	65 ± 2	68 ± 2	71 ± 2	71 ± 2
40 min	64 ± 2	68 ± 2	71 ± 2	71 ± 2*
50 min	65 ± 2	66 ± 2	72 ± 2*	72 ± 2*
60 min	65 ± 2	67 ± 2	72 ± 2	74 ± 3*

Note: Values are mean ± SEM.
*$P < .005$ compared with Group 1.
†$P < .05$ compared with Group 2.
(Courtesy of Jellish WS, Abodeely A, Fluder EM, et al: The effect of spinal bupivacaine in combination with either epidural clonidine and/or 0.5% bupivacaine administered at the incision site on postoperative outcome in patients undergoing lumbar laminectomy. *Anesth Analg* 96(3):874-880, 2003.)

TABLE 4.—Short-term Postanesthesia Care Unit Recovery Outcomes

	Group 1 Spinal: Bupivacaine Epidural: Clonidine Local: Bupivacaine	Group 2 Spinal: Bupivacaine Epidural: Clonidine Local: Saline	Group 3 Spinal: Bupivacaine Epidural: Saline Local: Bupivacaine	Group 4 Spinal: Bupivacaine Epidural: Saline Local: Saline
Peak pain scores				
Admit	0.0 ± 0.1	0.4 ± 0.3	0.7 ± 0.3	2.1 ± 0.6*†‡
10 min	0.2 ± 0.2	0.8 ± 0.3	1.1 ± 0.4	2.7 ± 0.6*†‡
20 min	0.2 ± 0.2	1.0 ± 0.4	1.1 ± 0.4	3.1 ± 0.6*†‡
30 min	0.4 ± 0.2	1.0 ± 0.4	1.4 ± 0.4	3.2 ± 0.5*†‡
40 min	0.5 ± 0.2	0.9 ± 0.3	1.9 ± 0.4*	2.8 ± 0.4*†
50 min	0.3 ± 0.2	1.0 ± 0.4	1.8 ± 0.3*	2.2 ± 0.4*†
60 min	0.1 ± 0.1	1.0 ± 0.4	2.0 ± 0.4*	2.3 ± 0.4†
Steward recovery scores				
Admit	5.6 ± 0.1	5.4 ± 0.1	5.8 ± 0.1†	5.8 ± 0.1†
10 min	5.8 ± 0.1	5.6 ± 0.1	5.9 ± 0.1	6.0 ± 0.0
20 min	5.9 ± 0.1	5.7 ± 0.1	5.8 ± 0.1	6.0 ± 0.0
30 min	5.9 ± 0.1	5.8 ± 1.0	5.9 ± 0.1	6.0 ± 0.0
40 min	5.9 ± 0.1	5.8 ± 0.1	5.9 ± 0.1	6.0 ± 0.0
50 min	5.9 ± 0.1	5.9 ± 0.1	6.0 ± 0.0	6.0 ± 0.0
60 min	5.9 ± 0.1	5.9 ± 0.1	6.0 ± 0.0	6.0 ± 0.0
No. receiving rescue dose of fentanyl (%)	3 (10.0)	5 (20.0)	11 (37.0)	21 (70)*†‡
Frequency of nausea, n (%)	0 (0)	2 (6.7)	1 (3.3)	0 (0)
Frequency of emesis, n (%)	0 (0)	0 (0)	0 (0)	0 (0)
Time to first rescue dose, h	5.4 ± 0.7	3.7 ± 0.5	2.6 ± 0.5*	1.7 ± 0.6*
Time to first movement, h	2.4 ± 0.1	2.7 ± 0.2	2.0 ± 0.2†	2.3 ± 0.1
Amount of rescue fentanyl, μg	5.2 ± 3.6	12.5 ± 5.5	39.2 ± 10.8*	77.6 ± 10.8*†‡

Note: Values are mean ± SEM
*$P < .005$ compared with Group 1.
†$P < .05$ compared with Group 2.
‡$P < .05$ compared with Group 3.
(Courtesy of Jellish WS, Abodeely A, Fluder EM, et al: The effect of spinal bupivacaine in combination with either epidural clonidine and/or 0.5% bupivacaine administered at the incision site on postoperative outcome in patients undergoing lumbar laminectomy. *Anesth Analg* 96(3):874-880, 2003.)

ciated with many unwanted side effects, such as respiratory depression, urinary retention, drowsiness, and pruritis. These side effects have also been reported in association with the epidural administration of narcotics. Neuropathic pain is experienced by many patients who require laminectomy or diskectomy. This burning, radiating pain is poorly responsive to opioids, whether administered systemically or intraspinally. Clonidine has been shown to be effective in relieving neuropathic pain. The effect of the addition of epidural clonidine and/or bupivacaine injected at the incision site on postoperative outcomes was evaluated in patients undergoing spinal anesthesia.

Methods.—A total of 120 patients scheduled for lumbar spine surgery were given bupivacaine spinal anesthesia supplemented by 150 µg epidural clonidine with or without incisional bupivacaine; epidural placebo plus incisional bupivacaine; or placebo with incisional saline.

Results.—No difference was found between the groups in IV fluids, blood loss, incidence of intraoperative bradycardia, and hypotension (Table 2). Postanesthesia care unit pain scores were lower and the demand for analgesia was less in patients who received both the clonidine and subcutaneous bupivacaine. Patients who received epidural clonidine also had improved postoperative hemodynamic outcomes (Table 3). No differences were found between the groups in hospital discharge, urinary retention, and other variables (Table 4).

Conclusions.—The addition of epidural clonidine as a supplement to spinal anesthesia seems to provide improved postoperative pain relief and hemodynamic stability in patients undergoing lower spine surgery without perioperative complications.

▶ This study demonstrates again the efficacy of spinal anesthesia for lumbar laminectomy. Spinal anesthesia has been described for lumbar spine procedures since the 1930s and has become increasingly popular over the last decade. In this study, the administration of epidural clonidine and local infiltration of bupivacaine at the operative site give additional benefits in terms of improved immediate postoperative hemodynamics, longer postoperative analgesia, and a decreased requirement for systemic narcotic administration compared with spinal anesthesia alone. These advantages are produced without unwanted side effects, such as urinary retention, which is associated with the addition of spinal or epidural narcotics. The authors' recommendations to add epidural clonidine and local infiltration with bupivacaine seem well founded.

S. Black, MD

Comparison of Epidural, Continuous Femoral Block and Intraarticular Analgesia After Anterior Cruciate Ligament Reconstruction

Dauri M, Polzoni M, Fabbi E, et al (Univ of Rome 'Tor Vergata'; Motor Science Univ, Rome)

Acta Anaesthesiol Scand 47:20-25, 2003   12–7

Introduction.—Moderate to severe postoperative pain is common in patients undergoing anterior cruciate ligament reconstruction (ACLR). Locoregional analgesia approaches are considered to provide faster patient recovery and less side effects versus IV administration of opioids. Three locoregional techniques of pain management after ACLR were compared in a prospective, randomized trial.

Methods.—Sixty consecutively enrolled adults, ASA class I-II, were randomly assigned to 1 of 3 groups: epidural (EPI) received epidural ropivacaine 0.2% plus sufentanil 0.2 µg/mL at 5 mL/h; continuous femoral block (CFB) received a continuous infusion of the same analgesic mixture through a femoral catheter; and intra-articular (IA) received a continuous intra-articular infusion of ropivacaine 0.2% plus sufentanil 0.2 µg/mL at 5 mL/h. All participants were allowed patient-controlled analgesia boluses of 5 mL of local anesthetic. Analgesia was evaluated for 36 hours at completion of surgery via a visual analogue scale and a verbal scale, along with the number of patient-controlled boluses administered and the amount of supplementary IV ketorolac, if administered.

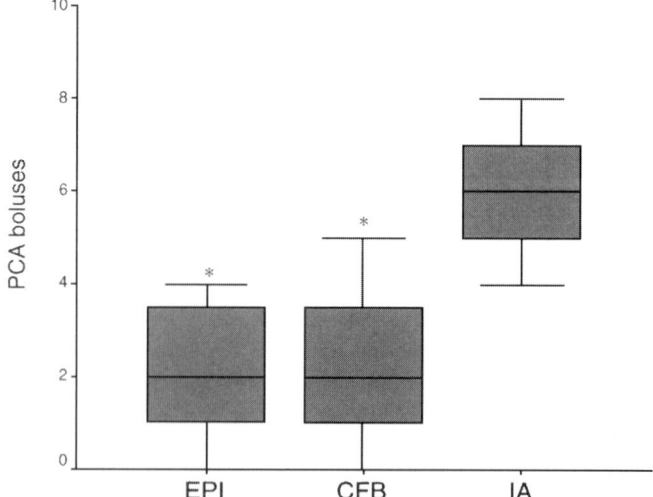

FIGURE 2.—Patient-controlled analgesia boluses among the 3 groups. The *box* represents the 25th to 75th percentiles, while the median is represented by the *solid line*. *Error bars* mark extreme values. *Asterisk* indicates *P* < .001 versus IA. *Abbreviations: PCA,* Patient-controlled analgesia; *EPI,* epidural; *CFB,* continuous femoral block; *IA,* intra-articular. (Courtesy of Dauri M, Polzoni M, Fabbi E, et al: Comparison of epidural, continuous femoral block and intraarticular analgesia after anterior cruciate ligament reconstruction. *Acta Anesthesiol Scand* 47:20-25, 2003.)

TABLE 2.—Adverse Effects

	Nausea	Vomitus	Pruritus	Urinary Retention	Sedation	Hypotension	Headache
EPI (n=20)	4	0	5	8	3	1	2
CFB (n=20)	10	1	1	0	4	0	0
IA (n=20)	6	1	5	0	2	0	0
P-value	0.122	0.596	0.168	<0.001	0.676	0.362	0.126

Numbers in cells represent incidence of effect.
Abbreviations: EPI, Epidural ropivacaine 0.2% and sufentanil 0.2 µg mL; *CFB*, continuous femoral block ropivacaine 0.2% and sufentanil 0.2 µg mL; *IA*, intra-articular ropivacaine 0.2% and sufentanil 0.2 µg.
(Courtesy of Dauri M, Polzoni M, Fabbi E, et al: Comparison of epidural, continuous femoral block and intraarticular analgesia after anterior cruciate ligament reconstruction. *Acta Anesthesiol Scand* 47:20-25, 2003.)

Results.—The visual analogue scale and verbal scale scores were significantly higher in the IA group during the 24 hours after surgery, compared to the EPI and CFB groups. The need for ketorolac was higher in group IA during the postoperative period (Fig 2). Adverse effects were similar in all groups with the exception of urinary retention, which was significantly more common in the EPI group (Table 2).

Conclusion.—Both epidural and continuous femoral neck block offer sufficient pain relief in patients who undergo ACLR. Intra-articular analgesia appears to be unable to provide satisfactory pain relief regarding the analgesic requirements of patients undergoing ACLR.

▶ With the increasing use of low molecular weight heparin in orthopedic surgery patients, continuous femoral plexus block appears to be the best choice among the 3 modalities studied. The significantly higher incidence of urinary retention with epidural analgesia reinforces that opinion.

S. E. Abram, MD

Continuous Interscalene Brachial Plexus Blockade Provides Good Analgesia at Home After Major Shoulder Surgery—Report of Four Cases
Nielsen KC, Greengrass RA, Pietrobon R, et al (Duke Univ, Durham, NC)
Can J Anesth 50:57-61, 2003   12–8

Introduction.—Continuous interscalene brachial plexus blockade (CIBPB) in a hospital setting can provide excellent surgical conditions and postoperative analgesia for patients undergoing major shoulder surgery. Four patients were reported for whom the efficacy and advantages of CIBPB for postoperative analgesia at home were examined.

Methods.—Four patients (mean age, 45 years; range, 47-68 years) scheduled for unilateral open rotator cuff repair under CIBPB with IV sedation were visited by a home infusion services nurse the day before surgery. Nurses assessed the home environment and provided information about the infusion pump and routine postoperative care. The CIBPB was performed with a 30 to 40 mL solution of 0.5% ropivacaine with epinephrine 1:400,000 incrementally injected. With the needle maintained in the same position (Fig-

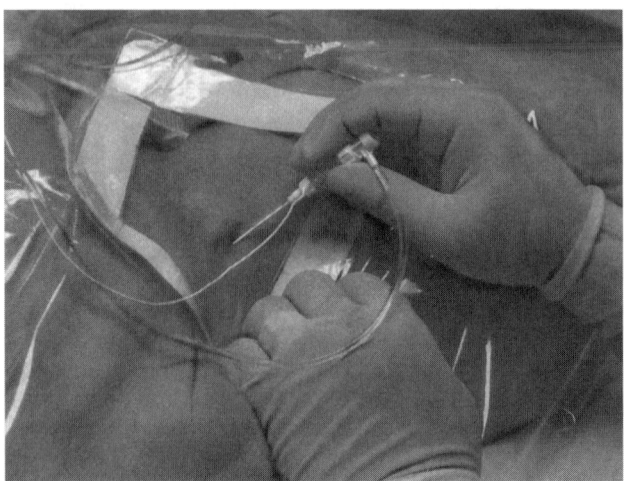

FIGURE.—Needle positioning and anterolateral orientation of the bevel during continuous interscalene brachial plexus blockade placement for surgery on the left shoulder. (Courtesy of Nielsen KC, Greengrass RA, Pietrobon R, et al: Continuous interscalene brachial plexus blockade provides good analgesia at home after major shoulder surgery—Report of four cases. *Can J Anesth* 50:57-61, 2003.)

ure), a 20-gauge standard end-hole epidural catheter was threaded 5 cm beyond the tip of the needle.

After surgery, patients were transferred to the postanesthesia care unit, then home with an automated infusion pump administering 0.2% ropivacaine at 10 mL/h for 72 hours. Before discharge, patients and their attendant were given verbal and written instructions regarding local anesthetic toxicity and precise contact information for an anesthesiologist or nurse. Outcomes were determined both preoperatively and postoperatively, including verbal analogue pain scores, verbal analogue nausea scores, side effects, cognitive function (Mini-Mental State Questionnaire), sleep (hours per night), and patient satisfaction (Likert scale).

Results.—The verbal analogue scores for the initial 3 postoperative days were low. Two patients reported 1 episode of nausea. No complications were linked with either local anesthetic toxicity or catheter use. Cognitive functioning improved during the first 3 postoperative days. Sleep improved from a mean of 5 hours before surgery to 7 hours during the initial 3 postoperative nights. Patient satisfaction was high and cost savings were significant.

Conclusion.—The use of CIBPB in the 72 hours after major shoulder surgery can provide good analgesia with minimal opioid requirement, cost savings, and possibly improvement in outcome measures.

▶ I selected this abstract to highlight the use of continuous regional blockade, not only in a hospital setting but also at home.

M. Wood, MD, FRCA

Neurologic Complications of 405 Consecutive Continuous Axillary Catheters
Bergman BD, Hebl JR, Kent J, et al (Mayo Clinic, Rochester, Minn; Associated Anesthesiology, Saint Paul, Minn)
Anesth Analg 96:247-252, 2003   12–9

Background.—Continuous axillary brachial plexus block is used in the perioperative management of patients undergoing complex surgical procedures in the upper extremity, including major orthopedic surgery requiring early painful postoperative mobilization with continuous motion devices, postoperative sympathectomy in patients undergoing upper-extremity replantation procedures, and the diagnosis and treatment of chronic pain syndromes. In theory, the use of continuous axillary brachial plexus block may increase the risk of neurologic complications because of catheter-induced mechanical trauma or local anesthetic toxicity. The frequency of complications with current techniques and applications was reviewed.

Methods.—A retrospective review was conducted of 405 placements of continuous axillary catheters in 368 patients. A preexisting condition was present in 10% of complications, including 30 patients with a preoperative ulnar neuropathy. In 305 cases (75.3%), the axillary catheter was placed to facilitate rehabilitation after major elbow surgery. Catheter placement was typically performed postoperatively after documentation of the patient's normal neurologic examination.

Results.—The local anesthetic infusion contained bupivacaine in 88.7% of patients, and mepivacaine in 11.1% of patients. The mean infusion rate was 10 ± 2 mL/h. Catheters were indwelling for a mean of 55 ± 32 hours. In 31 patients, the axillary catheter was replaced because of inadequate analgesia or technical problems. Nine complications developed in 8 patients, for an overall frequency of 2.2%. Included in these complications were one each of localized infection, axillary hematoma, and retained catheter fragment requiring surgical excision. In addition, signs and symptoms of systemic (preseizure) local anesthetic toxicity were reported in 2 patients. New neurologic deficits were reported in 4 patients postoperatively. The neural dysfunction was not anesthesia related in 2 patients. In all 4 of these patients, the continuous catheter was placed after major elbow surgery.

Conclusions.—The risk of neurologic complications associated with continuous axillary blockade is similar to the risk associated with single-dose blockade techniques.

▶ The risk-benefit ratio for continuous brachial plexus blocks appears to be acceptable for patients at risk of long-term severe pain (patients with preexisting pain undergoing amputation, patients with a history of complex regional pain syndrome, patients requiring early aggressive joint mobilization, patients who need reimplantation or extensive vascular repair). One technical comment: infraclavicular block provides similar analgesia to axillary block with more stability and less movement of the catheter. Whether this translates to a lower failure rate or fewer complications is not known. This might make a nice study.

S. E. Abram, MD

Patient-Controlled Epidural Analgesia in Children: Can They Do It?
Birmingham PK, Wheeler M, Suresh S, et al (Northwestern Univ, Chicago)
Anesth Analg 96:686-691, 2003   12–10

Background.—Continuous epidural infusions are widely used in children. However, the treatment of pain using patient-controlled epidural analgesia (PCEA) has not been extensively studied. Use of PCEA offers children flexibility and a degree of control that can improve overall pain relief, patient satisfaction, and family acceptance. Issues that have been debated concerning this method include whether the epidural catheter should be inserted while the patient is awake, sedated, or after general anesthesia has been induced. Some authors believe it is important to attempt neuraxial anesthesia in patients before general anesthesia is induced to avoid nerve injury. The experience of PCEA in 128 children having surgical procedures was reported.

Methods.—The children (youngest age, 5.2 years) underwent a total of 132 procedures that involved moderate to severe postoperative pain. The child's cognitive ability and cooperation were assessed by the attending anesthesiologist along with input from the parents. Catheters were placed after anesthetic induction in over 80% of the patients, although when the catheter was placed at the thoracic level, it was generally done before induction.

Results.—Analgesia was sufficient with the initial settings for 89 patients (67.4%) and was ultimately sufficient after changes in the settings or solutions in 119 cases (90.1%). Pain scores of 6 or greater on a 10-point scale were reported by 32.6% of the patients at some point during treatment (Fig 1), and 76.7% of these received adequate treatment by changing the infusion rate, demand dose, or both, reducing the pain score to under 3 on a 5-point scale or under 6 on the 10-point scale. Five patients achieved satisfactory analgesia when the epidural infusion solution was changed, and the remaining 5 patients required conversion to IV patient-controlled analgesia to control their pain.

The demand option was used an average of 18.0 times daily, with a range of 3 to 52 times. Catheters were left in most patients with fevers of 38.5°C or greater without producing adverse effects. Most of the patients (78%) were cared for safely on regular wards, with monitoring achieved by continuous pulse oximetry. Epidural demand doses were self-administered, avoiding the possibility of increased serious adverse side effects when someone other than the patient operates the demand option. None of the patients required treatment or intervention for sedation or respiratory depression.

Overall, 90.1% of the patients had satisfactory analgesia for as long as 103 hours without desaturation, clinical evidence of toxicity, or serious ad-

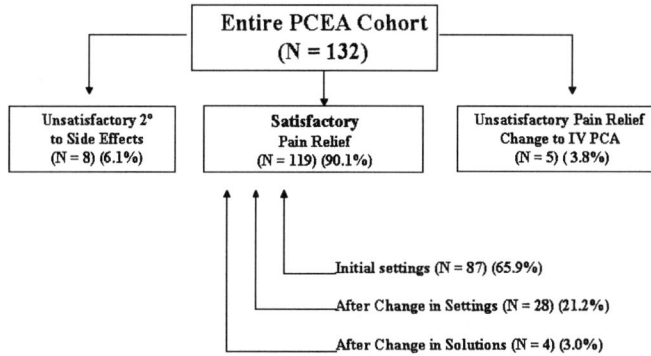

FIGURE 1.—Pain control algorithm. Total satisfactory pain control was achieved in 90.1% of children: 65.9% with the initial settings, 21.2% more with changes in patient-controlled epidural analgesia (*PCEA*) settings and an additional 3.0% with a change in solution. Unsatisfactory pain control in 3.8% of children and side effects in 6.1% necessitated a change to IV patient-controlled analgesia (*IV PCA*). (Courtesy of Birmingham PK, Wheeler M, Suresh S, et al: Patient-controlled epidural analgesia in children: Can they do it? *Anesth Analg* 96:686-691, 2003.)

verse effects. Adverse effects did induce a change to IV patient-controlled analgesia in 8 patients.

Conclusion.—These children, the youngest of whom was aged 5.2 years, were able to understand and willing to use PCEA. The results in the younger children resembled those achieved with patients aged 9 years or older ($P = .90$ and $P = .75$). To avoid exceeding the recommended limits, careful attention to the total hourly local anesthetic dose was required. The incidence of adverse side effects was small, indicating that PCEA should be considered for the management of pediatric postoperative pain. Study of PCEA's advantages (superior analgesia, less drug consumption overall, better patient and/or parent acceptance) and factors such as choice of solution, catheter insertion site, tip position, and optimal patient subpopulations are needed.

▶ This prospective report clearly shows that PCEA is a safe and effective means of providing pain relief in pediatric patients after major surgical procedures. Younger children had as good results as older children and were as likely to utilize the demand mode. The authors did note that the child and parents were evaluated preoperatively for appropriateness of this technique. Not all young children were felt to be good candidates. Use of PCEA did not result in automatic transfer to the ICU or other special units and was not associated with significant complications.

As compared to PCEA in adults, differences in clinical practice were noted by the authors. First, children are far more likely to have the epidural catheter placed after induction of general anesthesia, although thoracic epidurals appeared to be placed prior to induction when possible in this series. Secondly, in small children, careful attention must be paid to setting limits of infusions to avoid local anesthetic toxicity, which is rarely a concern in adults and larger children.

S. Black, MD

Chronic Pain Management

A Cross-Sectional Study Correlating Degeneration of the Cervical Spine With Disability and Pain in United Kingdom Patients

Peterson C, Bolton J, Wood AR, et al (Canadian Mem Chiropractic College, Toronto; Anglo-European College of Chiropractic, Bournemouth, England)
Spine 28:129-133, 2003   12–11

Introduction.—The association between spinal degeneration and patient symptoms is controversial, despite several trials that have examined these relationships. A prospective cross-sectional investigation was performed to ascertain the association between degeneration of all the joints in the cervical spine and to identify the effects of impending litigation on pain and disability levels in patients with and without trauma.

Methods.—Radiographic and questionnaire data were obtained from 180 consecutive patients with neck pain. Neck severity was determined by means of 2 time-dependent scales. The Neck Disability Index and questions concerning chronicity, etiology, and associated litigation were completed by all participants. Radiographs were examined for the number of levels of degeneration and the severity of degeneration in the disks as well as the uncovertebral and facet articulations.

Results.—Seventy-one patients (40.57%) reported neck pain caused by injury. Only 5.1% had associated litigation. There was no statistically significance difference in pain severity or disability levels between patients who did and did not have cervical degeneration. The number of levels of cervical degeneration and the severity of the degeneration in the disks, facets, and uncovertebral joints were not associated with the levels of pain and disability.

Patients with neck pain due to injury tended ($P = .055$) to experience more pain in the preceding week and significantly more disability ($P < .001$). Significant differences were observed between those with and without injury in pain intensity ($P < .025$), reading ($P < .001$), headaches ($P < .025$), ability to drive ($P < .01$), and concentration ($P < .01$). Women reported significantly more pain ($P < .01$) and disability ($P < .001$), compared to men; women did not have more degeneration in any joints.

Conclusion.—In patients with neck pain, there was no significant difference in reported pain and disability levels between those who did and did not have evidence of cervical spine degeneration. Patients whose neck pain was caused by trauma reported significantly more pain and disability, compared to those whose pain had other causes. This was not caused by more spinal degeneration or overriding litigation issues.

▶ This study is not unusual in its findings. Many studies have failed to link radiographic findings with pain complaints, yet we frequently judge the validity of patients' pain complaints on the severity of the degenerative changes seen radiographically. Many previous studies have also failed to find correlations between litigation status and pain severity or response to treatment. Nevertheless, we often suspect that patients involved in litigation are exaggerating their symptoms in an effort to maximize compensation. The study suggests that radiographic findings are unlikely to demonstrate the source of pain in injured patients.

S. E. Abram, MD

Risk Assessment of Hemorrhagic Complications Associated With Nonsteroidal Antiinflammatory Medications in Ambulatory Pain Clinic Patients Undergoing Epidural Steroid Injection
Horlocker TT, Bajwa ZH, Ashraf Z, et al (Mayo Clinic, Rochester, Minn; Beth Israel Deaconess Med Ctr, Boston)
Anesth Analg 95:1691-1697, 2002   12–12

Introduction.—Nonsteroidal anti-inflammatory drugs (NSAIDs) are considered a contraindication to epidural steroid injection because of the risk of hemorrhagic complications. Thus, outpatients scheduled for an epidural steroid injection for chronic pain relief may be asked to discontinue NSAIDs or to undergo costly platelet function tests. The risk of spinal hematoma was prospectively studied in patients administered epidural steroid injections.

Methods.—The study population included 1035 patients undergoing 1214 epidural steroid injections in ambulatory pain centers. Patients were asked if they had a history of excessive bleeding or easy bruising and whether they had used an antiplatelet medication the previous week. Data considered in the analysis were the regional technique, level of needle placement, needle gauge and approach, elicitation of a paresthesia during needle/catheter placement, the occurrence of mild spinal bleeding, and neurologic symptoms experienced after the injection.

Results.—The most common diagnoses represented were acute radiculopathy (49%) and spinal stenosis (32%). Only 15% of patients reported a history of bleeding or bruising; one third reported NSAID use. Most (80%) epidural steroid injections were administered at the lumbar level with a midline (93%) approach and using a needle of 18-gauge or less. Blood was noted during needle or catheter placement in only 63 (5.2%) patients, and there were no spinal hematomas.

Significant independent risk factors for minor hemorrhagic complications on multivariate analysis were increased age, multiple needle passes, and injection volume less than 8 mL, but not the use of NSAID therapy. Postinjection bruising at the needle site was associated with a history of bleeding/bruising. The frequency of transient neurologic deficits after the injection was significantly associated with female gender, no local anesthetic, and less experience on the part of the physician.

Conclusion.—Results of this study of patients with chronic pain are in agreement with those performed in obstetric and surgical populations. Epidural steroid injections are safe in patients receiving NSAIDs, although factors such as increased age may increase the risk of minor hemorrhagic complications.

▶ The lack of serious hemorrhagic complications among patients on NSAIDs who underwent epidural steroid injections is somewhat encouraging. However, since the incidence of such complications is extremely low, it is impossible to determine whether these drugs do indeed increase the risk. With increasing numbers of patients on platelet inhibitors, such as clopidogrel and ticlopidine (and more to come with television advertising), vigilance is needed to avoid neuraxial blocks in these individuals.

S. E. Abram, MD

Lateral Branch Blocks as a Treatment for Sacroiliac Joint Pain: A Pilot Study
Cohen SP, Abdi S (Walter Reed Army Med Ctr, Washington, DC; New York Univ; Harvard Med School, Boston)
Reg Anesth Pain Med 28:113-119, 2003   12-13

Background.—Some patients with chronic low back pain suffer significant pain as a result of sacroiliac (SI) joint disease, for which corticosteroid injection can sometimes provide good relief, even if only briefly. Radiofrequency (RF) denervation of the SI joint has also been shown to ease pain, although the failure rate with this technique is over 60%. Nerve blocks on the various branches of the dorsal rami may permit the diagnosis of low back pain coming from the facet joints. Patients who obtain significant pain relief from diagnostic medial branch blocks may also derive substantial long-term benefit from RF denervation.

No studies have yet demonstrated whether L4 and L5 dorsal rami blocks and S1–3 lateral branch blocks (LBBs) can diagnose SI joint pain or whether RF denervation has a role. The efficacy of RF lesioning of the nerves innervating the SI joint to relieve pain was evaluated.

Methods.—In the 18 patients assessed, SI joint pain had been confirmed. Nerve blocks of the L4-5 primary dorsal rami and S1–3 lateral branches that innervated the affected joint were performed (Fig 1). RF denervation was then done for patients who obtained at least 50% pain relief from the blocks.

Results.—Thirteen patients (72%) had greater than 50% pain relief with the LBBs, with 2 having relief that extended for several months. These 2 patients did not have RF neurotomy. Two patients were lost to follow-up. Thus, 9 patients had RF denervation, and 8 of them obtained significant pain relief that lasted at least 9 months. The 1 patient who did not achieve a 50% or better relief of pain reported 40% relief. One patient was able to decrease the amount of opioids being taken. One hundred percent relief was achieved in only 2 of the 9 patients.

In the 8 patients who had successful RF denervation and the 2 with prolonged LBB effects, the visual analogue scale pain scores declined an average of 5.2 with SI joint blocks. The 6 patients who had negative outcomes had a

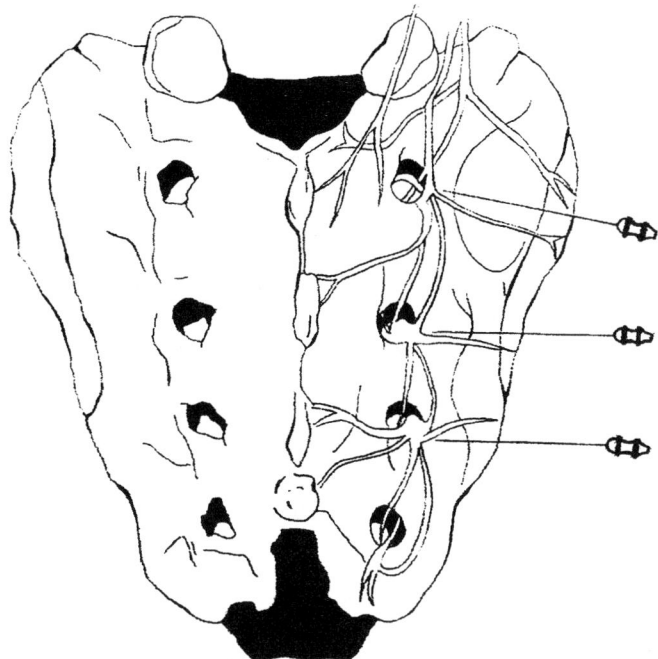

FIGURE 1.—Schematic drawing showing the S1–3 lateral branches innervating the sacroiliac joint and overlying ligaments. The needles depict the approximate location for the diagnostic lateral branch block. (Courtesy of Cohen SP, Abdi S: Lateral branch blocks as a treatment for sacroiliac joint pain: A pilot study. *Reg Anesth Pain Med* 28:113-119, 2003.)

mean reduction of 4.1. No side effects or complications attended any of the procedures

Conclusion.—LBBs and SI joint injections produced comparable degrees of pain relief for most of the patients assessed. Of those who had pain relief with LBB, RF denervation may also have provided benefit. Over 90% of the patients had some relief with the nerve blocks, although only 72% obtained significant relief. No reliable, long-term treatments are yet available for SI joint pain.

▶ RF denervation of facet joints that have been shown to act as pain generators is a relatively successful procedure. Denervation of the SI joint has previously been shown to have a high failure rate. The authors describe an alternate technique that appears to be reasonably effective.

S. E. Abram, MD

The Sacroiliac Joint: A Potential Cause of Pain After Lumbar Fusion to the Sacrum

Katz V, Schofferman J, Reynolds J (San Francisco Spine Inst, Daly City)
J Spinal Disord Tech 16:96-99, 2003   12–14

Background.—From 13% to 30% of cases of chronic low back pain seen in specialty spine practices can be attributed to the sacroiliac joint (SIJ). Generally the pain is unilateral or bilateral, occurs below the waist, and radiates to the ipsilateral groin, buttock, thigh, or foot or abdomen, in rare cases. When the history suggests the SIJ is involved, fluoroscopically guided intra-articular SIJ injection with local anesthetic is required to confirm or exclude the diagnosis. Physical examination and imaging methods are generally not useful.

If the pain is reduced by more than 75% within 15 to 45 minutes of the injection, painful SIJ is highly probable. Adding corticosteroids to the injectate and achieving relief lasting for over 1 week is further confirmation. Painful SIJ was suspected in patients who had previous lumbar fusion to the sacrum and later complained of low back and gluteal pain. A retrospective review of these patients was given.

Methods.—The 34 patients (13 men and 21 women) ranged in age from 30 to 81 years and reported low back pain after lumbosacral fusion. All were given SIJ injections, including glucocorticosteroid, with the percentage and duration of pain relief documented.

Results.—Over 75% pain relief was reported by 59% of the patients within 15 to 45 minutes of the injection, and for 11 of these 20 patients, the relief lasted 14 days or more. For 6 patients, the degree of relief exceeded 20% but was less than 75%, although 1 patient had pain relief that lasted for 30 days. Eight patients (24%) had no pain relief either during the local anesthetic phase or long term. A total of 12 patients had pain relief for over 10 days, with a range of 14 to 180 days and a mean of 76 days.

The 11 patients who achieved over 75% immediate pain relief plus at least 10 days of extended relief were diagnosed as having definite painful SIJ. Ten patients were diagnosed with possible SIJ pain dysfunction, 9 of whom had over 75% relief immediately but no prolonged relief and 1 who had between 20% and 75% relief plus over 14 days of extended relief. SIJ pain was excluded as a diagnosis in the 13 patients who had either no response or little response with no long-term relief.

Conclusion.—Among patients who have undergone lumbar fusion to the sacrum, painful SIJ dysfunction was noted to cause pain in the low back, gluteal area, groin, leg, or foot. Thus, painful SIJ can be included in the differential diagnosis of these patients. The diagnosis can be confirmed by fluoroscopically guided SIJ injection to obtain pain relief.

▶ The authors postulate that patients who have fusions that include the lumbosacral junction develop hypermobility and degeneration of the SIJ. It is likely that similar mechanical forces produce premature degeneration of facet joints at the segments just above the level of fusion.

S. E. Abram, MD

Nerve-Root Injections for the Relief of Pain in Patients With Osteoporotic Vertebral Fractures
Kim D-J, Yun Y-H, Wang J-M (Ewha Womans Univ Hosp, Seoul, Korea)
J Bone Joint Surg Br 85:250-253, 2003   12–15

Background.—Vertebral fracture is a common complication of osteoporosis and a cause of significant disability. Most fractures heal within a few weeks or months, but some are not responsive to conservative treatment. Surgery is usually not indicated unless there is a neurologic deficit or gross deformity. Vertebroplasty with percutaneous injection of polymethylmethacrylate into the vertebral bodies has been proposed for the augmentation of osteoporotic vertebral bodies, and significant pain relief is achieved in most patients. However, many patients require treatment with a less-invasive method. The efficacy of nerve-root injection of steroids for the management of radicular pain caused by osteoporotic vertebral fractures was investigated.

Methods.—The study group was composed of 58 patients with pain from osteoporotic vertebral fractures that were unresponsive to conservative treatment. The mean age of the 53 women and 5 men was 72.5 years. All the patients were given a nerve-root injection with lidocaine, bupivacaine, and DepoMedrol. The mean duration of follow-up was 13.5 months. Pain scores were assessed before treatment, at 1 and 6 months after treatment, and at the end of follow-up.

Results.—The mean pain scores before treatment and at 1 and 6 months after treatment were 85, 24.9, and 14.1; at the end of follow-up the mean pain score was 17.4. According to the modified criteria used to grade the results, 6 patients were considered to have an excellent result, 42 a good result, and 10 a fair result. There was evidence of a newly developed compression fracture in 3 patients. There were no complications related to the procedure.

Conclusions.—Nerve-root injections are effective for the reduction of pain in patients with osteoporotic vertebral fractures. This treatment should be considered in these patients before percutaneous vertebroplasty or operative treatment is performed.

▶ The use of selective nerve root injection with steroid may be a reasonable treatment option before initiating vertebroplasty, which clearly has more associated risks. However, this study does not establish the technique as effective. The medical literature has far too many studies like this one, which is not much more than anecdotal in its approach, and far too few randomized controlled trials. If the pain exhibited by a patient with an osteoporotic vertebral body fracture is clearly radicular, either a translaminar or a transforaminal steroid injection would seem reasonable.

S. E. Abram, MD

Kryorhizotomy: An Alternative Technique for Lumbar Medial Branch Rhizotomy in Lumbar Facet Syndrome
Bärlocher CB, Krauss JK, Seiler RW (Univ of Berne, Switzerland)
J Neurosurg: Spine 98:14-20, 2003   12–16

Introduction.—One of the potential sources of low back pain is lumbar zygapophyseal or facet joint degeneration (or lumbar facet syndrome [LFS]). The mechanical pain of LFS is characterized by pain that is a dull, deep ache

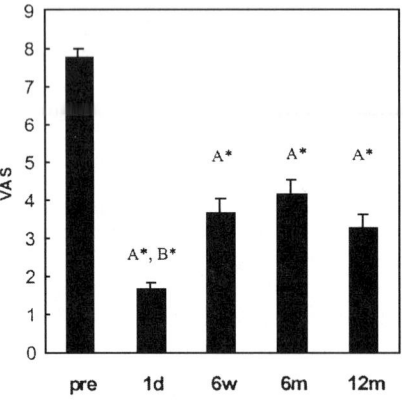

A* = significant vs. Preoperatively (P<0.001)
B* = significant vs. 6 weeks and 6 months (P<0.05)

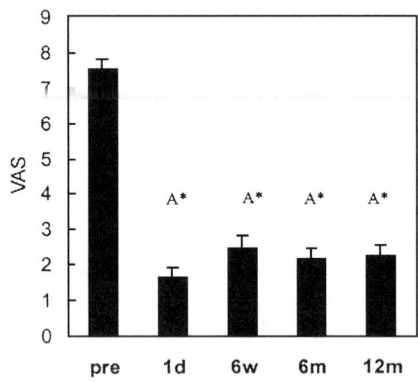

A* = significant vs. Preoperatively (P<0.001)

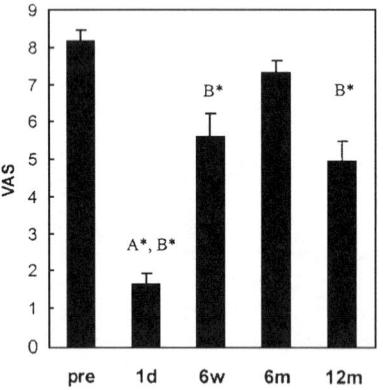

A* = significant vs. All others
B* = significant vs. Preoperatively

FIGURE 4.—Bar graphs demonstrating prekryorhizotomy and postkryorhizotomy visual analogue scale pain scores. **Top Left,** Mean visual analogue scale (*VAS*) scores in all 50 patients (responders and nonresponders). **Top Right,** Mean scores in responders only (31 patients; 5 patients with beneficial rekryorhizotomy after 6 weeks were included). **Bottom,** Mean VAS scores in nonresponders only (19 patients), including 6 patients who underwent a rigid stabilization after 6 months with marked amelioration of pain postoperatively. (Courtesy of Bärlocher CB, Krauss JK, Seiler RW: Kryorhizotomy: An alternative technique for lumbar medial branch rhizotomy in lumbar facet syndrome. *J Neurosurg: Spine* 98:14-20, 2003.)

that may be difficult to localize. The efficacy of treatment of LFS by percutaneous lumbar facet kryorhizotomy was prospectively assessed.

Methods.—Between December 1998 and January 2000, kryorhizotomy was performed in 50 patients with chronic low back pain in whom pain was relieved by controlled diagnostic medial branch blocks of the lumbar zygapophyseal (facet) joints. Patient outcome was determined by the visual analogue pain scale and evaluation of work capacity. All outcome measures were reassessed at 6 weeks, 6 months, and 1 year postoperatively.

Results.—At 1-year follow-up, 31 of 50 patients (62%) had a good response to lumbar facet kryorhizotomy (Fig 4). Good results of 50% or more were observed in 85% of patients (*P* < .01) without previous spinal surgery; only 46% had previous spinal surgery. In 5 patients (16%) in whom a good initial benefit was seen yet who experienced increased pain within 6 weeks after kryorhizotomy, the beneficial result was recovered after an early repeated procedure. No side effects were reported. Nineteen (38%) of 50 procedures were not considered successful. In 6 of 19 cases, a rigid stabilization of the involved segment produced permanent pain relief.

Conclusion.—Percutaneous lumbar kryorhizotomy was beneficial in patients with LFS who had not undergone previous spinal surgery. Kryorhizotomy has practically no risk and appears to be a valuable alternative to lumbar medical branch neurotomy.

▶ Although facet rhizotomy using cryoablation is mentioned in a few pain textbooks, there have been no series of these procedures published prior to this report. The main disadvantage of the procedure is the large size of the probe, which is passed through a 12-gauge angiocath sheath.

S. E. Abram, MD

Disc Stimulation and Patterns of Referred Pain
O'Neill CW, Kurgansky ME, Derby R, et al (Spinal Diagnostics and Treatment Ctr, Daly City, Calif)
Spine 27:2776-2781, 2002   12–17

Introduction.—Experimental trials have shown that noxious stimulation of interspinous ligaments, facet joints, and paravertebral muscles produces referred pain into the extremity, with the distal extent of radiation dependent on the intensity of stimulation. Analogous investigations have not been performed on the lumbar intervertebral disks. The pattern of pain response to noxious stimulation of the intervertebral disks was examined in a prospective, within-subjects, observational experimental study.

Methods.—Data were prospectively gathered from a prospective series of patients enrolled in a concomitant outcome trial on the intradiskal electrothermal annuloplasty (IDET) procedure for the treatment of low back pain. The efficacy of the IDET procedure was not the focus of this trial. Twenty-five consecutive patients meeting all inclusion criteria filled out a pain diagram before undergoing the IDET annuloplasty procedure. The location, in-

TABLE 1.—Number of Patients With Certain Pattern of Presented and Reproduced Pain

Pain Drawing Pain Location	Low Back Only (Including Buttocks/Hip)	Low Back and Thigh	Low Back, Thigh, Lower Leg
Low back only (including buttocks/hip)	9	9	—	—
Low back and thigh	11	6	5	
Low back, thigh, lower leg	5	1	1	3

Abbreviation: IDET, Intradiskal electrothermal annuloplasty.
(Courtesy of O'Neill CW, Kurgansky ME, Derby R, et al: Disc stimulation and patterns of referred pain. *Spine* 27:2776-2781, 2002.)

tensity, and familiarity of any pain provoked during disk heating were correlated with patient symptoms and duration of heating.

Results.—During the disk-heating procedure, 68% of patients reported the exact reproduction of their usual pain, both in quality and location of pain (Table 1). No patients reported any unfamiliar pain during the procedure. The pattern of pain reproduction was consistent, with pain originating proximally and progressing distally as stimuli intensity increased.

Conclusion.—Noxious stimulation of the intervertebral disk may produce low back and referred extremity pain in patients with these symptoms. The distal extent of pain produced results from the intensity of stimulation. Disk stimulation can reproduce pain that extends to below the knee.

▶ This study confirms data from diskography and from mechanical stimulation of the disk during surgery under local anesthesia demonstrating correlation between clinical pain and evoked pain and the existence of diskogenic pain referred to the lower extremity. Of particular interest is the finding that higher intensities of noxious stimulation are needed to evoke more distal sites of referred pain.

S. E. Abram, MD

Lumbar Disc Herniation Regression After Successful Epidural Steroid Injection
Buttermann GR (Midwest Spine Inst, Stillwater, Minn)
J Spinal Disord Tech 15:469-476, 2002   12–18

Background.—Most patients' symptoms are reduced during the typical course of lumbar herniated nucleus pulposus (HNP), and many patients have a reduction in the size of their disk herniation. Successful conservative treatment results in a spontaneous decrease in HNP size in 66% to 80% of cases. Typically, the largest disk herniations show the greatest decrease in size and in the patients' symptoms. A comparison of patients who had conservative treatment with those having epidural steroid injection (ESI) was undertaken to define the proportion and degree of HNP regression and to determine whether ESI is helpful or whether improvement results from the natural history of the disorder.

Methods.—Thirty-eight patients who had improved without invasive treatment (Non-Inv group) and 20 patients who did not improve until after ESI (ESI group) underwent follow-up MRI scans. The Non-Inv group had improved without invasive treatment within 6 weeks of the onset of symptoms; the ESI patients showed no such improvement. No differences were noted at presentation between the 2 groups on questionnaires, including a back and leg visual analogue scale, the Oswestry disability scale, and a pain diagram.

Results.—Both groups evidenced significant improvements between the baseline and the 1- to 3-month follow-up evaluations, and there was no difference between the groups after 1 to 2 years. No significant correlation was found between the percentage of HNP size change and improved follow-up outcome scales. On regression analysis, improved Oswestry disability score correlated with decline in HNP size for sequestered and extruded herniation types. Size declines were more likely to occur in larger HNPs.

Sequestered and extruded HNPs were larger than contained HNPs on the baseline imaging studies and were smaller than contained HNPs on follow-up MRI. Patients in the Non-Inv group tended to have more resorbed extruded and sequestered disk herniations on follow-up MRI scans than those in the ESI group. In addition, patients who had more rapid decline in their symptoms tended to have more disk herniations that showed a high MRI T2 signal. Regardless of treatment, clinical improvement was similar in the 2 groups at follow-up.

Conclusion.—It was hypothesized that patients having ESI improved because the steroid decreased the inflammation of the nerve roots while not decreasing the size of the disk herniations. Thus, those who did not respond within 6 weeks had an inflammatory component not present in the patients who did respond quickly. Alternatively, because of the natural history of HNP, the patients who had ESI could simply have been exhibiting a spontaneous regression that took longer than in the other patients. The clinical improvement appeared to be independent of ESI therapy.

It is possible that the ESI triggered an easing of the symptoms of HNP during the normal course of regression and long-term spontaneous resolution. Those HNPs that were larger at the onset of the study showed the greatest decrease in size, particularly if they had been sequestered or extruded. Patients who do not experience resolution quickly may benefit from the use of ESI to ease symptoms while the disorder works through its natural course.

▶ Several studies have documented regression of herniated disks over time. Regression is more likely with large herniations and with disk extrusions as opposed to contained herniations. This study indicates that ESIs neither increase the rate of disk reabsorption nor interfere with the process.

S. E. Abram, MD

Midterm Outcome After Vertebroplasty: Predictive Value of Technical and Patient-Related Factors

Hodler J, Peck D, Gilula LA (Washington Univ, St Louis)
Radiology 227:662-668, 2003   12–19

Background.—Vertebroplasty has been used increasingly for the treatment of osteoporotic fractures and malignant disease of the lumbar, thoracic, and in rare cases, cervical vertebral bodies. Treatment time is relatively short, and vertebroplasty is not as technically demanding as surgical techniques, including posterior and interbody fusion. Another advantage of this technique is that percutaneous vertebroplasty can be performed in vertebrae that are unsuitable for surgical fixation. However, the side effects of vertebroplasty can be severe. Most of these side effects are associated with leakage of polymethylmethacrylate (PMMA) into the spinal canal or the intervertebral foramina. Different types of PMMA leakage and patient-related factors were evaluated in relation to clinical midterm (1-24 months) outcome after vertebroplasty.

Methods.—A review was conducted of standardized 4-view radiographs obtained during 363 vertebroplasties in 181 treatment sessions in 152 patients, including 121 patients with osteoporotic fractures, 30 with malignant disease, and 1 with hemangioma. Four types of PMMA leakage and other potential predictors were related to postprocedural pain response and midterm outcome after vertebroplasty. Statistical analysis was performed with χ^2 and Kruskal-Wallis tests. The mean duration of follow-up was 8.8 months.

Results.—At discharge, pain was absent after 106 of the 181 vertebroplasty sessions (58.5%), better after 50 procedures (27.6%), and unchanged after 25 procedures (13.8%). In 258 of the 363 treated vertebral levels, at least one type of leakage was found. None of the evaluated factors, including leakage of PMMA, were found to be significantly related to postprocedural pain response. However, response to pain at midterm outcome was strongly related to postprocedural treatment success.

Conclusions.—Leakage of small to moderate amounts of PMMA from the vertebral body has no significant effect on therapeutic success. The best predictor of midterm clinical outcome after vertebroplasty is immediate postprocedural pain.

▶ The lack of correlation between treatment success and volume of PMMA injected suggests that there is a mechanism of analgesic action other than stabilization of the collapsed vertebra. The rapidity with which analgesia occurs may also be compatible with another mechanism of action, such as sensory denervation of the injured vertebral body.

S. E. Abram, MD

A Giant Herniated Disc Following Intradiscal Electrothermal Therapy

Cohen SP, Larkin T, Polly DW Jr (Walter Reed Army Med Ctr, Washington, DC; Uniformed Services Univ of the Health Sciences, Bethesda, Md)
J Spinal Disord Tech 15:537-541, 2002   12–20

Background.—Offered as an alternative to surgery for some patients with single- or 2-level discogenic back pain, intradiscal electrothermal therapy (IDET) may work via collagen modification, cauterization of granulation tissue, or coagulation of nociceptors. Success rates of over 60% have been reported without serious complications. A patient with a preexisting, contained disk herniation developed neurologic symptoms after IDET.

Case Report.—Man, 29, an active-duty soldier, underwent 2-level IDET for L4-L5 and L5-S1 discogenic pain. The patient was 6 foot 6 inches tall and weighed 152 kg. The low back pain radiating to his left thigh had been present for 1.5 years. He had undergone chiropractic therapy, nonsteroidal anti-inflammatory drug therapy, and physical therapy but had minimal results. Thirteen months before having IDET, an MRI scan of the lumbar spine revealed a contained L5-S1 herniated disk with no nerve root impingement, a small L4-L5 disk bulge, and degenerative changes at both levels.

After various treatments without success, IDET was performed as an outpatient procedure. The patient was then given a lumbar support brace and instructions to avoid all activities more strenuous than light walking and gentle leg stretches for 1 month. After 5 days, the patient returned, complaining of worsening low back pain with new radiation into his left foot. No strenuous activities or precipitating event could be recalled. Nonfocal sensory changes were present, and the patient was given a week of steroids, increasing opioid doses, and acetaminophen around the clock.

After several weeks, he returned with weakness in his leg plus trouble performing even nonstrenuous military duties. A very large L5-S1 left paracentral herniated disk effacing the left S1 nerve root was found on MRI. Follow-up discography 4 months after IDET showed that the L4-L5 level was not contributing to the pain, and the patient had an uncomplicated, single-level, bilateral transforaminal lumbar interbody fusion at L5-S1 one month later. Over 28 mL of material was removed from the disk site at L5-S1. Radicular and axial symptoms were nearly totally gone after 2 years, with no neural compression and a solid interbody arthrodesis.

Conclusion.—The patient had been originally diagnosed with discogenic pain from the L4-L5 and L5-S1 levels. After IDET, only the L5-S1 disk caused symptoms. Whether the giant herniated disk resulted from the IDET or was caused by disease progression is not clear.

▶ It is not clear whether the appearance of a large disk protrusion was the result of progression of the patient's degenerative disk disease or whether the procedure produced further damage to the annulus, causing rapid progression of radicular symptoms. IDET is a procedure whose risk-benefit ratio has yet to be established.

S. E. Abram, MD

Percutaneous Vertebroplasty and Kyphoplasty for Painful Vertebral Body Fractures in Cancer Patients
Fourney DR, Schomer DF, Nader R, et al (Univ of Texas, Houston; Johns Hopkins Univ, Baltimore, Md)
J Neurosurg: Spine 98:21-30, 2003   12–21

Background.—Destructive vertebral lesions are a common source of morbidity, especially pain, among patients with cancer. Minimally invasive vertebroplasty and kyphoplasty can be used to stabilize the fractured vertebral body and obtain pain relief. The safety and efficacy of percutaneous vertebroplasty and kyphoplasty for the treatment of painful vertebral body fractures were examined in patients with cancer.

Study Design.—Fifty-six patients with cancer, aged 30 to 82 years, who underwent percutaneous vertebroplasty or kyphoplasty for intractable spinal pain were studied. The procedures were performed at the University of Texas M D Anderson Cancer Center between October 2000 and February 2002. The median symptom duration was 3.2 months. The median follow-up was 4.5 months.

Findings.—Significant pain relief was reported after 84% of procedures and no change after 5 procedures (Table 3). Reductions in self-reported pain remained significant for up to 1 year of follow-up. Analgesic consumption

---

TABLE 3.—Pain Outcome After 58 Treatment Sessions Involving Vertebro-
and/or Kyphoplasty*

	Number of Treatment Sessions (%)			
Pain Relief	VP	KP	VP & KP	Total
complete	8 (23)	1 (7)	3 (38)	12 (21)
improved	22 (63)	11 (73)	4 (50)	37 (64)
no change	3 (9)	1 (7)	1 (13)	5 (9)
worse	0	0	0	0
data unavailable	2 (6)	2 (13)	0	4 (7)
total	35 (60)	15 (26)	8 (14)	58

*Results refer to an analysis of documented visual analogue scale pain scores within the first 24 hours. Multiple results during that period were averaged.
Abbreviations: VP, Vertebroplasty; KP, kyphoplasty.
(Courtesy of Fourney DR, Schomer DF, Nader R, et al: Percutaneous vertebroplasty and kyphoplasty for painful vertebral body fractures in cancer patients. *J Neurosurg: Spine* 98:21-30, 2003.)

was reduced at 1-month follow-up. Asymptomatic cement leakage was detected during vetebroplasty, but not during kyphoplasty. There were no procedure-related complications or deaths.

Conclusions.—Percutaneous vertebroplasty and kyphoplasty are safe and provide effective, durable pain relief for many patients with intractable pain caused by cancer-related vertebral body fractures.

▶ Until the development of these techniques, little could be done for patients with metastatic disease who developed compression fractures of the vertebral bodies. Much of the published experience with these procedures has been in patients with compression fractures related to osteoporosis. This study confirms the efficacy of vertebroplasty and kyphoplasty in patients with metastatic disease involving the vertebral bodies. It is surprising that patients experience relief almost immediately after the procedure. This leads to speculation that the procedures may have an effect on nociceptive afferent fibers within the vertebral body.

S. E. Abram, MD

Prevention of Postherpetic Neuralgia With Varicella-Zoster Hyperimmune Globulin
Hügler P, Siebrecht P, Hoffmann K, et al (Miners' Assoc Hosp, Bottrop, Germany; Ruhr-Univ Bochum, Germany; Ruprecht-Karls-Univ, Heidelberg, Germany)
Eur J Pain 6:435-445, 2002   12–22

Background.—Postherpetic neuralgia (PHN) may develop in 9% to 14% of all patients after recovery from an acute attack of herpes zoster. The effect of a prophylactic IV injection of varicella-zoster hyperimmune globulin (VZV-IG) on patients at high risk of developing PHN was assessed in this prospective, placebo-controlled, double-blind clinical trial.

Study Design.—Forty patients older than 50 years with a dermatologic diagnosis of herpes zoster were studied. PHN was defined as pain in the dermatome affected by VZV of at least 15% points on a visual analogue scale (VAS). All patients received IV acyclovir therapy and were randomly as-

Frequency of postherpetic neuralgia in each group on day 42

			PHN	No PHN	Totals
Groups	Placebo	Number	14	6	20
		Percent	70.0%	30.0%	100.0%
	Varitect	Number	7	13	20
		Percent	35.0%	65.0%	100.0%

FIGURE 4.—Table of the outcome parameter 'postherpetic neuralgia' (*PHN*). (Courtesy of Hügler P, Siebrecht P, Hoffman K, et al: Prevention of postherpetic neuralgia with varicella-zoster hyperimmune globulin. *Eur J Pain* 6:435-445, 2002. Copyright European Federation of Chapters of the International Association for the Study of Pain.)

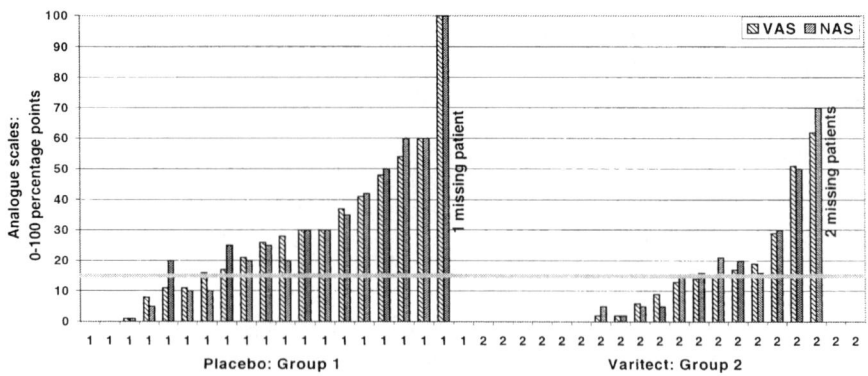

FIGURE 6.—Subjective pain intensity (visual analogue scale [*VAS*], numerical analogue scale [*NAS*]) on day 42. All patients in both groups arranged by pain intensity (VAS) are represented. *Gray line*: limit of postherpetic neuralgia. (Courtesy of Hügler P, Siebrecht P, Hoffman K, et al: Prevention of postherpetic neuralgia with varicella-zoster hyperimmune globulin. *Eur J Pain* 6:435-445, 2002. Copyright European Federation of Chapters of the International Association for the Study of Pain.)

signed to receive either VZV-IG or albumin (placebo). The primary outcome was the incidence of PHN on day 42 by VAS. Secondary outcomes included the McGill Pain-Rating Questionnaire, the revised multidimensional pain scale (RMSS), and the Freiburg symptom list (FBL).

Findings.—The frequency of PHN was 70% in the placebo group and 35% in the VZV-IG treatment group (Figs 4 and 6). The McGill Questionnaire found that the variability in the perception of pain was greater in the placebo group. There were no significant differences between the 2 groups in the FBL. The patients in the placebo group reported their pain as more "obstinate" on the RMSS than those in the treatment group.

Conclusions.—A single prophylactic injection of VZV-IG reduced the incidence and intensity of postherpetic pain in many patients at risk for PHN. Despite this success, completely effective therapy for PHN remains elusive.

▶ The prevention of severe, persistent neuropathic pain in patients with shingles is an important treatment goal. Elderly patients and those with severe pain during the acute phase of herpes zoster infections are at greatest risk. The use of antivirals early in the course of the disease appears to be helpful in reducing the duration and severity of pain, but a significant number of patients develop severe PHN in spite of antiviral therapy initiated promptly. The use of hyperimmune globulin appears to be effective in further reducing the incidence and severity of PHN.

The answer to this common and often devastating problem may lie in the public health domain. It is possible to monitor cell-mediated immunity to the varicella-zoster virus and to boost immunity in older individuals whose levels are low and who are at risk for developing herpes zoster infections and PHN.[1]

If this proves to be an effective prophylactic measure, it should become a regular part of the routine health care of every individual older than 50.

S. E. Abram, MD

Reference

1. Levin MJ, Smith JG, Kaufhold RM, et al: Decline in varicella-zoster virus (VZV)-specific cell-mediated immunity with increasing age and boosting with high-dose VZV vaccine. *J Infect Dis* 188:1336-1344, 2003.

Pregabalin for the Treatment of Postherpetic Neuralgia: A Randomized, Placebo-Controlled Trial
Dworkin RH, Corbin AE, Young JP Jr, et al (Univ of Rochester, NY; Pfizer Global Research and Development, Ann Arbor, Mich)
Neurology 60:1274-1283, 2003   12–23

Background.—Postherpetic neuralgia (PHN) is the most common complication of herpes zoster in immunocompetent patients. For many years, tricyclic antidepressants were considered first-line therapy for PHN, and more recently anticonvulsant, opioid, and topical analgesics have been found to have significant beneficial effects. However, many patients are refractory to treatment because of inadequate pain relief or intolerable side effects, and there is a need for additional safe and effective treatments for these patients. Pregabalin has been found to be effective in animal models of neuropathic and nociceptive pain. The safety and efficacy of pregabalin were evaluated in the treatment of PHN.

Methods.—A total of 173 patients with PHN, which was defined as pain for 3 or more months after healing of herpes zoster rash, were enrolled in this multicenter, parallel-group, double-blind, placebo-controlled study. The patients were randomly assigned to receive 8 weeks of treatment with pregabalin or placebo. Patients who received pregabalin were further assigned to receive either 600 mg/d or 300 mg/d. The primary outcome measure was the mean of the last 7 daily pain ratings. Secondary outcome measures included additional pain ratings, sleep interference, quality of life, mood, and patient and clinician ratings of global improvement.

Results.—The pregabalin-treated patients reported greater decreases in pain than patients treated with placebo. Pain was significantly reduced in the pregabalin-treated patients after the first full day of treatment and throughout the course of the study. There were also significant improvements on the McGill Pain Questionnaire total, sensory, and affective pain scores. The proportions of patients with at least 30% and at least 50% decreases in mean pain scores were greater in the pregabalin than in the placebo group (63% vs 25% and 50% vs 20%). Patients in the pregabalin group also experienced improved sleep compared with those in the placebo group. Side effects from pregabalin were generally mild to moderate in intensity.

Conclusions.—Treatment with pregabalin is safe and effective in relieving pain and improving sleep in patients with PHN.

▶ As with many other trials of newer anticonvulsants for neuropathic pain, treatment failure with gabapentin was an exclusion criterion. What we practitioners really want to know is: What drugs are effective for the gabapentin-resistant patient? Obviously this is not the question drug manufacturers want to address.

S. E. Abram, MD

Characteristics and Associated Features of Persistent Post-Sympathectomy Pain
Kapetanos AT, Furlan AD, Mailis-Gagnon A (Toronto Western Hosp; Toronto Western Research Inst; Inst for Work & Health, Toronto; Univ of Toronto)
Clin J Pain 19:192-199, 2003   12–24

Introduction.—Late complications are reported among patients who undergo surgical sympathectomy (SS) for hyperhidrosis, but few studies have examined late complications in patients who have had this procedure for treatment of neuropathic pain. A series of consecutive patients seen for neuropathic pain was retrospectively reviewed to determine the patterns and characteristics of postsympathectomy pain.

Methods.—Patients eligible for inclusion in the study had undergone SS for the indication of neuropathic pain and continued to experience considerable pain after the procedure. Charts were reviewed for demographic data, nature of the pain before and after SS, sensory findings, and the incidence of complications such as compensatory hyperhidrosis (CH) and abnormal gustatory sweating (GS).

Results.—The records of 17 patients (13 women and 4 men) with a mean age of 37 years at the time of SS were examined. Five patients experienced temporary pain relief for an average duration of 4 months. Eight patients continued to have the same or worse pain in addition to a new or expanded pain, and 1 patient was free of the original pain but experienced a new debilitating pain. In 3 patients, pain was unchanged after SS. Seven of 11 patients who were asked about pathologic GS reported experiencing this complication. CH was present in 11 of 13 patients asked about this complication.

Abnormal sweating (CH) developed at a median of 5 days after SS. In patients with GS, the condition was described as profuse, usually involving the underarm and antecubital fossa as well as the face. Three of 4 patients who had SS for lower extremity pain experienced both CG and GS.

Conclusion.—Postsympathectomy pain may be more severe and debilitating than the initial pain complaint, and serious pain complications were common in this patient series. Patients and clinicians should be aware of these complications when SS is being considered so that potential benefits can be weighed against known risks.

▶ This report provides the pain management physician useful information regarding the downside of SS. Over half the patients who failed to obtain relief from the procedure experienced new, distressing symptoms, and, in a review cited by the authors,[1] 25% of all patients who undergo this procedure develop new pain problems as a result of the procedure.

S. E. Abram, MD

Reference

1. Furlan AD, Mailis A, Papagapiou M: Are we paying a high price for surgical sympathectomy? A systematic literature review of late complications. *J Pain* 1:245-257, 2000.

Lamotrigine Monotherapy for Control of Neuralgia After Nerve Section
Sandner-Kiesling A, Seitlinger GR, Dorn C, et al (Karl Franzens-Univ, Graz, Austria)
Acta Anaesthesiol Scand 46:1261-1264, 2002   12–25

Background.—Nerve sections can cause neuropathic pain, which often responds to antidepressants or anticonvulsants. Six patients were described who were treated with the novel anticonvulsant lamotrigine (LTG) for control of neuralgia after nerve section.

Study Design.—The 6 patients had neuralgia caused by nerve section that did not respond to surgical or pharmacologic pain relief. After a 1-week washout period, therapy was initiated with 25 mg of LTG and increased by 25 mg every 6 days. After the dose reached 100 mg/d, 50-mg increments were added every 6 days, when necessary, up to a maximum of 300 mg/d. Patients completed a weekly pain diary that included adverse events.

Findings.—No breakthrough medication was required by any of these 6 patients during maintenance therapy with 75 to 300 mg/d of LTG of 1 to 23 months' duration. Pain intensity was reduced 33% to 100%, and pain frequency was reduced 80% to 100%. No adverse events were recorded during maintenance therapy.

Conclusions.—After failure of primary therapy for neuropathic pain caused by nerve section, long-term LTG therapy reduces both the intensity and frequency of pain without adverse effects. Controlled clinical studies should be performed to further evaluate this promising therapy.

▶ In the United States, gabapentin is often the first-line anticonvulsant selected for posttraumatic mononeuropathy. In all but one of the cases reported, LTG was the first anticonvulsant used. While it is helpful to know that LTG is effective in some cases of mononeuropathy, it would be very useful to know how effective it is for patients who have failed treatment with other anticonvulsants. My own experience is that this drug is generally not very useful for patients who have failed therapy with gabapentin.

S. E. Abram, MD

Gabapentin Effect on Neuropathic Pain Compared Among Patients With Spinal Cord Injury and Different Durations of Symptoms

Ahn S-H, Park H-W, Lee B-S, et al (Yeungnam Univ, Daegu, Korea; Natl Rehabilitation Hosp, Seoul, Korea; Ajou Univ, Suwon, Korea)

Spine 28:341-347, 2003

12–26

Introduction.—Chronic pain is reported frequently by patients who have sustained spinal cord injury (SCI), and in many cases the pain is severe and neuropathic in nature. Neuropathic pain resulting from SCI is characterized by sensations of burning, stabbing, or numbness and is often refractory to treatment. Gabapentin is effective in relieving some types of neuropathic pain, but there are few studies of the drug's use in the treatment of neuropathic pain after traumatic SCI.

Methods.—Thirty-one patients with SCI or cauda equina syndrome participated in a study of the effects of gabapentin on neuropathic pain. All had failed to gain adequate relief with conventional analgesics. The duration of symptoms was less than 6 months in 13 patients (group 1) and more than 6 months in 18 patients (group 2). After an 18-day titration period, patients entered a 5-week maintenance period of gabapentin treatment. The initial dose was 300 mg/d, with 300 mg increases every 3 days until a dose of 1800 mg/d was reached. Further increases to 2400 mg/d and 3600 mg/d were allowed if required, and dosages were decreased if adverse events occurred. Conventional analgesics were continued at a therapeutic level.

Results.—Groups 1 and 2 were similar in mean age and in number of patients without cauda equina or conus medullaris lesions. Twenty-five patients (81%) completed the study, 20 of them maintained with a dosage of 1800 mg/d, 3 with 1200 mg/d, 1 with 2400 mg/d, and 1 with 3600 mg/d. At the end of the study, the mean pain and sleep interference scores, rated on a visual analogue scale, were significantly lower in both groups. Pain reduction reached a plateau after 4 weeks of therapy. Somnolence, the most common adverse effect, appeared to be dose dependent. Most adverse effects were mild or moderate in intensity.

Conclusion.—Gabapentin decreased neuropathic pain refractory to conventional analgesics, particularly in patients whose duration of symptoms was less than 6 months. The drug was beneficial, however, in those with a longer duration of symptoms. No serious side effects were attributed to gabapentin.

▶ Pain of SCI is one of the most difficult problems faced by pain management physicians. This study, along with several previous noncontrolled reports, attests to the efficacy of gabapentin in SCI patients. However, there is room for skepticism. The study is not controlled, and there is no guarantee that patients would not have improved to the same degree had they been given placebos. This is particularly true for the group with the short pain duration. Another drawback to this study is the lack of stratification according to type of pain.

There are several different pain syndromes encountered among SCI patients, and it would be helpful to know which ones are most responsive.

S. E. Abram, MD

Gabapentin in Neuropathic Pain Syndromes: A Randomised, Double-Blind, Placebo-Controlled Trial
Serpell MG, for the Neuropathic Pain Study Group (Gartnavel Gen Hosp, Glasgow, Scotland; et al)
Pain 99:557-566, 2002   12–27

Introduction.—Neuropathic pain is often resistant to standard treatments such as nonsteroidal anti-inflammatory drugs and opioids. Recent studies have reported that anti-epileptics are effective in some types of neuropathic pain; the anti-epileptic gabapentin became the first such agent to be licensed in the United Kingdom for the treatment of all neuropathic pain conditions. Patients with a wide range of neuropathic pain syndromes were enrolled in an investigation of the safety and efficacy of gabapentin.

Methods.—The randomized study was conducted in 35 hospital outpatient pain clinics in the United Kingdom and the Republic of Ireland. Eligible patients were adults with a definite diagnosis of neuropathic pain and at least 2 of 4 nonspecific symptoms: allodynia, burning pain, shooting pain, or hyperalgesia. In a double-blind manner, 153 patients were assigned to gabapentin and 152 to placebo. Gabapentin was administered in 3 divided doses, initially titrated to 900 mg/d over 3 days, followed by 2 increases to a maximum of 2400 mg/d if required by the end of week 5. Patients kept pain diaries and were assessed for treatment effect on individual pain symptoms and quality of life.

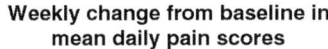

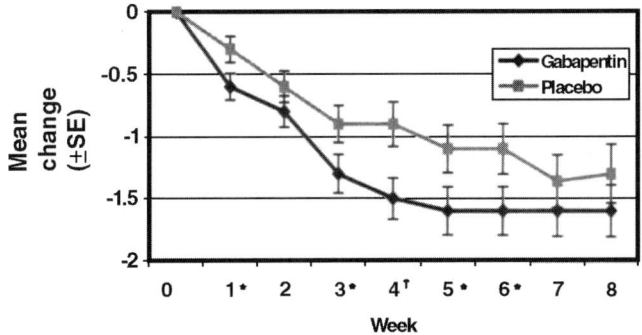

FIGURE 3.—Weekly change from baseline in mean daily pain scores. *Asterisk* indicates $P \leq .05$ versus placebo. *Single dagger* indicates $P \leq .01$ versus placebo Crank based analysis of covariance. (Courtesy of Serpell MG, for the Neuropathic Pain Study Group: Gabapentin in neuropathic pain syndromes: A randomised, double-blind, placebo-controlled trial. *Pain* 99:557-566, 2002.)

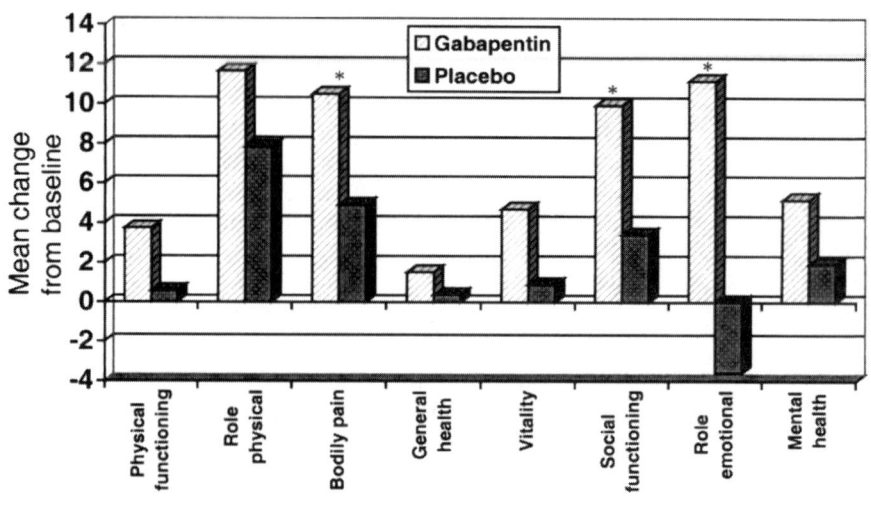

*P < 0.05 (ANCOVA).

FIGURE 5.—Summary of changes in domains of the Short Form-36 Health Survey. Scores represent mean change (SE) from baseline to final calculable score adjusted for specific covariates (baseline score and cluster/study center). A positive change indicates improvement. *Asterisk* indicates $P \leq .05$ versus placebo (Mantel-Haenszel). (Courtesy of Serpell MG, for the Neuropathic Pain Study Group: Gabapentin in neuro-pathic pain syndromes: A randomised, double-blind, placebo-controlled trial. *Pain* 99:557-566, 2002.)

Results.—Allodynia was reported at baseline by 69% of patients, burning pain by 80%, shooting pain by 86%, and hyperalgesia by 71%. At week 5, 28 patients had withdrawn from the gabapentin group; of those remaining, 101 were taking 2400 mg/d, 18 were taking 1800 mg/d, and 27 were taking 900 mg/d. Over the 8-week study period, the average daily pain score had decreased by 21% in the gabapentin-treated group and by 14% in the placebo group (Fig 3). Other measures of pain and quality of life (Fig 5) also showed gabapentin to be significantly more effective than placebo. Gabapentin was well tolerated; most adverse events (dizziness and somnolence) were mild and transient.

Conclusion.—Gabapentin, at doses ranging from 900 to 2400 mg/d, improved symptoms for patients with a variety of neuropathic pain syndromes. The drug appeared to be equally effective in treating different types of pain and was well tolerated.

▶ While the percent reduction in mean pain ratings was small in this study, the results are meaningful. Since the mean includes patients who experienced no relief, it is likely that the responders did substantially better than the mean 21% reduction would indicate. One important aspect of this study is that one third of patients had previously failed therapy with anticonvulsants. This may indicate that gabapentin is effective for patients who have failed other anti-epileptics. However, insufficient data are provided to prove or disprove that assumption.

S. E. Abram, MD

Gabapentin in Postamputation Phantom Limb Pain: A Randomized, Double-Blind, Placebo-Controlled, Cross-Over Study

Bone M, Critchley P, Buggy DJ (Leicester Gen Hosp, England; Mater Misericordiae Hosp, Dublin)
Reg Anesth Pain Med 27:481-486, 2002   12–28

Introduction.—Severe phantom limb pain after surgical amputation occurs in 50% to 67% of amputees at 6 months post procedure. It is challenging to treat. Gabapentin has been shown to be effective in several syndromes of neuropathic pain. The analgesic efficacy of gabapentin in phantom limb pain was assessed in a randomized, double-blind, placebo-controlled, cross-over investigation.

Methods.—Nineteen patients with phantom limb pain attending a multidisciplinary pain clinic were enrolled. Any other anticonvulsant therapy was discontinued. All treatments lasted 6 weeks, separated by a 1-week washout period. Codeine/paracetamol was permitted as rescue analgesia. The daily dose of gabapentin was titrated in increments ranging from 300 mg to 2400 mg or the maximum tolerated dose. Patients were evaluated at weekly intervals. The major outcome measure was visual analogue scale pain intensity difference, compared with baseline at completion of each treatment. Secondary measures included indexes of sleep interference, depression (Hospital Anxiety and Depression scale), and activities of daily living (Bartel Index).

Results.—The mean patient age was 56 years (range, 24-68 years; 16 men). Of 19 patients evaluated, 14 completed both arms of the trial. Both placebo and gabapentin treatments resulted in decreased visual analogue scale scores versus baseline (Table 2). The pain intensity difference was sig-

TABLE 2.—Weekly Visual Analogue Scale Pain Scores (Derived From Daily Visual Analogue Scale Pain Scores) and Categorical Pain (Baseline-End of Therapy)

Variable	Placebo Arm	Gabapentin Arm	P Value for Gabapentin v Placebo
Baseline before placebo/gabapentin	6.7 ± 1.9	6.1 ± 1.8	$P=.19$
Week 1	5.3 ± 2.6	4.3 ± 2.2	$P=.30$
Week 2	4.1 ± 2.0*	3.9 ± 2.5†	$P=.80$
Week 3	4.8 ± 2.9	3.3 ± 2.3†	$P=.13$
Week 4	4.4 ± 2.1*	4.1 ± 2.7	$P=.24$
Week 5	4.7 ± 2.9*	3.2 ± 2.5†	$P=.13$
Week 6	5.1 ± 2.2	2.9 ± 2.2	$P=.025$
Categorical pain baseline	1.8 ± 0.9	1.5 ± 0.9	$P=.49$
Categorical pain end of therapy	1.6 ± 1.2	1.45 ± 1.0	$P=.80$

Note: All data shown are mean ± standard deviation. From 19 randomized patients, 14 completing both arms fully.

Placebo arm VAS: *Repeated measures analysis of variance with Dunnet's post hoc test comparing each week with baseline: Baseline placebo versus week 2, $P < .01$; baseline placebo versus week 4, $P < .05$; baseline placebo versus week 5, $P < .05$; baseline versus other weeks, NS.

Gabapentin arm visual analogue scale: †Repeated measures analysis of variance with Dunnet's post hoc test comparing each week with baseline: Baseline gabapentin versus week 2, $P < .05$; baseline gabapentin versus week 3, $P < .01$; baseline gabapentin versus week 5, $P < .01$; the median (range) final dose of gabapentin in the gabapentin arm was 2400 mg (1800 to 2400).

(Courtesy of Bone M, Critchley P, Buggy DJ: Gabapentin in postamputation phantom limb pain: A randomized, double-blind, placebo-controlled, cross-over study. *Reg Anesth Pain Med* 27:481-486, 2002.)

TABLE 3.—Weekly Pain Intensity Difference Scores (Derived From Daily Visual Analogue Scale Pain Scores as Visual Analogue Scale T_0 T_x)

VAS PID	Placebo Arm	Gabapentin Arm
Week 1	1.4 ± 0.8	1.6 ± 1.0
Week 2	2.6 ± 1.2	2.2 ± 1.2
Week 3	1.9 ± 1.1	2.8 ± 1.2
Week 4	2.3 ± 1.1	2.0 ± 1.2
Week 5	2.0 ± 1.3	2.9 ± 1.5
Week 6	1.6 ± 0.7	3.2 ± 2.1*

Note: All data shown as mean ± standard deviation. From 19 randomized patients, 14 completing both arms fully.

*$P = .03$, Mann-Whitney U test. Baseline Gabapentin versus week 6, $P < .01$. Baseline versus other weeks, NS. The median (range) final dose of gabapentin in the gabapentin arm was 2400 mg (1800 to 2400).

(Courtesy of Bone M, Critchley P, Buggy DJ: Gabapentin in postamputation phantom limb pain: A randomized, double-blind, placebo-controlled, cross-over study. *Reg Anesth Pain Med* 27:481-486, 2002.)

nificantly greater for placebo than for gabapentin (3.2 vs 1.6; $P = .03$) (Table 3). No significant differences were observed between placebo and gabapentin therapy in numbers of tablets of rescue medication needed, sleep interference, Hospital Anxiety and Depression scale, or Bartel index. Gabapentin was well tolerated and there were few reports of side effects.

Conclusion.—Gabapentin monotherapy was superior to placebo after 6 weeks of treatment in relieving postamputation phantom limb pain. There were no significant between-group differences in mood, sleep interference, or activities of daily living. A type II error cannot be excluded for these variables.

▶ While the degree of pain reduction seen with gabapentin seems modest, the results are encouraging, since few interventions have been shown to provide significant benefit for patients with this condition. It would be useful to look at the individual pain scores of patients in the study. Since there was a fairly high standard deviation, there would be some patients with minimal pain relief and others with substantial benefit.

S. E. Abram, MD

Gabapentin Markedly Reduces Acetic Acid–Induced Visceral Nociception
Feng Y, Ciu M, Willis WD (Peking Univ, Peoples Republic of China; Univ of Texas, Galveston; Allergan Inc., Irvine, Calif)
Anesthesiology 98:729-733, 2003   12–29

Introduction.—Gabapentin is a novel, well-tolerated anticonvulsant drug that has recently been used clinically as an antihyperalgesic agent in the treatment of certain neuropathic pain states. The ability of gabapentin to inhibit responses to peritoneal irritation–induced visceral pain was assessed, along with the effect of gabapentin on spinal cord amino acid release.

Methods.—The acetic acid–induced writhing assay was used in Sprague-Dawley rats to ascertain the extent of antinociception. Animals received an

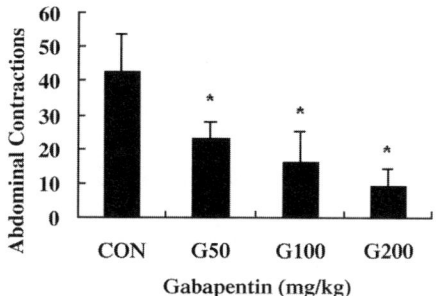

FIGURE 1.—Gabapentin attenuated abdominal contractions in a dose-related fashion following intra-peritoneal injection of 0.6% acetic acid (mean ± standard deviation). *Asterisk* indicates $P < .05$ versus control group. *Abbreviations: CON,* Saline control; *G50,* 50 mg/kg gabapentin; *G100,* 100 mg/kg gabapentin; *G200,* 200 mg/kg gabapentin. (Courtesy of Feng Y, Ciu M, Willis WD: Gabapentin markedly reduces acetic acid–induced visceral nociception. *Anesthesiology* 98:729-733, 2003. Copyright American Society of Anesthesiologists Inc. Used with permission of Lippincott-Raven Publishers.)

intraperitoneal injection of acetic acid 40 minutes after intraperitoneal administration of vehicle or gabapentin (50, 100, or 200 mg/kg). CSF dialysate was obtained by microdialysis from spinal subarachnoid space in anesthetized rats.

Acetic acid–induced release of amino acids into the dialysate—including glutamate, aspartate, serine, glutamine, and glycine—after intraperitoneal injection of acetic acid was assessed by measurement of changes in the concentrations of these amino acids. The influences of pretreatment with saline or gabapentin (100 mg/kg intraperitoneally) on amino acid release were compared.

Results.—Gabapentin reduced writhing responses in a dose-related fashion (Fig 1). Dialysate concentrations of glutamate, aspartate, and serine increased significantly after intraperitoneal injection of acetic acid. Glutamine and glycine concentrations were not significantly increased. Rats pretreated with 100 mg/kg gabapentin versus saline showed suppression of the acetic acid–induced increases in glutamate, aspartate, and serine concentrations.

Conclusion.—Gabapentin effectively restricts acetic acid–induced nociception. The antinociceptive effects of gabapentin correlate with the suppression of noxious-evoked release of excitatory amino acids in the spinal cord.

▶ Clinicians have been concentrating their trials of gabapentin and other anticonvulsants on patients with neuropathic pain. This study should stimulate interest in this drug for the management of visceral pain. Chronic pancreatitis and pancreatic cancer are conditions that involve both visceral pain and injury to visceral afferent nerves and would appear to be reasonable conditions to treat with gabapentin.

S. E. Abram, MD

Efficacy of Intravenous Magnesium in Neuropathic Pain

Brill S, Sedgwick PM, Hamann W, et al (Univ Hosp Lewisham, London; St George's Hosp Med School, London; Guy's and St Thomas' Hosp, London)
Br J Anaesth 89:711-714, 2002   12–30

Background.—Postherpetic neuralgia (PHN) is a complication of acute herpes zoster. It is characterized by severe pain and paresthesia in the area of the skin affected by the initial herpes infection. PHN is an increasing clinical problem in the elderly population, with a prevalence reaching 75% in patients older than 70 years who have previously had a herpes zoster infection. The typical features of PHN include burning, aching, or itching and continuous pain, often occurring in association with hyperalgesia and allodynia. Studies have indicated that the N-methyl-D-aspartate (NMDA) receptor is involved in the development of hypersensitivity, and NMDA is known to be a critical factor in the establishment of several chronic pain states. Magnesium is known to block the NMDA receptor. The analgesic properties of magnesium sulfate were evaluated in patients with PHN.

Methods.—In this double-blind, placebo-controlled, crossover study, magnesium sulfate or saline was administered as an IV infusion in 7 patients with PHN. Spontaneous pain was recorded, and qualitative sensory testing with cotton wool was performed before and after the infusion.

Results.—Pain scores during the infusion were significantly lower for magnesium compared with placebo at 20 and 30 minutes, but not at 10 minutes. The magnesium sulfate infusion was safe and well tolerated by all the patients.

Conclusions.—These findings support the concept that the NMDA receptor is involved in the control of PHN, and that the NMDA receptor–blocking mechanism of magnesium sulfate can be used as the basis for effective pain control in some patients with PHN.

▶ This study suggests that magnesium may be useful in treating certain neuropathic pain states. Unfortunately, other NMDA antagonists, such as dextromethorphan, have not been very helpful for most patients with established neuropathic pain. It is possible that Mg^{++} may have provided pain relief in the study patients through other antinociceptive or antihyperalgesic effects. Such a hypothesis is supported by the fact that other NMDA antagonists have relieved allodynia but not spontaneous pain in other types of neuropathy. One drawback of this ion is that it is poorly absorbed from the gastrointestinal tract, and oral administration produces an osmotic diarrhea.

S. E. Abram, MD

Venlafaxine Versus Imipramine in Painful Polyneuropathy: A Randomized, Controlled Trial

Sindrup SH, Bach FW, Madsen C, et al (Univ of Southern Denmark, Odense)
Neurology 60:1284-1289, 2003   12–31

Background.—Patients with polyneuropathy are often given tricyclic antidepressants (TCAs) as first-line treatment, although contraindications and

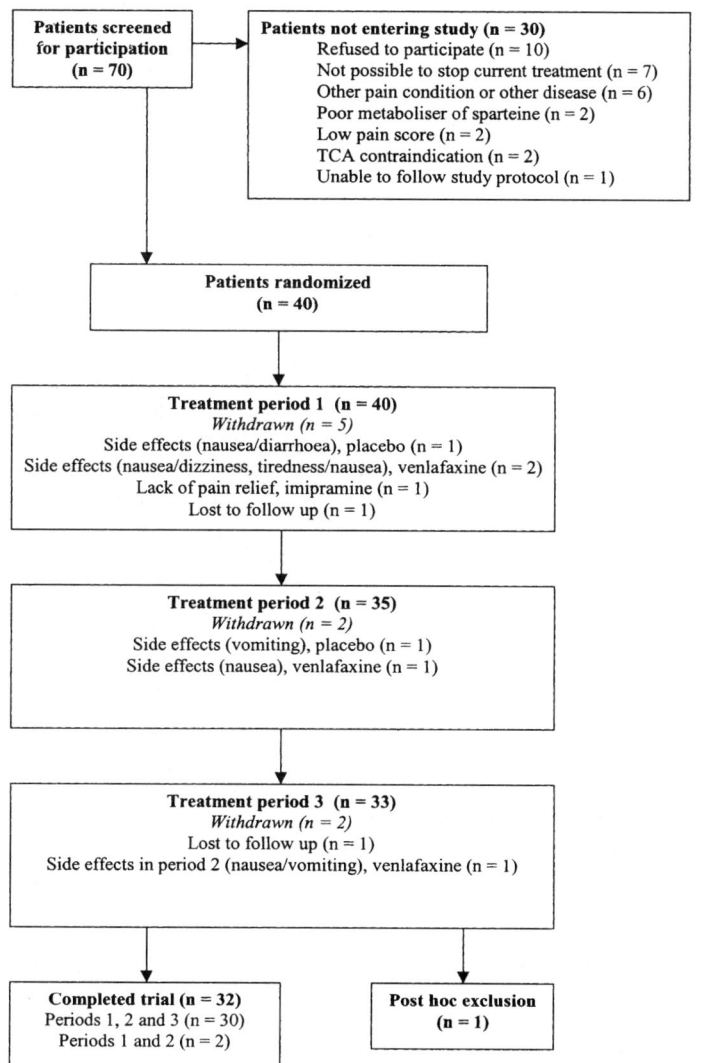

FIGURE 1.—Patient flow in study. (Courtesy of Sindrup SH, Bach FW, Madsen C, et al: Venlafaxine versus imipramine in painful polyneuropathy: A randomized, controlled trial. *Neurology* 60:1284-1289, 2003. Copyright American Academy of Neurology. Used with permission of Lippincott-Raven Publishers)

side effects limit their usefulness. Selective serotonin reuptake inhibitors are generally ineffective or at least less effective than TCA for this disorder. Venlafaxine, a serotonin that is a weak noradrenaline reuptake inhibitor, was proposed as a possible choice to relieve pain in polyneuropathy and was compared for that function with the TCA imipramine.

Methods.—A randomized, double-blind, placebo-controlled study design with a 3-way crossover was chosen. Twenty-nine patients completed all 3 study periods, each of which was 4 weeks long (Fig 1). The dosages used were 225 mg for venlafaxine and 150 mg for imipramine. Patients rated pain paroxysms, presence of constant pain, and pain evoked by touch and pressure using a numeric rating scale ranging from 0 to 10 points.

Results.—Compliance with the venlafaxine regimen was 97%, imipramine 96%, and placebo 98%. Lower pain scores were obtained during venlafaxine and imipramine use than during placebo use, but the values with venlafaxine and imipramine showed no significant differences. Both venlafaxine and imipramine reduced pain paroxysms, pressure-evoked pain, and constant pain; few instances of touch-evoked pain occurred and did not show any alteration, regardless of regimen. The consumption of paracetamol during the fourth treatment week was affected by the treatment; the consumption during imipramine use was less than with placebo.

A trend toward greater relief with venlafaxine than with placebo was noted. Complete, good, or moderate pain relief was reported more often with imipramine than with placebo. Venlafaxine tended to achieve this degree of pain relief less often than imipramine. Imipramine was also found to be more helpful in obtaining clinically relevant pain relief among patients with diabetic neuropathy compared with venlafaxine. For venlafaxine, the number needed to treat to obtain 1 patient with moderate or better pain relief was 5.2; the number for imipramine was 2.7.

Conclusion.—The efficacy of venlafaxine was shown to be comparable to that of imipramine for the relief of pain in patients with polyneuropathy.

▶ In general, selective serotonin reuptake inhibitors have not been as effective as TCAs in treating neuropathic pain. This is unfortunate, as the selective serotonin reuptake inhibitors tend to be better tolerated and are much less likely to cause weight gain. In this study, both venlafaxine and imipramine provide statistically significant pain reduction compared to placebo. However, the effect is not very robust for either drug. Nevertheless, venlafaxine may be a reasonable choice for patients unable to tolerate tricyclics.

S. E. Abram, MD

Chronic Post-sternotomy Pain
Kalso E, Mennander S, Tasmuth T, et al (Helsinki University Central Hosp)
Acta Anaesthesiol Scand 45:935-939, 2001   12–32

Background.—Chronic postoperative pain can persist for years and has been reported after thoracotomies, hysterectomies, repair of inguinal hernia, and mastectomies. The incidence of severe, incapacitating postoperative pain associated with these procedures is about 3% to 5%. Significant post-operative pain is also caused by sternotomy, and patients with chronic post-sternotomy pain are often referred to pain clinics. However, epidemiologic studies on chronic poststernotomy pain are scarce. The incidence and pos-sible risk factors of chronic pain after sternotomy operations performed for coronary bypass grafting or thymectomy were examined.

Methods.—This study included 2 groups of patients who were studied for persistent pain after sternotomy. A questionnaire was sent to 71 patients with myasthenia gravis who had undergone a thymectomy during 1985-1996, and to 720 patients who had undergone coronary bypass grafting (CABG) in 1994. Patients were asked about the presence of pain and other symptoms in the chest, shoulders, arms, or legs that they believed to be asso-ciated with their surgery. The patients were also asked about the quality of the pain and its evolution over time. The patients' records were checked for details about surgery, anesthesia, and the state of coronary disease.

Results.—The response rate was 87%. The interval between the surgery and the interview varied from 6 months to 12 years in the patients with my-asthenia gravis, and from 2 to 3 years in the CABG group. In the patients with myasthenia gravis, 27% reported chronic poststernotomy pain, which was moderate to severe in 48% of the patients. In the CABG patients, 28% of the patients continued to have poststernotomy pain, which was moderate to severe in 38% of the patients. One third of the patients who had postster-notomy pain reported sleep disturbances as a result of the pain.

Conclusions.—Chronic poststernotomy pain may have a significant ad-verse effect on the patient's quality of life. Additional studies are needed to determine whether the incidence of this problem can be reduced by minimiz-ing complications, improving postoperative care, and starting early ad-equate pain management.

The Incidence of Chronic Post-sternotomy Pain After Cardiac Surgery: A Prospective Study
Meyerson J, Thelin S, Gordh T, et al (Univ Hosp, Uppsala, Sweden)
Acta Anaesthesiol Scand 45:940-944, 2001   12–33

Background.—Some patients who undergo cardiac surgery will experi-ence poststernotomy pain. The characteristics, incidence, and clinical course of this pain are not well known. The incidence of chronic poststernotomy pain in patients undergoing sternotomy for cardiac surgery was determined in general and according to the specific surgical procedure.

Methods.—A group of 349 consecutive patients was included in this pro-spective study. The patients were evaluated by postal questionnaire for chronic poststernotomy pain 1 year after surgery. Patients were asked to de-scribe and score any persistent pain after the surgical procedure and to rate their pain on a visual analogue scale. The patients were then classified into 3 subgroups according to surgical procedure. The first group was composed of

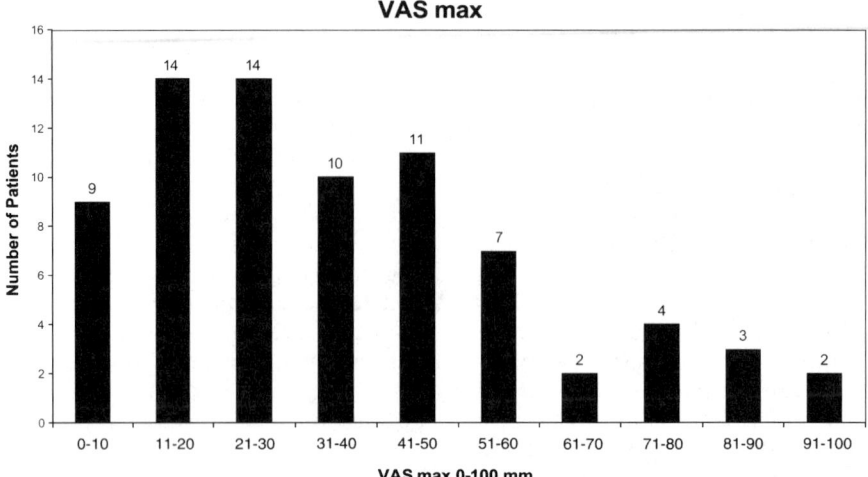

FIGURE 2.—Post-sternotomy pain. Distribution of ratings of maximum pain on the visual analogue scale (VAS$_{max}$) n = 76. (Courtesy of Meyerson J, Thelin S, Gordh T, et al: The incidence of chronic post-sternotomy pain after cardiac surgery: A prospective study. *Acta Anaesthesiol Scand* 45:940-944, 2001.)

patients who underwent coronary bypass grafting (CABG) procedures, including internal thoracic artery grafting (ITAG). The second group was composed of patients who underwent CABG without grafting, and the third group included patients who underwent valve replacement without CABG.

Results.—Responses were obtained from 318 patients (91%) of whom 90 (28%) reported chest discomfort other than the discomfort they experienced before surgery. Scoring on the visual analogue scale indicated that 41 patients (13%) reported maximum pain intensity of 30 mm or greater (indicative of moderate pain), and that 14 of these patients (4%) scored 54 mm or greater (indicative of severe pain) (Fig 2). No statistically significant differences in pain incidence and intensity were observed when comparing the patients according to the type of surgery.

Conclusions.—A high overall incidence (28%) of noncardiac poststernotomy pain after cardiac surgery was documented. The intensity of pain was modest in most patients, but 4% of patients reported severe pain. The incidence of pain after sternotomy was not only associated with harvest of the internal thoracic artery, and additional etiologic factors must be sought.

▶ These 2 studies (Abstracts 12–32 and 12–33) indicate that chronic pain after sternotomy is a very common problem. The incidence is the same after 3 years as it is after 6 months to 1 year, indicating that treatment success is very low once the condition becomes chronic. Pain associated with sternotomy is caused by a variety of somatic and neuropathic conditions. In addition, persistent pain of cardiac origin, not considered in these studies, is fairly common. The appearance of significant cardiac disease creates substantial psychological stressors for many patients. These patients need careful evaluation with treatment directed toward the specific physical and psychological pathology identified.

S. E. Abram, MD

Effect of Thoracic Epidural Analgesia on Refractory Angina Pectoris: Long-term Home Self-treatment
Richter A, Cederholm I, Jonasson L, et al (Univ Hosp, Linköping, Sweden; Högland Hosp, Eksjö, Sweden)
J Cardiothorac Vasc Anesth 16:679-684, 2002   12–34

Introduction.—For patients with refractory angina, any treatment that improves the quality of life (QOL) without worsening coronary artery disease is desirable. The effects of long-term home self-treatment with thoracic epidural analgesia (TEA) on angina, QOL, and safety were assessed in a prospective, consecutive pilot investigation.

Methods.—Between January 1998 and January 2000, 37 consecutive patients with refractory angina were treated with TEA by using a subcutaneously tunneled epidermal catheter. Patients were educated to provide self-treatment at home with intermittent injections of bupivacaine. The clinical outcome of TEA was evaluated by using the Canadian Cardiovascular Society anginal classification, number of anginal attacks per week, nitroglycerin consumption per week, and overall self-rated QOL assessed by visual analogue scale (0-100) according to the EroQol 5D. Data were obtained until January 2001. Follow-up ranged between 1 and 3 years.

Results.—All except 1 patient improved symptomatically. The improvement was maintained throughout treatment, which ranged between 4 days to 3 years (Fig 2). The Canadian Cardiovascular Society angina class diminished from 3.6 to 1.7, the frequency of anginal attacks dropped from 46 to 7 per week, nitroglycerin intake dropped from 32 to 5 per week, and the overall self-rated QOL evaluated by visual analogue scale rose from 24 to 76 (all $P < .001$). No serious catheter-associated complications were observed. However, 51% of the catheters became displaced, and a new one had to be inserted during the evaluation period.

Conclusion.—Long-term self-administered home treatment with TEA appears to be an effective and safe adjuvant treatment for patients with refractory angina. It provides symptomatic relief of angina and improves QOL.

▶ This report indicates that simple techniques requiring no sophisticated equipment and minimal involvement of health care personnel can be very effective. The protocol used is similar to those employed in some of the early reports of home-based epidural analgesia for cancer pain.[1] The most troublesome difficulties with the technique are catheter displacement and fibrosis around the catheter tip, both of which require catheter replacement. For patients who experience repeated difficulties maintaining functional catheters,

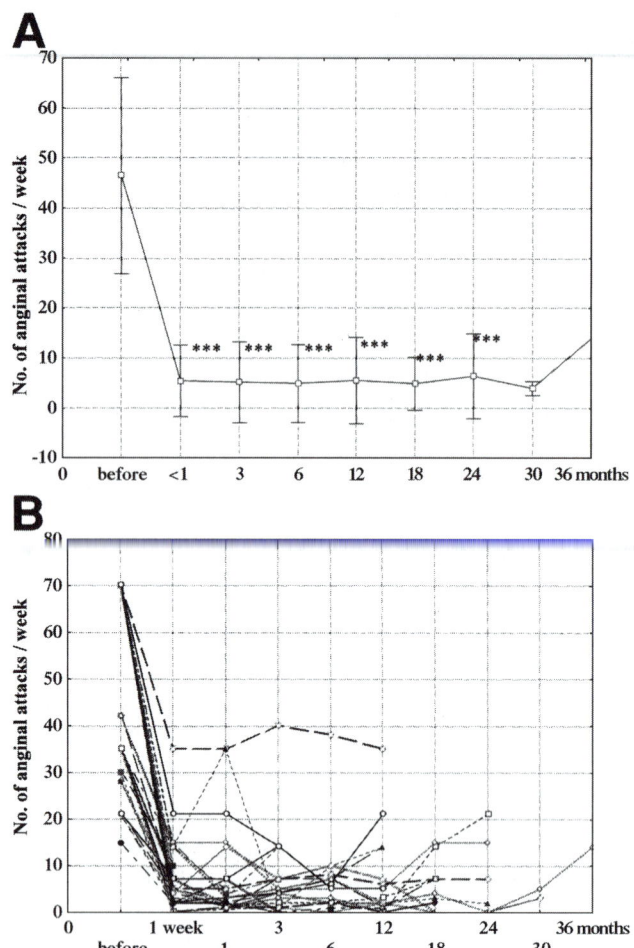

FIGURE 2.—A, The number of anginal attacks per week (mean, SD) before and during thoracic epidural analgesia (TEA) treatment. *Stars* indicate significant differences compared with before (***P* < .001). At 30 and 36 months, there are only 2 and 1 patients. No statistical test was done in these intervals. B, Individual plots of each patient's number of anginal attacks a week (mean, SD) before and during TEA treatment. (Courtesy of Richter A, Cederholm I, Jonasson L, et al: Effect of thoracic epidural analgesia on refractory angina pectoris: Long-term home self-treatment. *J Cardiothorac Vasc Anesth* 16:679-684, 2002.)

an implanted intrathecal drug delivery device may be a reasonable though considerably costlier alternative.

S. E. Abram, MD

Reference

1. Hogan QH, Maddox JD, Abram SE, et al: Epidural opiates and local anesthetics for the management of cancer pain. *Pain* 46:271-279, 1991.

Prevalence and Characteristics of Chronic Pain Among Chemically Dependent Patients in Methadone Maintenance and Residential Treatment Facilities

Rosenblum A, Joseph H, Fong C, et al (Natl Development of Research Insts, New York; New York State Office of Alcoholism and Substance Abuse Services, New York and Albany; Beth Israel Med Ctr, New York)

JAMA 289:2370-2378, 2003   12–35

Introduction.—Studies of the prevalence of chronic pain suggest that more than 70 million adults in the United States are affected. Pain may be even more prevalent in the chemically dependent population, and the experience of pain may interact with substance use disorders in complex ways. Patients from methadone maintenance treatment programs (MMTPs) and from short-term inpatient substance abuse programs were surveyed to determine the prevalence and characteristics of chronic severe pain.

Methods.—Representative samples of 390 patients from 2 MMTPs and 531 patients from 13 inpatient programs, all in New York State, completed questionnaires. Data collected included demographic information; substance abuse history and treatment; pain severity, type, duration, and impact on quality of life; and medication used to treat pain. Psychiatric distress was measured with a 6-item version of the Symptoms Checklist-90.

Results.—The mean age of the MMTP patients was 43 years; 38% were women, 25% were white, 36% were black, and 33% were Hispanic. Heroin (88%), alcohol (77%), and cocaine (34%) were the most frequently reported problem substances. The mean methadone dose was 78.2 mg/d. Inpatients had a mean age of 36 years; 20% were women, 44% were white, 31% were black, and 16% were Hispanic. Alcohol (74%), cocaine (54%), and heroin (15%) were the most frequently reported problem substances.

Chronic severe pain was experienced by 36% of MMTP patients and 24% of inpatients; pain during the previous week was reported by 80% and 78%, respectively. Pain severity and pain duration were correlated, particularly among MMTP patients. Pain interfered with physical and psychosocial functioning in 65% of MMTP patients and in 78% of inpatients with chronic pain.

Among those with chronic pain, inpatients were significantly more likely than MMTP patients to have used illicit drugs and alcohol to treat pain and less likely to have been prescribed pain medications. Multivariate correlates of chronic pain in MMTP patients were age, chronic illness, lifetime psychiatric illness, psychiatric distress, and time in treatment. For inpatients, correlates of chronic pain were race, drug craving, chronic illness, and psychiatric distress.

Conclusion.—The prevalence of chronic, severe pain is high among patients in substance abuse treatment, especially those in MMTPs. Chronic pain may contribute to illicit drug use, and the undertreament of pain is a significant concern in populations with chemical dependency.

▶ The prevalence of severe pain among opioid dependent individuals in a chemical dependency treatment program is clearly higher than in the general population. Among patients in the MMTP, the average dose was substantial (mean, 78 mg/d). There was a significant correlation between time in the program and pain prevalence. While some patients indicated that preexisting pain was the reason for first using controlled or illegal substances, this was not the case for the great majority. The prevalence of severe pain among individuals without a preexisting painful condition was 32%. These data suggest that a likely mechanism for severe pain among these people is opioid-induced hyperalgesia. The pathophysiology of this condition is now well understood. Animal models indicate that daily opioid administration can produce tolerance and hyperalgesia in 5 to 7 days. Indeed, transient hyperalgesia can be seen following a single dose of a short-acting opioid. Persistent exposure of spinal opioid receptors leads to sensitization of spinal neurons mediated by activation of protein kinase C, which acts to enable the N-methyl-D-aspartate (NMDA) receptor. Chronic opioid exposure also leads to activation of spinal cord glial cells, with subsequent increased production of proinflammatory cytokines, which further sensitize neurons. Of note is the fact that methadone has NMDA antagonist effects. Despite this, patients in MMTPs typically exhibit hyperalgesia.[1] Either the NMDA antagonist effect is insufficiently robust to prevent this occurrence or other non-NMDA mechanisms—eg, glial activation—are involved.

S. E. Abram, MD

Reference

1. Doverty M, White JM, Somogyi AA, et al: Hyperalgesic responses in methadone maintenance patients. *Pain* 90:91-96, 2001.

Catheter-Associated Masses in Patients Receiving Intrathecal Analgesic Therapy
McMillan MR, Doud T, Nugent W (Foothills Regional Pain Ctr, Seneca, SC; Mountain Med Imaging, Seneca, SC)
Anesth Analg 96:186-190, 2003   12–36

Introduction.—Intraspinal drug infusion for the treatment of chronic pain conditions carries a risk of neurologic injury from the development of catheter-associated masses. The exact incidence and prevalence of this complication is unknown, but in the cohort of patients reported here, 3 of 7 examined were found to have these masses.

Methods.—When the index case was discovered, all patients in the authors' practice who were receiving intrathecal drug therapy were being treated with reconstituted crystalline preservative-free morphine sulfate or fentanyl citrate in saline (preservative-free bupivacaine was added in some cases). The duration of treatment for the 7 patients ranged from 3 months to 47 months.

When the first catheter-associated intrathecal mass was recognized, the remaining patients underwent screening radiocontrast lumbar myelography and CT scanning. Not screened were additional patients whose therapy duration was less than 3 months. Patients found to have catheter-associated masses but no serious neurologic complications could elect to have the intrathecal system removed, continue intrathecal therapy with another drug, or discontinue therapy leaving the pump and/or catheter in place.

Results.—Two patients with catheter-associated masses had failed back surgery syndrome and 1 had osteoarthritis of the knee. The mean duration of therapy among patients with masses was 19.6 months. Their mean morphine dose (11.8 mg/d) was greater than that of patients without masses (1.26 mg/d). Patients with masses were also younger than those without masses (mean, 51 vs 73 years). The mass regressed after therapy stopped in 1 patient and remained stable in another; these patients had no additional treatment-related complications or neurologic impairment. The third patient with a catheter-associated mass required decompression laminectomy for symptoms of spinal cord compression and was left with permanent functional left lower-leg paresis.

Conclusion.—Patients receiving long-term intrathecal analgesic drug therapy are at risk for the development of catheter-associated masses. The lesions may be asymptomatic or result in permanent neurologic deficits. Use of CT myelography allows for early detection of the masses and intervention if required.

▶ Granulomas that develop at the tip of implanted spinal catheters have been reported in patients receiving high concentrations and high doses of morphine and hydromorphone. These masses can produce serious complications, including paraplegia. Initial symptoms are often new-onset pain, usually producing symptoms within dermatomes adjacent to the mass. This report raises the possibility that the incidence may be higher than previously estimated. It would seem reasonable to screen any patient receiving at least 10 mg/mL hydromorphone or 25 mg/mL morphine intrathecally.

S. E. Abram, MD

Experimental Pain Management

Phase I Safety Assessment of Intrathecal Ketorolac
Eisenach JC, Curry R, Hood DD, et al (Wake Forest Univ, Winston-Salem, NC; Univ of California, San Diego, La Jolla)
Pain 99:599-604, 2002   12–37

Background.—In animal studies, intrathecally administered cyclooxygenase (COX) inhibitors produce antinociception and are not associated with toxicity. This phase I study used an open-label, dose-escalating design to assess the neurotoxicity of intrathecal ketolorac in humans.

Study Design.—The study group consisted of 20 healthy adult volunteers. These participants had baseline neurologic, blood pressure, heart rate, oxyhemoglobin saturation, and end-tidal carbon dioxide assessments. Then the first 5 volunteers received 0.25 mg, the next 5 received 0.5 mg, the next 5 received 1 mg, and the final 5 received 2 mg of preservative-free intrathecal ketrorolac. Assessments were repeated for the next 24 hours. Volunteers were questioned as to side effects and were followed up for 6 months. Efficacy was evaluated by a Peltier-controlled thermode heat stimulus applied to the volar forearm and lateral calf.

Findings.—Ketorolac injection did not affect blood pressure, but there was a small dose-dependent reduction in heart rate during the first hour. Ketorolac did not affect sensory or motor function or reflexes. One participant had a mild headache 24 hours later that resolved spontaneously. Ketorolac administration did not reduce pain report to heat stimuli.

Conclusions.—Intrathecal injection of the COX inhibitor ketorolac was well tolerated in healthy adult volunteers. It did not appear to affect the response to noxious heat stimuli. These findings suggest that intrathecal ketorolac is safe to use in further studies to determine its analgesic properties.

▶ It is unclear whether spinally administered nonsteroidal anti-inflammatory drugs (NSAIDs) will be of clinical importance for either acute or chronic pain management. Spinal NSAIDs are capable of reducing phase 2 pain behavior in the rat formalin test, indicating that prostaglandins probably play a role in spinal sensitization. However, the effect is not very robust, and there is a ceiling effect as the dose is increased. As indicated by the results of heat pain testing in this study, it is unlikely that intrathecal NSAIDs will provide significant antinociceptive effects. On the other hand, there is some clinical evidence that preoperatively administered NSAIDs have a preemptive effect. If so, the spinal route may be a reasonable way to block spinal sensitization induced by surgical trauma, as the very small doses required would avoid the renal, gastrointestinal, and hemostatic complications of systemic NSAIDs.

S. E. Abram, MD

Loss of T-Type Calcium Current in Sensory Neurons of Rats With Neuropathic Pain
McCallum JB, Kwok W-M, Mynlieff M, et al (Med College of Wisconsin, Milwaukee; Marquette Univ, Milwaukee, Wis; VA Med Ctr, Milwaukee, Wis)
Anesthesiology 98:209-216, 2003   12–38

Introduction.—Chronic pain due to peripheral pathology or posttraumatic neuropathy is maladaptive, challenging to treat, and poorly understood at the cellular level. Calcium channels have an important role in neuronal processes. Although sensory neurons are rich in low-voltage–activated calcium channels (LVACCs), the physiologic function of these channels is not known. Their possible role in rebound burst firing may make them vulnerable to increased excitability after neuropathic injury. Pharmacologically isolated LVACCs after neuropathic injury in male rats were characterized and compared to sham-operated rats with the use of fluorescent markers to identify cells with axons projecting to the injury site.

Methods.—A CCI model of rat peripheral neuropathy was used. Pharmacologic methods were employed to isolate LVACC in cells from the dorsal root ganglia of neuropathic and sham-operated rats, including the blockage of high-voltage–activated calcium channels with fluoride and selective toxins. The LVACCs were assessed with conventional whole cell patch clap electrophysiology techniques.

Results.—After chronic constriction injury of the peripheral axon, LVACC was significantly diminished compared to sham animals, as demonstrated by a 60% decrease in peak current density and a 80% decrease in total calcium influx (Fig 6). A depolarization shift in the voltage dependence of activation and an increase in the incidence of deactivation and inactivation seemed to produce this decrease in LVACC. Either Ni^{2+} or milbefradil,

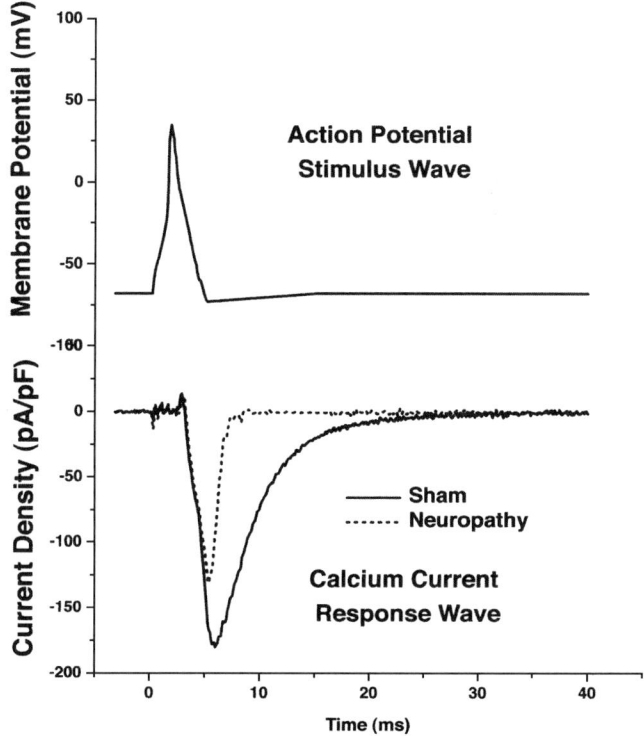

FIGURE 6.—Whole cell low voltage–activated CA^{2+} flux was significantly reduced in cells from neuropathic rats compared to sham animals. In response to an action potential waveform, peak current density declined from -45.2 ± 13.4 pA/pF (n = 21) to -20.1 ± 4.6 pA/pF (n = 16) after neuropathy, and the area under the wave representing total Ca^{2+} flux dropped from -199.6 ± 91.4 pA/pF to -40.4 ± 5.7 pA/pF ms after neuropathy. Likewise, duration of Ca^{2+} flux was reduced from 9.9 ± 1.3 ms to 5.2 ± 0.4 ms. (Courtesy of McCallum JB, Kwok W-M, Mynlieff M, et al: Loss of T-Type calcium current in sensory neurons of rats with neuropathic pain. *Anesthesiology* 98:209-216, 2003. Copyright American Society of Anesthesiologists Inc. Used with permission of Lippincott-Raven Publishers.)

blockers of LVACC, applied to the bath of normal dorsal root ganglion cells during current clamp significantly and reversibly increased excitability.

Conclusion.—The loss of LVACC may contribute to the reduced spike frequency adaptation and increased excitability after injury to the sensory neurons. Through reduced Ca^{2+} influx, the cells become less stable and more likely to initiate or transmit bursts of action potentials. Consequently, modulation of Ca^{2+} currents of the dorsal root ganglion may be a possible therapeutic intervention.

▶ Nerve injury models in animals have demonstrated allodynia and hyperalgesia that can be blocked by N-methyl-D-aspartate (NMDA) antagonists or by agents that block glial cell activation. Unfortunately, this knowledge has not yet translated to appreciable success in treating posttraumatic neuropathic pain in humans. The demonstration of significant changes in the activity of voltage-activated calcium channels in experimentally induced sciatic mononeuropathy opens new doors of investigation that may lead to novel agents capable of blocking or reversing the changes that lead to chronic neuropathic pain.

S. E. Abram, MD

Miscellaneous

Attacking Pain at its Source: New Perspectives on Opioids
Stein C, Schäfer M, Machelska H (Freie Universität Berlin)
Nature Med 9:1003-1008, 2003   12–39

Background.—Opioids have been the most powerful drugs used to manage severe acute and chronic pain but are associated with serious side effects. The new opioids activate opioid receptors outside the CNS and can avoid unwanted effects that are centrally mediated. Among the new research approaches now arising are selective targeting of opioid peptide–containing cells to sites of pain and gene transfer to improve opioid synthesis.

Peripheral Opioid Receptors and Targeting.—Peripheral opioid receptors have been confirmed on C and A fibers; vanniloid receptor-1–positive visceral fibers; and neurons that express isolectin B4, substance P, or calcitonin gene–related peptide. The inhibitory effect of opioids on peripheral sensory neurons appears to involve primarily calcium channel modulation and suppression of tetrodotoxin-resistant sodium channels. Tissue injury, such as inflammation, neuropathy, or bone damage, enhances peripheral opioid analgesia. Endogenous opioid ligands expressed within inflamed tissue may yield an additive or synergistic interaction at the peripheral opioid receptor. Tolerance does not appear to develop in this situation. In addition, circulating opioid-producing immune cells seem to home in on damaged tissue to secrete their opioids and then continue on to the regional lymph nodes.

Mechanisms and Investigations.—Opioids are released from immunocytes under the regulation of interleukin-1β and corticotropin-releasing hormone (CRH). Triggers to this process include environmental stress and endogenous CRH. The central blockade of pain decreases the migration of opioid-producing immunocytes to the injured sites, which indicates a reduced need for peripheral pain-control cells. Immunosuppression and blockade of the extravasation of opioid-containing leukocytes can extinguish CRH- and stress-induced analgesia. Other sources of opioids are the pituitary and adrenal glands, keratinocytes that have been stimulated by endothelin-1, and sensory neurons that are stimulated to overexpress by gene transfer. Among the new opioid ligands found to act exclusively in the periphery without central side effects are loperamide, asimadoline, arylacetamide, and peptidic kappa-opioid receptor agonists. Peripheral opioids were found to be effective in a wide variety of animal models, addressing visceral as well as neuropathic pain. Clinically, the intra-articular administration of the μ agonist morphine has been shown to reduce pain scores or supplemental analgesic consumption (or both) in patients having knee surgery; its action was dose dependent and reflected a peripheral mechanism of action without side effects. Other clinical areas in which peripheral opioids were successful in controlling pain without side effects are spinal fusion surgery, dental surgery, corneal abrasion repair, urinary bladder surgery, and laparoscopic tubal ligation. The injection of agonists into noninflamed areas along nerve trunks has proved ineffective.

Conclusions.—The development of new, peripherally selective opioid drugs is needed to address problems of abuse with the centrally acting opioids. Among the advantages already identified are the absence of central side effects; anti-inflammatory effects; lack of tolerance and constipation; lack of the gastrointestinal, renal, and thromboembolic complications that accompany nonsteroidal anti-inflammatory drugs; and efficacy against neuropathic pain.

▶ Research on the mechanisms of pain is past its infancy, but there is still much work to do. However, I predict that there will be an explosion of new information over the next 5 to 10 years, resulting in novel therapy for pain.

M. Wood, MD, FRCA

Repeated Failure of Epidural Analgesia: An Association With Epidural Fat?

Lang SA, Korzeniewski P, Buie D, et al (Univ of Calgary, Alta, Canada; Univ of Saskatchewan, Saskatoon, Canada)
Reg Anesth Pain Med 27:494-500, 2002   12–40

Introduction.—Many factors have been linked to inadequate epidural analgesia. A case of repeated failure of epidural analgesia in a patient with epidural lipomatosis was reported.

> *Case Report.*—Woman, 44, underwent elective small-bowel resection. An L_{1-2} epidural catheter was inserted for postoperative analgesia. She gave no indication of having pain at the time of emergence from general anesthesia or during the first 2 hours in the

recovery room. Assessment of the level of hypoesthesia to ice while she was comfortable in the recovery room indicated a functional epidural catheter (cephalad level of T_{10}).

At 2 hours after recovery room admission, the patient complained of increasing pain. An additional 6 mL of 0.25% bupivacaine was placed in the catheter. The patient's pain decreased but remained substantial. There was little evidence of sensory block above the T_{10} level and a T_{10} catheter was placed in the epidural space. Testing verified proper placement of the catheter. A test dose of 5 mL of 0.25 % bupivacaine provided prompt and complete pain relief. The level of hypoesthesia did not exceed the T_{10} level.

About 1 hour later, the patient complained again of increasing discomfort. There was no evidence of sensory block. The patient had no response to a bolus of 8 mL of 1% lidocaine. Thorough examination did not indicate any cause for the pain other than a malfunctioning epidural catheter. A third epidural catheter was inserted at the T_{8-9} level. Placement of the catheter in the epidural space was confirmed by a test dose of 10 of mL 0.5% bupivacaine. The level of hypoesthesia to ice was limited to a narrow bilateral band from T_7–T_9.

Analgesia failed 2 hours after placement of the third catheter, which was removed. The patient's pain was subsequently managed with IV patient-controlled analgesia morphine. MRI showed extensive epidural fat dorsal to the spinal cord from C_5–C_7 and from T_3–T_9. An imaging diagnosis of epidural lipomatosis was made.

Conclusion.—Repeated failure of epidural analgesia together with restricted segmental conduction block after administration of a large amount of local anesthetic should lead to consideration of epidural lipomatosis.

▶ Epidural lipomatosis is most often encountered in patients who have a history of treatment with corticosteroids. The condition can first be seen as a radiculopathy, and there are case reports of unsuccessful treatment with epidural steroid injections initiated without prior imaging. In 1 of those cases, exacerbation of symptoms occurred following steroid epidurals. MRI scan demonstrated an increase in the amount of epidural fat.[1]

S. E. Abram, MD

Reference

1. Sandberg DI, Lavyne MH: Symptomatic spinal epidural lipomatosis after local epidural corticosteroid injections (case report). *Neurosurgery* 45:162-165, 1999.

13 Clinical Trials

Self-Management of Asthma in General Practice, Asthma Control and Quality of Life: A Randomised Controlled Trial
Thoonen BPA, Schermer TRJ, van den Boom G, et al (Univ Med Centre Nijmegen, The Netherlands)
Thorax 58:30-36, 2003   13–1

Background.—The finding that airway inflammation is the main causative process in asthma has led to recommendations that inhaled corticosteroids be introduced early in the management of this disease. However, asthma morbidity is still significant, and poor compliance with prescribed inhaled medications is an important cause of uncontrolled disease. Patients with mild asthma treated by a general practitioner may be appropriate candidates for intermittent treatment as long as adequate control of their asthma is maintained.

Most studies in the literature have reported that self-management is effective in patients with more severe asthma or those with frequent exacerbations, but it is not known whether guided self-management could also be effective in patients with milder asthma. The effectiveness of asthma self-management in general practice was investigated.

Methods.—A group of 19 general practices were randomly assigned to either usual care or self-management for their asthma patients. These patients were included after confirmation of the general practice diagnosis. Follow-up was 2 years. The patients kept diary cards and visited the lung function laboratory every 6 months. The main outcome measures were number of successfully treated weeks, limited-activity days, asthma-specific quality of life, forced expiratory volume in 1 second (FEV_1), FEV_1 reversibility, concentration of histamine provoking a fall in FEV_1 of 20% or more (PC_{20} histamine), and amount of inhaled steroids.

Results.—The study enrolled 214 patients of whom 62% were female. The mean percentage of successfully treated weeks per patient in the usual care group was 72% (74 of 103 weeks), compared with 78% (81 of 105 weeks) of the self-management group. The mean number of limited activity days was 1.2 in the self-management group compared with 3.9 in the usual care group. The estimated increase in asthma quality of life score was 0.10 points per visit in the usual care group and 0.21 points per visit in the self-management group. There was no change in FEV_1, FEV_1 reversibility, or

PC_{20}. Patients in the self-management group had a savings of 217 puffs of inhaled steroid per patient compared with those in the usual care group.

Conclusion.—It appears that self-management decreases the burden of illness as perceived by asthma patients and is at least as effective as the treatment usually provided by primary care physicians in the Netherlands. Thus, self-management should be considered a safe basis for intermittent treatment with inhaled corticosteroids.

▶ This study shows that self-management is at least as effective as a primary care physician in helping patients control asthma symptoms and is much better in reducing limited number of days and even medication usage. It is important to understand some of the mechanics of this study. Patients in the self-management practices made 4 individual training visits during which they received tailored education and instructions and how to use their personalized self-treatment plans. These plans covered items on how to adjust corticosteroid dosage in response to increasing or decreasing peak expiratory flow. The patients were then followed up for 2 years. The group that had the self-management had fewer days of limited activity by a factor of 65% and fewer emergency room visits and less medication usage.

Are we in the era where patients are going to take much more control of their own mediation and medicine use and responsibility for their health? If so, we will probably have a major reduction in health care cost and a major increase in well-being. It seems to me that is one of the only ways that society can afford medical care demographics as America changes to older and older populations over the next 35 years.

This study is one that showed that you can reduce health care resource use dramatically and disability days dramatically by self-care for asthma. What does that mean for preoperative preparation and postoperative pain therapy? I think we already have seen some of those changes. Educated patients will be discharged much faster and do just as well, if not better, than those who are uneducated about perioperative expectations.

M. F. Roizen, MD

Randomized Prospective Comparison of Forced Air Warming Using Hospital Blankets Versus Commercial Blankets in Surgical Patients

Kabbara A, Goldlust SA, Smith CE, et al (Case Western Reserve Univ, Cleveland, Ohio)

Anesthesiology 97:338-344, 2002   13–2

Background.—Hypothermia is defined as a core temperature of less than 36°C and may develop in patients undergoing major surgery. One of the most effective methods for maintaining normothermia in a patient intraoperatively is forced-air warming. However, the cost of disposable forced-air warming blankets may limit the widespread use of this technique. It has been demonstrated that forced-air warming with hospital bed sheets is twice as effective as with commercial blankets in heating standardized thermal bodies using identically warmed 38°C forced air and the Bair Hugger Model 500 Warming Unit. However, no data are available on the use of this hospital blanket-warming technique with surgical patients. The effectiveness of forced-air warming using hospital blankets versus warming with a Bair Hugger warming unit to create a tent of warm air was evaluated.

Methods.—This study was conducted among adult patients undergoing major surgery. The patients were randomly assigned to receive forced-air warming with either a commercial Bair Hugger blanket (control group, 44 patients) or standard hospital blankets (experimental group, 39 patients). The set points were 43°C for the control group and 38°C for the experimental group. Distal esophageal temperatures were monitored. Patients were contacted the following day to determine any problems with the warming technique to which they were assigned.

Results.—The surface area covered was 36% ± 12% in the experimental group and 40% ± 10% in the control group. The final temperatures at the end of surgery were similar at 36.2 ± 0.6°C in the experimental group and 36.4 ± 0.7°C in the control group. The number of patients with esophageal temperatures below 36°C at the end of surgery was similar in the 2 groups (12 of 39 in the experimental group [31%] vs 12 of 44 in the control group [27%]). Most patients were satisfied with their anesthetic and warming technique, with 38 of 39 patients in the experimental group and 44 of 44 patients in the control group expressing satisfaction. No thermal injuries occurred in either group.

Conclusion.—Standard hospital blankets heated to 38°C with forced air were just as effective as commercial blankets heated with forced air at 43°C for adequately warming surgical patients intraoperatively. However, this experimental technique should not be used until additional safety evaluations have been conducted.

▶ Since most forced-air warmers are provided by the company that provides the disposable air-warming hospital blanket, using the forced-air warming with hospital blankets may not be any less expensive. There is blanket laundry, etc. My belief is this may not be any advantage at all when one gets to finally calculating the full cost.

M. F. Roizen, MD

Laryngeal Morbidity and Quality of Tracheal Intubation: A Randomized Controlled Trial
Mencke T, Echternach M, Kleinschmidt S, et al (Univ of Saarland, France)
Anesthesiology 98:1049-1056, 2003   13–3

Background.—The part of the airway most often injured as a complication of anesthesia is the larynx. Among the most common injuries are vocal cord paralysis and hematoma or granuloma of the vocal cords. In addition, postoperative hoarseness (PH) is often seen, with prolonged or permanent hoarseness found in 1% of patients. The risk factors contributing to laryngeal injury have been identified, but the quality of tracheal intubation has not been evaluated as one of them. The complications occurring with an induction technique of propofol, fentanyl, and a neuromuscular blocking agent were compared with those accompanying the same regimen without a neuromuscular blocking agent, focusing specifically on vocal cord sequelae and PH.

Methods.—Forty patients were randomly assigned to receive a propofol-fentanyl induction regimen with atracurium and 40 the same regimen without atracurium. The Copenhagen Score was used to measure intubation conditions. A standardized interview evaluated PH 24, 48, and 72 hours after anesthesia. Stroboscopy was used to assess the vocal cords before surgery and 24 and 72 hours afterward. Follow-up examinations were continued until PH or vocal cord sequelae had resolved.

Results.—There were no significant intergroup differences regarding intubation time, number of attempts, or Cormack grades. Significantly higher rates of excellent intubating scores and clinically acceptable scores were obtained with the atracurium than without. Among those receiving atracurium, the incidence of PH was significantly less than among those in whom saline solution was used. PH was only seen in the postanesthesia period among the atracurium group but lingered into the postoperative period in the saline solution group. The number of days with PH was 6 with atracurium and 25 with saline solution. The saline solution group also had significantly more cases of vocal cord sequelae than the atracurium group. The number of days with vocal cord sequelae was 50 for the saline solution group and 5 for the atracurium group. The intubating score and the development of PH were closely correlated, with 11% of patients with excellent intubating scores having PH, 29% of those with good scores, and 57% of those with poor scores. Vocal cord sequelae were seen in the same pattern, with 11% of those with excellent intubating scores having sequelae, 22% of those with good scores, and 50% of those with poor scores.

Conclusions.—The addition of atracurium to an induction technique with propofol and fentanyl significantly reduced the incidence of PH and vocal cord sequelae. With excellent intubating scores, both PH and vocal cord sequelae were noted significantly less frequently than with poor scores. Thus, the quality of the tracheal intubation and the use of atracurium were shown to influence the incidence of laryngeal morbidity.

▶ Do the conditions for ease of intubation affect laryngeal morbidity, such as vocal cord sequelae or hoarseness? The answer appears to be yes. Care should be given to the "timing of intubation" and the use of muscle relaxants.

M. Wood, MD, FRCA

A Randomized, Controlled Trial of the Use of Pulmonary-Artery Catheters in High-Risk Surgical Patients

Sandham JD, for the Canadian Critical Care Clinical Trials Group (Univ of Calgary, Alta, Canada; et al)

N Engl J Med 348:5-14, 2003   13–4

Background.—Some observational studies have suggested that the use of pulmonary artery (PA) catheters to guide therapy is associated with an increased mortality rate. However, trials that examined this issue to date have been hindered by methodologic problems, including selection bias, noncompliance by physicians, and crossover from standard care (without the use of a PA catheter) to use of a PA catheter. Therapy guided with a PA catheter was compared with standard therapy among high-risk, elderly patients undergoing surgery followed by a stay in the ICU.

Methods.—To address concerns in previous trials, this study used a multicenter, randomized, controlled clinical trial involving blinded assessment of outcomes. The study group comprised 1994 high-risk patients aged 60 years or older with American Society of Anesthesiologists (ASA) class III or IV risk who were scheduled for urgent or elective major surgery followed by a stay in an ICU. Outcomes were assessed by observers blinded to the treatment group assignments. The primary outcome was the in-hospital mortality rate from any cause. The patients were randomly assigned to the use of a PA catheter (997 patients) or no use of a PA catheter (997 patients) during surgery.

Results.—A total of 77 patients (7.7%) in the no-PA-catheter group died in the hospital, compared with 78 patients (7.8%) in the group in which a PA catheter was used. There was a higher rate of pulmonary embolism in the

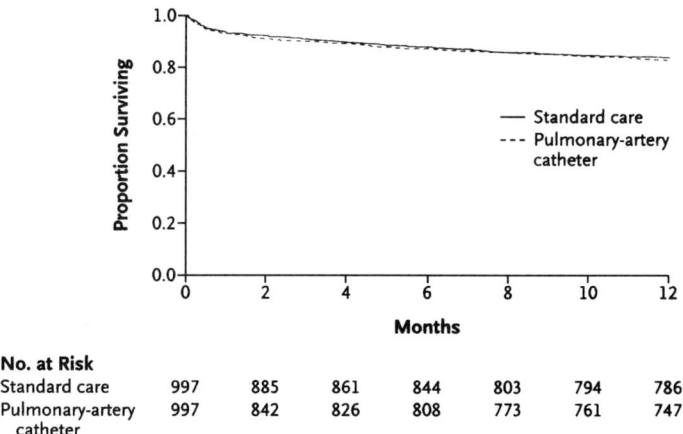

No. at Risk

Standard care	997	885	861	844	803	794	786
Pulmonary-artery catheter	997	842	826	808	773	761	747

FIGURE 1.—Kaplan-Meier survival curves to 1 year. Data for 6 patients in the standard care group and 7 patients in the catheter group for whom exact dates of death were unavailable are included in the number at risk up to the last follow-up contact when the patient was still alive. (Reprinted by permission of *The New England Journal of Medicine* from Sandham JD, for the Canadian Critical Care Clinical Trials Group: A randomized, controlled trial of the use of pulmonary-artery catheters in high-risk surgical patients. *N Engl J Med* 348:5-14, 2003. Copyright 2003, Massachusetts Medical Society. All rights reserved.)

catheter group than in the standard care group (8 events vs no events). The survival rates at 6 months were similar (88.1% in the standard care group and 87.4% in the PA catheter group) (Figs 1 and 2 and Table 2). The median duration of hospital stay was 10 days for each group.

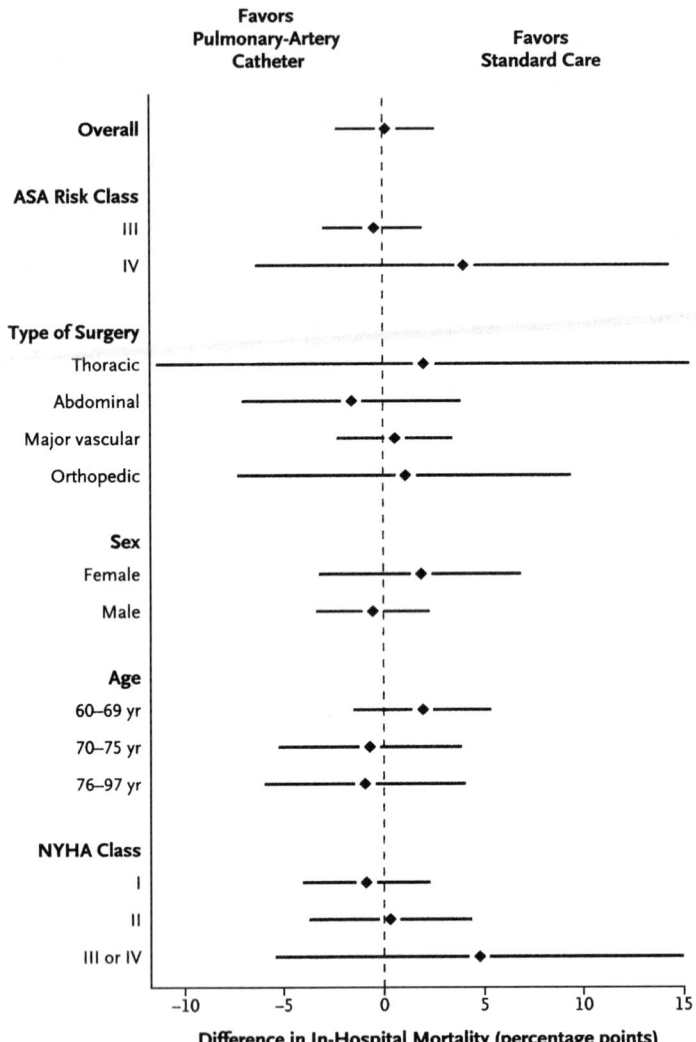

FIGURE 2.—Estimated differences in in-hospital mortality in the catheter group as compared with the standard care group, overall and according to American Society of Anesthesiologists (*ASA*) risk class, type of surgery, sex, age, and New York Heart Association (*NYHA*) class. Positive differences indicate excess mortality in the catheter group as compared with the standard care group, whereas negative differences indicate lower mortality in the catheter group. *Bars* represent 95% confidence intervals. (Reprinted by permission of *The New England Journal of Medicine* from Sandham JD, for the Canadian Critical Care Clinical Trials Group: A randomized, controlled trial of the use of pulmonary-artery catheters in high-risk surgical patients. *N Engl J Med* 348:5-14, 2003. Copyright 2003, Massachusetts Medical Society. All rights reserved.)

TABLE 2.—In-Hospital Mortality and Perioperative and Postoperative Morbidity

Variable	Standard-Care Group	Catheter Group	P Value
Length of hospital stay — days			
Median	10	10	0.41
Interquartile range	7-15	7-15	
In-hospital mortality — no. (%)	77 (7.7)	78 (7.8)	0.93
Myocardial infarction — no. (%)	33 (3.4)	40 (4.3)	0.41
Congestive heart failure — no. (%)	108 (11.2)	119 (12.6)	0.36
Supraventricular tachycardia — no. (%)	88 (9.1)	84 (8.9)	0.95
Ventricular tachycardia — no. (%)	2 (0.2)	2 (0.2)	1.00
Pulmonary embolism — no. (%)	0	8 (0.9)	0.004
Renal insufficiency — no. (%)	95 (9.8)	70 (7.4)	0.07
Hepatic insufficiency — no. (%)	26 (2.7)	23 (2.4)	0.84
Sepsis from central venous catheter or			
pulmonary-artery catheter — no. (%)	13 (1.3)	12 (1.3)	0.95
Wound infection — no. (%)	83 (8.6)	66 (7.0)	0.23
Pneumonia — no. (%)	70 (7.3)	63 (6.7)	0.70
Adverse events due to pulmonary-artery			
catheters or central venous catheters			
— no. (%)			
Pulmonary infarction	0	1 (0.1)	1.00
Hemothorax	0	2 (0.2)	0.24
Pulmonary hemorrhage	0	3 (0.3)	0.12
Pneumothorax	4 (0.4)	8 (0.9)	0.36
Arterial puncture	1 (0.1)	3 (0.3)	0.37

Note: There were 997 patients in each group, but because surgery was canceled for some patients for a variety of reasons, the total number of patients for all variables except length of hospital stay and in-hospital mortality was 965 for the standard care group and 941 for the catheter group.

(Reprinted by permission of *The New England Journal of Medicine* from Sandham JD, for the Canadian Critical Care Clinical Trials Group: A randomized, controlled trial of the use of pulmonary-artery catheters in high-risk surgical patients. *N Engl J Med* 348:5-14, 2003. Copyright 2003, Massachusetts Medical Society. All rights reserved.)

Conclusion.—This randomized controlled trial found no benefit associated with therapy using a PA catheter versus standard care (surgery without the use of a PA catheter) for elderly, high-risk surgical patients requiring a stay in the ICU after surgery.

▶ This is probably one of the most important articles to be published in the last 5 years in regard to clinical trials and patient outcome. Debate has raged for many years as to the value of therapy directed by the insertion of a PA catheter: The patient is high risk and should a PA catheter be placed? Others have suggested that the use of a PA catheter is associated with increased mortality. In this specific study, no benefit was found in the use of a PA catheter in high-risk surgical patients. What about the use of perioperative echocardiography? Is this technology less invasive, less likely to be associated with increased mortality and to be associated with improved outcome? It remains to be seen whether perioperative echocardiography or surface echocardiography becomes a routine alternative to monitoring and goal-directed therapy.

M. Wood, MD, FRCA

A Prospective Study to Determine Whether Cover Gowns in Addition to Gloves Decrease Nosocomial Transmission of Vancomycin-Resistant Enterococci in an Intensive Care Unit

Srinivasan A, Song X, Ross T, et al (Johns Hopkins Med Institutions, Baltimore, Md)
Infect Control Hosp Epidemiol 23:424-428, 2002   13–5

Background.—Enterococci are now the second most common nosocomial infection of the bloodstream. In 1999, 25% of these isolates were vancomycin resistant, a 47% increase from 1994. Bacteremia with vancomycin-resistant enterococci (VRE) is associated with higher morbidity rates, longer length of hospital stay, and higher hospital costs than is bacteremia with vancomycin-sensitive enterococci. Current guidelines of the Hospital Infection Control Practices Advisory Committee (HICPAC) of the Centers for Disease Control and Prevention (CDC) recommend the use of gowns and gloves for some interactions with patients colonized or infected with VRE to prevent nosocomial transmission of VRE. The effect of disposable cover gowns on preventing nosocomial transmission of VRE was assessed.

Methods.—This prospective study was conducted in a 16-bed ICU at a university teaching hospital. The study group included all patients who were at risk of acquiring VRE and were admitted to the ICU from August 1998 to January 1999. All the patients had at least 2 perirectal cultures. VRE isolation was changed from gowns and gloves to gloves alone. The main outcome measures were the VRE acquisition rates and risk factors for VRE acquisition.

Results.—The rate of VRE acquisition was 1.80 cases per 100 days at risk in the gown and gloves period compared with 3.78 in the gloves only period. Proportional hazards modeling, adjusted for length of stay, showed that the gloves-only precaution with a hazard ratio of 2.5 was the only independent risk factor for VRE acquisition.

Conclusions.—These findings support the current HICPAC recommendations for the use of cover gowns to reduce the nosocomial transmission of VRE.

▶ The study demonstrated dramatic results favoring the use of disposable gowns. I must say, I was a little surprised by the findings. No doubt, the quality of care an individual patient on "infection precautions" receives is inferior compared with a patient not on "infection precautions." The number of bedside assessments and time per assessment decreases, thus some "streamline" the process by not dressing in all the requested attire. However, this study supports the "more is better" mantra.

J. D. Lang, Jr, MD

Testosterone Gel Supplementation for Men With Refractory Depression: A Randomized, Placebo-Controlled Trial

Pope HG Jr, Cohane GH, Kanayama G, et al (McLean Hosp, Belmont, Mass; Harvard Med School, Boston; Harvard School of Public Health, Boston)
Am J Psychiatry 160:105-111, 2003   13–6

Background.—Testosterone supplementation may relieve depressive symptoms in men. Until recently, however, such supplementation had to be administered parenterally. The efficacy of testosterone transdermal gel was investigated in men with refractory depression and low or borderline testosterone levels.

Methods.—Twenty-three men, aged 30 to 65 years, with refractory depression and morning serum total testosterone levels of 350 mg/dL or less were enrolled in the study. One patient responded to an initial 1-week, single-blind placebo trial. The remaining 22 were randomly assigned to 1% testosterone gel, 10 g/d, or identical-appearing placebo. The patients continued their current antidepressant regimens. Ten patients receiving testosterone and 9 receiving placebo completed the full 8 weeks of the study.

Findings.—Testosterone recipients showed significantly greater improvements in scores on the Hamilton Depression Rating Scale compared with placebo recipients. Improvements occurred on both the vegetative and affective subscales. Scores on the Clinical Global Impression severity scale also showed significant improvement. However, scores on the Beck Depression Inventory were not significantly different between groups. One testosterone recipient reported increased difficulty in urinating, which suggests exacerbation of benign prostatic hyperplasia.

Conclusion.—Testosterone gel may have antidepressant effects in depressed men with low testosterone levels. Further research is needed to verify these preliminary findings.

▶ You will be seeing more and more hormone replacement therapies for men, I believe, in the future. The place for hormone replacement therapy in women is still debated, and that in men is probably not a very big place. But this study is one of the "buts." The authors showed in this study that testosterone supplementation appears to have a large antidepressant effect in this population of depressed men who have low testosterone levels.

Remember that testosterone can have unwanted side effects, such as an increase in aggressive behavior patterns, increased cancer risk (especially prostate cancer), and perhaps some other problems. But I believe that this study, combined with others that have been orally reported, show improvements in libido, sense of well being, even bone mass, and may increase our likelihood of seeing patients receiving testosterone gel preoperatively. Should we discontinue these medications? We don't know the answer to that.

M. F. Roizen, MD

14 Anesthesia Outside the Operating Room

Conscious Analgesia/Sedation With Remifentanil and Propofol Versus Total Intravenous Anesthesia With Fentanyl, Midazolam, and Propofol for Outpatient Colonoscopy
Rudner R, Jalowiecki P, Kawecki P, et al (Silesian Univ, Katowice, Poland)
Gastrointest Endosc 57:657-663, 2003   14-1

Background.—Colonoscopy is a necessary but often uncomfortable procedure for investigation of disorders of the lower gastrointestinal tract. Patients undergoing colonoscopy will often have pain and vasovagal reactions, necessitating the administration of analgesic and sedative agents or both. Because colonoscopy is now performed as an outpatient procedure, the anesthetic and sedative agents must guarantee the comfort and safety of patients and also provide for rapid recovery of full psychomotor function to enable discharge from the endoscopy unit as soon as possible. Conscious sedation is the technique most widely used for sedation in colonoscopy. The combined administration of an opiate and benzodiazepine provides excellent sedation and analgesia during colonoscopy; however, a sedative regimen involving the use of midazolam with opiates is not ideal. The hypothesis was tested that, for colonoscopy, analgesia/sedation with remifentanil and propofol might be more effective compared with anesthesia by IV administration of midazolam, fentanyl, and propofol.

Methods.—The study group for this prospective, randomized trial was composed of 100 adult patients who received either conscious analgesia/sedation (sedation group, 50 patients) or total IV anesthesia (TIVA group, 50 patients). Analgesia/sedation was achieved by infusion of remifentanil (0.20 to 0.25 µg/kg per minute) and propofol in titrated doses. TIVA was induced by IV administration of fentanyl (2 µg/kg), midazolam (0.05 mg), and propofol (dosage titrated). Cardiorespiratory parameters and bispectral index were monitored and recorded, and the quality of the analgesia was assessed with a numerical pain rating scale (NRS). The level of recovery and the return of psychomotor efficiency were evaluated with the Aldrete scale and a Modified Post Anesthesia Discharge Scoring (MPADS) system.

Results.—The 2 groups were similar in terms of demographic data, initial parameters, and duration of colonoscopy. All the patients in the TIVA group reported that they found the colonoscopy procedure to be painless (NRS score of 0). The average pain intensity score in the sedation group was 0.4. A significant difference was noted between the sedation and TIVA groups regarding the time from the end of the procedure until the maximum MPADS score was attained (-6.9 [4.0] vs 25.7 [8.4] minutes).

Conclusions.—It would appear from these findings that the combined administration of remifentanil and propofol for outpatient colonoscopy will provide sufficient analgesia, satisfactory hemodynamic stability, and minor respiratory depression. Additionally, this combination of remifentanil and propofol provides for rapid recovery and allows discharge of the patient as soon as 15 minutes after the procedure.

▶ This is a descriptive study from Poland published in a gastrointestinal journal. I selected it to highlight the move toward propofol sedation for outpatient colonoscopy rather than midazolam opioid sedation/analgesia; of course associated with propofol analgesia/anesthesia are many resultant consequences and implications such as billing, anesthesia manpower, and so on.

M. Wood, MD, FRCA

Risk Stratification and Safe Administration of Propofol by Registered Nurses Supervised by the Gastroenterologist: A Prospective Observational Study of More Than 2000 Cases
Heuss LT, Schnieper P, Drewe J, et al (Univ Hosp Basel, Switzerland)
Gastrointest Endosc 57:664-671, 2003   14–2

Introduction.—Conscious sedation is standard in patients undergoing gastrointestinal endoscopy. Propofol has been increasingly used as an alternative drug to prevent effects of the commonly used benzodiazepines. Propofol in the hands of nonanesthesiologists remains controversial. The safety profile of propofol as a single sedative agent, or in combination with other analgesics, for endoscopic procedures when administered by nurses under the supervision of nonanesthetists was examined in a university hospital gastroenterology department.

Methods.—All patients who underwent any endoscopic procedure between September 2000 and December 2001 were eligible for inclusion in this prospective observational investigation. The choice of sedation was voluntary. Data were collected regarding demographics, type of endoscopic procedure, and clinical characteristics. A structured personal history was used to create a 5-class risk stratification based on the criteria of the American Society of Anesthesiologists (Table 2). A total of 3475 procedures were performed in 2574 patients in whom propofol was administered by registered nurses.

Results.—There were no major complications due to the use of propofol. Overall reductions in the mean values for oxygen saturation (-2%) (Table 3), arterial pressure (-18%), and pulse rate (-10%) were identified. Severe

TABLE 2.—Initial Dose of Propofol to Induce Conscious Sedation and Total Dose Needed for the Procedure

	Mean Duration (Min)	P_{Init}	Dose Range	P_{Tot}	Dose Range
EGD					
ASA 1	13	1.31	0.23-3.91	1.90	0.67-6.52
ASA 2	13.5	1.15	0.17-5.97	1.75	0.57-8.29
ASA 3	14.5	0.92	0.14-5.60	1.51	0.56-8.40
ASA 4	17	0.72	0.22-1.82	1.30	0.57-2.55
ASA n.a.	14	1.08	0.21-2.40	1.59	0.57-5.00
Colonoscopy					
ASA 1	33	1.08	0.29-2.73	2.34	0.60-5.92
ASA 2	34	0.94	0.23-2.41	1.97	0.40-6.46
ASA 3	36	0.70	0.13-2.13	1.52	0.22-7.36
ASA 4	38	0.46	0.27-0.73	1.52	0.80-2.54
ASA n.a.	33	0.96	0.24-2.00	2.24	0.46-5.49

Note: Figures are milligram per kilogram of body weight based on American Society of Anesthesiologists classification.
Abbreviation: n.a., Not available.
(Courtesy of Heuss LT, Schnieper P, Drewe J, et al: Risk stratification and safe administration of propofol by registered nurses supervised by the gastroenterologist: A prospective observational study of more than 2000 cases. *Gastrointest Endosc* 57:664-671, 2003.)

respiratory depression necessitating intervention occurred in below 0.3% of all patients.

Conclusion.—The administration of propofol by registered nurses, with careful monitoring under the supervision of the gastroenterologist, was safe for conscious sedation during gastrointestinal endoscopy procedures in a large series of prospectively evaluated patients.

▶ As the authors point out, although sedation for gastrointestinal endoscopy is standard practice, the use of propofol by nonanesthesiologists is controversial. The package insert for Propofol (Diprivan 1%) in the United States states that for general anesthesia or monitored anesthesia care sedation, Diprivan

TABLE 3.—Adverse Effects: SaO_2 Less Than 90%

	$SaO_2 < 90\%$ n (%)	Emergency Intervention n (%)
Total	42 (1.6)	6 (0.2)
ASA 1	4 (0.8)	2 (0.4)
ASA 2	9 (1.3)	1 (0.1)
ASA 3	26 (2.5)	1 (0.1)
ASA 4	2 (3.8)	1 (1.9)
ASA n.a.	1 (0.3)	1 (0.3)
EGD	30 (1.9)	5 (0.3)
Colonoscopy	9 (1.3)	1 (0.1)
Combined	0 (0.0)	0 (0.0)
ERCP	2 (2.2)	0 (0.0)
EUS	1 (0.8)	0 (0.0)

Abbreviation: n.a., Not available.
(Courtesy of Heuss LT, Schnieper P, Drewe J, et al: Risk stratification and safe administration of propofol by registered nurses supervised by the gastroenterologist: A prospective observational study of more than 2000 cases. *Gastrointest Endosc* 57:664-671, 2003.)

should only be given by persons trained in the administration of general anesthesia. However, propofol is increasingly being used in the ICU and other areas out of the operating room. This article describes the adverse events that occurred when nurses used propofol for sedation in a gastrointestinal endoscopy area, but—important to note—in an academic tertiary medical center where help and rescue could be provided quickly.

M. Wood, MD, FRCA

15 Geriatric Medicine Issues

Recent Trends in Disability and Functioning Among Older Adults in the United States: A Systematic Review
Freedman VA, Martin LG, Schoeni RF (Polishner Research Inst, North Wales, Pa; Population Council, New York; Univ of Michigan, Ann Arbor)
JAMA 288:3137-3146, 2002   15–1

Background.—Disability and limitation are frequent accompaniments of aging and are associated with costs of care and treatment. It has recently been suggested that rates of disability are declining in this age group. This systematic review examined the evidence for US trends in the prevalence of self-rated age-related disability and limitations.

Study Design.—MEDLINE and AGELINE were searched for relevant articles published in English from 1990 through May 2002. Reference lists were reviewed and authors contacted to obtain further articles. Sixteen articles, based on 8 cross-sectional and cohort surveys, were selected for inclusion in this review.

Findings.—Of the 8 surveys, 2 were rated good, 2 were rated fair, 1 poor, and 1 mixed. Analysis of those surveys rated as at least fair demonstrated consistent declines in overall disability, activities of daily living disability, and functional limitations. Data on vision and cognition were inconsistent. No trends in disparities by age, sex, race, or education could be discerned.

Conclusion.—This systematic review suggested that the prevalence of disability declined for older US adults during the 1990s, by approximately −1.55% to −0.92% annually. The implications for future health care demands are not yet understood.

► This is perhaps the most important article I have seen on costs of medicine and relates to our health as well. What this article shows is that since the late 1980s, the rate of disability has been decreasing at 2% a year. The rate of mortality has been decreasing at the rate of 1% a year, and we have much further to go with these decreases. What does that mean? It means that we are less likely to be disabled in our old age and more likely to live longer. Fifty percent of these benefits are attributed to treatment of hypertension and 50% to multiple other factors. But we have much more to go; the data further indicate that we can continue this rate of decrease in disability and mortality for probably another 30 to 40 years.

This report has major implications for Medicare funding as well as for our own health. From a Medicare funding standpoint, if the rate of disability decreases by 1.5% a year, the Medicare and Social Security trust funds will last forever at their current rate of funding, or at least well past 2075. That obviously is great news, especially since the rate has been decreasing at 2% a year. This means that if Medicare trust funds are not raided and should they stand at the current rate of funding, they will be ample for most of us who are reading this article and this comment in the year 2003. Further, it gives us much hope.

It also appears that the average life span increasing at 1% per year means that we are aging only at a one third of the year for every year we are living. Let me give you an example: If you are 50 now and have a life expectancy of 80 and if these trends continue, your life expectancy may in fact expand to 90. Or if you are 50 and your genes and genetic heritage suggest you'll live to 95, current progress would suggest it is likely you'll live to 110 years of age. Now that seems outrageous, but that is what the current data indicate if we continue the current progress of the late 1980s and early 1990s. Now you see why I said this is perhaps the most important article you could read that was published in this last year.

M. F. Roizen, MD

Patient, Physician, and Family Member Understanding of Living Wills
Upadya A, Muralidharan V, Thorevska N, et al (Bridgeport Hosp, Conn; Yale Univ, New Haven, Conn)
Am J Respir Crit Care Med 166:1430-1435, 2002   15–2

Background.—Living wills are documents that are intended to convey the wishes of patients concerning medical care should they become acutely ill and unable to communicate with caregivers. However, there have been no published studies of whether patients, family members, and physicians understand the patient's living will and whether living wills, as currently written, are truly representative of a patient's end-of-life wishes. An understanding of living wills by patients, family members, and physicians was examined at 1 institution.

Methods.—This study was conducted at a community teaching hospital serving an inner-city population. Questionnaires were used to determine whether each cohort understood the patients' living wills in regard to endotracheal intubation and cardiopulmonary resuscitation (CPR).

Results.—A total of 4800 patients were admitted during the study period, 206 of whom reported having living wills, all of which precluded intubation and CPR in case of "terminal conditions." Of the 140 patients admitted to the general hospital wards, 17 (12%) wanted their living wills to preclude intubation or mechanical ventilation, and 12 (8.6%) did not want resuscitation under any conditions. Among physicians and family members, 7 of 120

(6%) of physicians and 4 of 108 family members indicated that they would not intubate or perform CPR even if there was a chance of recovery.

Of the 88 patients with complete data, 29 (33%) desired to have their living wills block intubation and mechanical ventilation only if their condition was judged to be terminal, and 46 patients (52%) want the living will to block intubation even if there was a 10% chance of recovery; 13 patients (15%) wanted intubation blocked even if the chance of recovery was greater than 50%. Similar findings were obtained regarding wishes for CPR.

Conclusion.—The data suggest significant differences in the understanding of living wills among patients, family members, and physicians. In this survey, the living will did not fully reflect the patient's understanding of receiving or not receiving life-sustaining treatment.

▶ This issue of living wills is complex. Interpretation can be extremely varied. We make significant efforts in our critical care and preoperative assessment didactic programs to educate our house staff. We also discuss this with our patients in the preoperative assessment clinic, as well as having a variety of literature available. We are not out to scare people but to educate them. Unfortunately, our numbers mimic those of Upadya et al in that way too few patients have living wills upon admission, and then, even if they exist, surrogate-physician dynamics and surrogates' understanding of the living will can be problematic. I also concur with this study on another point that was made in that, in many cases, physicians do not appropriately institute and apply living wills.

J. D. Lang, Jr, MD

Laparoscopic Cholecystectomy for Elderly Patients: Gold Standard for Golden Years?
Bingener J, Richards ML, Schwesinger WH (Univ of Texas, San Antonio)
Arch Surg 138:531-536, 2003   15–3

Background.—Laparoscopic cholecystectomy (LC) is known to have physiologic and cost advantages over the open approach. Recent research has questioned the efficacy of LC in persons older than 65 years. The safety and efficacy of LC in elderly patients were investigated.

Methods.—Between 1991 and 2001, 5884 consecutive patients, aged a mean 40 years, underwent attempted LC at 1 center. Three hundred ninety-five patients were older than 65 years. Sixty-four percent were male.

Findings.—Outcomes in patients aged 65 to 69 years were comparable to outcomes for younger patients previously reported. Patients in their 70s had a 40% incidence of complicated gallstone disease, such as acute cholecystitis, choledocholithiasis, or biliary pancreatitis. Patients in their 80s had a 55% of such disease. Overall, 1.4% of the patients died. The conversion rate was 17% in the first 5 years of the study period and 7% in the second half. Among patients with complicated disease, the conversion rate was 22%. For those with chronic cholecystitis, it was 2.5%. Mean length of hospitalization declined from 10.2 days in the first half of the study to 4.6 days in the second half.

Conclusions.—In this series, patients older than 70 years had a 2-fold increase in complicated biliary tract disease and conversion rates. However, mortality rate was low. Increased experience with LC had a favorable effect on outcomes over time. Further improvement in the outcomes of LC among the elderly will rely on early diagnosis and treatment before the onset of complications.

▶ The US population is aging dramatically, and its implications are increasingly being realized in health care. As the baby boomers age, the demand for health care will be dramatic, and I predict that there will be a shortage of physicians. We are asked to anesthetize more sick and elderly patients for relatively new procedures, such as LC, and are doing it very well.

M. Wood, MD, FRCA

16 Cardiopulmonary Resuscitation

A Double-Blind Randomized Trial: Prophylactic Vasopressin Reduces Hypotension After Cardiopulmonary Bypass
Morales DLS, Garrido MJ, Madigan JD, et al (Columbia Univ, New York)
Ann Thorac Surg 75:926-930, 2003   16–1

Background.—Vasopressor shock induced by cardiopulmonary bypass is usually mild and requires catecholamine vasopressor support at low doses to maintain perfusion pressure for the first few hours after bypass. However, a more severe state of distributive shock develops in approximately 8% of cases, and high-dose catecholamine vasopressor therapy is necessary in these patients. However, the administration of high-dose catecholamine vasopressors is associated with complications related to end-organ hypoperfusion and prevents early discharge from the ICU. The preoperative use of angiotensin-converting enzyme (ACE) inhibitors has been independently associated with an increased incidence of vasodilatory shock after cardiopulmonary bypass. This hypotension has been correlated with arginine vasopressin deficiency and can be corrected by its replacement. Whether initiation of vasopressin before cardiopulmonary bypass would ameliorate postbypass hypotension and catecholamine use by avoiding vasopressin deficiency was investigated.

Methods.—A total of 27 cardiac surgical patients receiving ACE inhibitor therapy were randomly assigned to receive either vasopressin (0.03 U/min) or an equal volume of normal saline beginning 20 minutes before cardiopulmonary bypass.

Results.—The prebypass mean arterial pressure and pulmonary artery pressure were not altered by vasopressin. After cardiopulmonary bypass, the vasopressin group had a lower peak norepinephrine dose than the placebo group (4.6 ± 2.5 vs 7.3 ± 3.5 µg/min), a shorter period on catecholamines (5 ± 6 vs 11 ± 7 hours), fewer hypotensive episodes (1 ± 1 vs 4 ± 2), and a shorter stay in the ICU (1.2 ± 0.4 vs 2.1 ± 1.4 days).

Conclusions.—The prophylactic administration in this cohort of cardiac surgical patients taking ACE inhibitor therapy at a dose without a vasopressor effect before cardiopulmonary bypass was found to reduce post–

301

cardiopulmonary bypass hypotension and vasoconstrictor requirements and to result in shorter duration of stay in the ICU.

Con: Vasopressin Is Not the Vasoconstrictor of Choice After Cardiopulmonary Bypass

Macfie A (Gartnavel Gen Hosp, Glasgow, Scotland)
J Cardiothorac Vasc Anesth 16:776-779, 2002   16–2

Background.—Arginine vasopressin (AVP) has been proposed as a rational therapy for patients in vasodilatory shock, in which catecholamine resistance is often present. However, the evidence for the safety and efficacy of vasopressin in vasodilatory shock is sparse, and vasodilatory shock may occur in 8% of cardiac surgical patients. Much of this evidence is in the form of case reports, retrospective analyses of case series, and small comparative studies with physiologic end points mainly from 1 research group. There is a need for large, multicenter, randomized controlled trials to assess the effect of AVP on outcome and organ dysfunction in this setting. This report discussed the pathophysiology of vasodilatory states after cardiopulmonary bypass (CPB) and provided a critical assessment of the evidence for the use of AVP in patients who have undergone CPB and are in a vasodilatory state.

Overview.—In the setting of CPB there is a release of a variable cascade of cytokines and other inflammatory mediators, which in turn induce the release of nitric oxide by the vascular endothelial cell surface. The systemic inflammatory response syndrome may be caused by contact stimulation by plastic surfaces, ischemia-reperfusion injury, endotoxemia, and surgical trauma. AVP has little effect on blood pressure in normal persons but significantly increases arterial pressure when the baroreceptor reflex is impaired. The therapeutic use of AVP in post-CPB vasodilatory shock would appear to be promising; several studies described in this report have yielded mixed results. Among the potential adverse effects of AVP are deficiencies of global and regional perfusion and pulmonary vasoconstriction. Gastrointestinal ischemia may result from the administration of AVP, and this may worsen the vasodilatory shock. AVP may increase the risk of thrombosis because it increases platelet aggregation, and it may cause water intoxication and may interact with other hormonal systems.

Conclusions.—At this time, AVP cannot be recommended as the vasoconstrictor of choice after CPB. It is unlikely that AVP will replace catecholamines as the vasoconstrictor of choice after CPB because the effects of AVP are unpredictable and difficult to titrate to effect.

Adverse Outcomes of Interrupted Precordial Compression During Automated Defibrillation
Yu T, Weil MH, Tang W, et al (Inst of Critical Care Medicine, Palm Springs, Calif; Univ of Southern California, Los Angeles)
Circulation 106:368-372, 2002   16–3

Background.—The ability to provide automated ECG rhythm analyses is one of the fundamental aspects of the operation of automated external defibrillators (AEDs). CPR is interrupted during this analysis, and current versions of AEDs prompt a "hands-off" interval of more than 10 seconds for rhythm analyses before advising the rescuer to deliver an electrical shock. It has been hypothesized that these interruptions would adversely affect outcomes of CPR. The effects of these interruptions in an animal model were evaluated.

Methods.—Ventricular fibrillation was induced in 20 male domestic swine weighing from 37.5 to 43 kg that were untreated for 7 minutes before initiation of CPR. Defibrillation was attempted with up to 3 sequential 150-J biphasic shocks; however, each attempt was preceded by 3-, 10-, 15-, or 20-second interruptions of chest compression (with 5 animals in each group), which corresponded to the interruptions mandated by commercially marketed AEDs for rhythm analysis and capacitor charge. This protocol was repeated at 1-minute intervals until successful resuscitation or for a total of 15 minutes.

Results.—Spontaneous circulation was restored in each of the 5 animals in which precordial compression was delayed for 3 seconds before each shock. However, spontaneous restoration of circulation was not obtained in any of the animals in which the delay was more than 15 seconds before the delivery of the first and subsequent shocks. Longer intervals of CPR interventions were required, and there was a correspondingly greater failure of resuscitation in close relation with increasing delays. There was an inverse relation between the duration of interruptions and the duration of subthresholds of coronary perfusion pressure. Arterial pressure and left ventricular ejection fraction after resuscitation were more severely impaired with increasing delays.

Conclusions.—This study of interrupted precordial compression during the use of AEDs found that the interruptions of precordial compression for rhythm analysis of more than 15 seconds before each shock adversely affected the outcome of CPR and increased the severity of postresuscitation myocardial dysfunction.

A Comparison of Vasopressin and Epinephrine for Out-of-Hospital Cardiopulmonary Resuscitation

Wenzel V, for the European Resuscitation Council Vasopressor During Cardiopulmonary Resuscitation Study Group (Leopold-Franzens Univ, Innsbruck, Austria; Free Univ, Berlin; Philipps Univ, Marburg, Germany)

N Engl J Med 350:105-113, 2004   16–4

Background.—There are more than a half million cases of sudden death annually in Europe and North America. More than half of these deaths occur in persons younger than 65 years, which is evidence of the need for optimal CPR strategies to improve the chances of survival. Epinephrine has been used during CPR for more than 100 years. However, in recent years its use has become controversial because epinephrine is associated with increased myocardial oxygen consumption, ventricular arrhythmias, and myocardial dysfunction in the period after resuscitation. Vasopressin is an alternative to epinephrine for vasopressor therapy during CPR, but the clinical experience with vasopressin in this setting is limited. Current international guidelines have recommended the use of epinephrine during CPR and advise that vasopressin should be considered a secondary alternative. The effects of vasopressin and epinephrine on survival were assessed in patients who had an out-of-hospital cardiac arrest.

Methods.—A total of 1186 adult patients who had an out-of-hospital cardiac arrest were randomly assigned to receive 2 injections of either 40 IU of vasopressin (589 patients) or 1 mg of epinephrine (597 patients) followed by additional treatment of epinephrine as necessary. The main outcome measure was survival to hospital admission, and the secondary outcome measure was survival to hospital discharge.

Results.—The clinical profiles of the 2 groups were similar. There was no significant difference between the 2 groups in the rates of hospital admission either among patients with ventricular fibrillation or among those with pulseless electrical activity. However, among patients with asystole, the use of vasopressin was associated with significantly higher rates of hospital admission (29% vs 20.3%) and hospital discharge (4.7% vs 1.5%). Among 732 patients in whom spontaneous circulation was not restored after 2 injections of the study drug, additional treatment with epinephrine resulted in significant improvement in survival to hospital admission and hospital discharge in the vasopressin group but not in the epinephrine group (hospital admission rate, 25.7% vs 16.4%; hospital discharge rate, 6.2% vs 1.7%). The groups were similar in terms of cerebral performance.

Conclusions.—This assessment of vasopressin and epinephrine in the setting of out-of-hospital CPR found that the effects of these drugs were similar in terms of management of ventricular fibrillation and pulseless electrical activity; however, vasopressin was shown to be more effective than epinephrine in patients with asystole. It would appear from these findings that vasopressin followed by epinephrine may be more effective than epinephrine alone in the treatment of refractory cardiac arrest.

Evidence Favoring the Use of an α_2-Selective Vasopressor Agent for Cardiopulmonary Resuscitation
Pellis T, Weil MH, Tang W, et al (Inst of Critical Care Medicine, Palm Springs, Calif; Univ of Southern California, Los Angeles; Loma Linda Univ, Calif)
Circulation 108:2716-2721, 2003   16–5

Background.—Both epinephrine and vasopressin are cited in the current International Guidelines on Emergency Cardiac Care as acceptable vasopressor drugs for the treatment of refractory ventricular fibrillation (VF). However, neither drug has been acknowledged to be of demonstrable benefit. The rationale for the use of vasopressor agents during CPR is the restoration of threshold levels of coronary perfusion pressure (CPP) and, therefore, myocardial blood flow. The restoration of these thresholds is the cardinal determinant of the success of resuscitation, particularly when untreated cardiac arrest is of 4 minutes or longer duration. Recent efforts to understand more clearly why only 1 of 8 patients initially resuscitated survive to discharge from the hospital have focused on impaired postresuscitation myocardial function. Both α_1-adrenergic and β-adrenergic agonists have been shown to increase the severity of global myocardial ischemic injury. The hypotheses that (1) combined α_1- and β-adrenergic blockade would improve initial resuscitation and postresuscitation myocardial and neurologic function and (2) the resulting α_2-actions of relatively brief duration would favor improved functions compared with more prolonged effect of nonadrenergic vasopressin were investigated.

Methods.—This study was conducted with 3 groups of 5 male domestic pigs weighing 37 ± 3 kg. Ventricular fibrillation was induced and left untreated for 7 minutes before initiation of precordial compression, mechanical ventilation, and attempted defibrillation. The pigs were randomized to receive central venous injections of equipressor doses of epinephrine, epinephrine in which both α_1- and β-adrenergic effects were blocked by previous administration of prazosin and propranolol, and vasopressin during CPR.

Results.—Resuscitation was successful in all but 1 animal. Injection of epinephrine resulted in significantly better cardiac output and fractional area change, together with more modest increases in troponin I after α_1- and β-adrenergic blockade. Postresuscitation neurologic function was improved after α_1- and β-adrenergic blockade compared with unblocked epinephrine and vasopressin.

Conclusions.—In an animal model of prolonged ventricular fibrillation, equipressor doses of epinephrine, epinephrine after α_1- and β-adrenergic blockade, and vasopressin were equally effective for the restoration of spontaneous circulation. However, combined α_1- and β-adrenergic blockade, which was representative of a predominantly selective α_2-vasopressor effect, provided improved postresuscitation cardiac and neurologic recovery.

Vasopressin, But Not Fluid Resuscitation, Enhances Survival in a Liver Trauma Model With Uncontrolled and Otherwise Lethal Hemorrhagic Shock in Pigs

Stadlbauer KH, Wagner-Berger HG, Raedler C, et al (Leopold-Franzens Univ, Innsbruck, Austria)

Anesthesiology 98:699-704, 2003   16–6

Background.—There has been much debate regarding resuscitation strategies in hemorrhagic shock, such as immediate versus delayed fluid resuscitation. A large clinical study of patients with penetrating torso trauma has reported that patients who received delayed fluid resuscitation had better chances of survival than patients who received immediate fluid resuscitation. Delayed fluid resuscitation may be beneficial when cardiocirculatory function has not collapsed but presents a dilemma in trauma patients who have cardiac arrest at the accident scene. Vasopressors are recommended in current international resuscitation guidelines in these patients when pulseless electrical activity or bradysystolic rhythm is imminent. A clinical study has reported that vasopressin may be useful for the management of patients with massive intra-abdominal bleeding. The effects of vasopressin and fluid resuscitation on survival in an animal model of liver trauma with uncontrolled and otherwise lethal hemorrhagic shock were compared.

Methods.—After induction of hemorrhagic shock, 23 pigs were randomly assigned to receive either 0.4 U/kg vasopressin (9 animals) or fluid resuscitation (7 animals) or placebo (7 animals). A continuous infusion of 0.08 U/kg per minute of vasopressin in the vasopressin group or normal saline was then administered in the fluid resuscitation and placebo groups, respectively. Bleeding was controlled after 30 minutes of experimental therapy by surgical intervention. Blood transfusion and rapid fluid infusion were then performed.

Results.—The vasopressin-treated animals had significantly higher maximum mean arterial blood pressure than animals in the fluid resuscitation and saline placebo groups (mean ± SD, 72 ± 26 vs 38 ± 16 vs 11 ± 7 mm Hg, respectively). Mean arterial blood pressure remained at approximately 40 mm Hg in all vasopressin-treated animals. Total blood loss was significantly higher in the pigs in the fluid resuscitation group compared with those in the vasopressin or saline placebo groups after 10 minutes of experimental therapy. All 7 pigs in the fluid resuscitation group and all 7 pigs in the placebo pigs died within approximately 20 minutes of experimental therapy, whereas 8 of 9 animals in the vasopressin group survived for more than 7 days.

Conclusions.—In this animal model of liver trauma with uncontrolled and otherwise lethal hemorrhagic shock, vasopressin but not fluid resuscitation or saline ensured survival with full recovery.

Therapeutic Hypothermia After Cardiac Arrest: An Advisory Statement by the Advanced Life Support Task Force of the International Liaison Committee on Resuscitation
Nolan JP, Morley PT, Vanden Hoek TL, et al (Resuscitation Council of Southern Africa; American Heart Association; European Resuscitation Council, Australia; et al)
Circulation 108:118-121, 2003   16–7

Background.—The induction of moderate hypothermia before cardiac arrest has been used successfully for 50 years to protect the brain against the global ischemia that can occur during open-heart surgery. There were reports in the early 1950s of the successful use of therapeutic hypothermia after cardiac arrest in human beings, but this technique was subsequently abandoned because of uncertainties regarding its benefits and difficulties with its use. Since those reports, the induction of hypothermia after the return of spontaneous circulation has been associated with improved functional recovery and reduced cerebral histologic deficits in a number of models of cardiac arrest. The most recent recommendations of the Advanced Life Support (ALS) Task Force of the International Liaison Committee on Resuscitation (ILCOR) regarding the use of therapeutic hypothermia after cardiac arrest were presented.

Overview.—The results of 2 prospective randomized trials comparing mild hypothermia with normothermia in comatose survivors of out-of-hospital cardiac arrest have been published. One study reported that 55% of patients in the hypothermia group has a favorable neurologic outcome at 6 months compared with 39% of patients in the normothermia group. The other study reported similar favorable outcomes in 49% of patients in the hypothermia group and 26% of patients in the normothermia group. However, the data available at this time are not sufficient to support the use of therapeutic hypothermia in patients with severe cardiogenic shock or life-threatening arrhythmias, pregnant patients, or patients with primary coagulopathy. However, thrombolytic therapy does not preclude the use of hypothermia because patients receiving thrombolytic therapy were included in these 2 trials.

Conclusions.—The recommendation of the ILCOR ALS Task Force regarding therapeutic hypothermia are that unconscious adults with spontaneous circulation after out-of-hospital cardiac arrest should be cooled to 32°C to 34°C for 12 to 24 hours when the initial rhythm is ventricular fibrillation, and that therapeutic hypothermia may also be beneficial for patients with other rhythms or with in-hospital cardiac arrest.

Cardiopulmonary Resuscitation After Near Drowning and Hypothermia: Restoration of Spontaneous Circulation After Vasopressin
Sumann G, Krismer AC, Wenzel V, et al (Leopold-Franzens-Univ, Innsbruck; Tyrol County Hosp, Austria)
Acta Anaesthesiol Scand 47:363-365, 2003   16–8

Background.—It is common clinical practice to avoid the use of vasopressor drugs during hypothermic CPR when the patient's core temperature is below 30°C. However, data from recent animal studies have challenged this practice. A case illustrating the beneficial effects of vasopression during prolonged CPR after a near drowning was presented.

Case Report.—A 19-year-old woman capsized with her kayak on a small creek in the Austrian Alps. The patient was trapped with her entire body below the surface of the water, which had a temperature of approximately 10°C, for about 15 minutes before rescue. The patient initially had asystole, severe accidental hypothermia, and wide, nonreactive pupils. CPR was initiated but asystole persisted after administration of 2 mg epinephrine IV. Vasopressin 40 IU was administered by an emergency medical technician 40 minutes after the initiation of treatment by the first physician, which resulted in an immediate return to sinus rhythm. Rewarming of the patient at the hospital was successful, but the patient died 15 hours later of refractory cardiocirculatory failure, massive gastrointestinal bleeding, and progressive edema of the lung and brain.

Conclusions.—This case report supports the opinion that vasopressors may be useful in restoration of spontaneous circulation in hypothermic cardiac arrest patients before rewarming. This strategy would obviate the need for prolonged mechanical cardiopulmonary resuscitation or the use of extracorporeal circulation. However, although cardiocirculatory failure, massive gastrointestinal bleeding, and progressive edema of the lung and brain are well-known complications of near-drowning, the profound vasopressor response associated with the combination of epinephrine and vasopressin cannot be definitively excluded as a contributing factor to multiorgan dysfunction.

▶ Vasopressin use in cardiac patients has increased dramatically in recent years. It is used regularly to vasoconstrict when catecholamines are failing[1-3] and has been added to the ACLS protocols.[4] But what of negative effects? It potentially can be a problem for saphenous vein grafts.[5] It may have negative effects on the coronary microcirculation.[6] I worry about spasm of the internal mammary artery after CPB and teach my residents to use nitroglycerin to reduce the incidence of this serious problem.[7-9] Yet, Morales and the Columbia group (Abstract 16–1), which has been a proponent of vasopressin use in CPB patients, describe a useful action of low-dose vasopressin in patients who have been taking ACE inhibitors preoperatively. This has been a consistent problem at our institution and is associated with vasodilatory shock after CPB.[1] Their results were impressive: (1) lower peak norepinephrine dose, (2) shorter duration of catecholamine use, (3) fewer hypotensive episodes, and (4) shorter intubation/ICU times in the treatment group. This study reminds us of the use of vasopressin in patients with vasodilatory shock and high cardiac output (sepsis, late phase of hemorrhagic shock). I have been using this protocol with some success but have found that often the drug is started postoperatively in the ICU by the surgeons in patients with low cardiac output syndromes. Many of these patients have had severe complications such as renal failure and skin necrosis. We must all be careful about the knee jerk use of any drug in a given situation—especially one with powerful and complex effects such as vasopressin.

But what of the use of vasopressin during resuscitation—an area related to cardiac anesthesia? Vasopressin has a long half-life of 17 to 35 minutes. This potentially could have long-term deleterious effects both after CPR and CPB. Macfiel outlines some of the concerns with vasopressin during the perioperative period. Caution is warranted: I know that is true with me.

The interest in vasopressin in the setting of CPR was driven by the observation that vasopressin levels were high in survivors and lower in nonsurvivors of CPR.[10] In animal studies, vasopressin maintained better coronary and cerebral perfusion pressures during CPR. Epinephrine in higher doses caused vasoconstriction but also had adverse effects on postresuscitation cardiac function mediated through α_1-adrenoreceptors, such as increased myocardial work, reduced subendocardial perfusion, and worse left ventricular function. Vasopressin may have potential benefits over epinephrine alone because of a greater vasoconstrictor effect in the presence of hypoxia and acidosis and being devoid of adrenergic action. The American Heart Association guidelines recommend a single dose of 40 IU of vasopressin as an alternative to 1 mg of epinephrine every 3 to 5 minutes during cardiac arrest. The largest prospective study to date comparing vasopressin with epinephrine in in-hospital cardiac arrests showed no increase in survival to hospital discharge with the use of vasopressin.[11] This is an important article that should be read by all interested in this subject.

Wenzel et al (Abstract 16–4), in a European Resuscitation Council study of 1500 patients, helps clarify this contentious issue. The current international guidelines for CPR recommend the use of epinephrine during cardiac resuscitation, with vasopressin considered only as a secondary alternative, because clinical data on vasopressin therapy have been limited. In this study, 1219 adults who had had an out-of-hospital cardiac arrest were randomized to receive 2 injections of either 40 IU of vasopressin or 1 mg of epinephrine, followed by additional treatment with epinephrine if needed. Survival to hospital admission was the primary end point, and the secondary end point was survival to hospital discharge. Rates of hospital admission were similar in the vasopressin group and the epinephrine group among patients with ventricular fibrillation (46.2% vs 43.0%; $P = .48$) and among those with pulseless electrical activity (33.7% vs 30.5%; $P = .65$). However, among patients with asystole, rates of hospital admission were higher with vasopressin than with epinephrine (29.0% vs 20.3%; $P = .02$), as were rates of hospital discharge (4.7% vs. =

1.5%; $P = .04$). Among 732 patients in whom 2 injections of the study drug failed to restore spontaneous circulation, additional treatment with epinephrine significantly improved the rates of survival to hospital admission and hospital discharge in the vasopressin group but not in the epinephrine group (hospital admission rate, 25.7% vs 16.4%, $P = .002$; hospital discharge rate, 6.2% vs 1.7%, $P = .002$). Cerebral function was similar in both groups.

This important article suggests that vasopressin has effects similar to those of epinephrine in the management of ventricular fibrillation and pulseless electrical activity, but vasopressin was superior to epinephrine in patients with asystole. Vasopressin followed by epinephrine may be more effective than epinephrine alone in the treatment of refractory cardiac arrest. An editorial follows in the same issue and suggests that practitioners should be encouraged to incorporate this information into their protocols "immediately."

Pellis et al (Abstract 16–5) took the next logical step comparing epinephrine (group 1) alone, α_2-agonist activity (group 2: epinephrine with α_1- and β-adrenergic blockade) and vasopressin (group 3) alone in CPR after ventricular fibrillation arrest in animals. This was done to reduce the global myocardial ischemic injury. It took more defibrillator shocks with group 1, but myocardial damage was lowest in the group. The study also confirms that epinephrine alone increases the incidence of ventricular ectopy. Similar problems were noted with vasopressin despite the higher coronary perfusion pressure noted in that group. This highlights the potential negatives of vasopressin alone and that coronary perfusion pressure, despite its popularity as a goal in the literature, is not the only goal during CPR. Unfortunately, for us in the field, protocols will now become more complicated and one size may not fit all.

Stadlbauer et al (Abstract 16–6) performed an excellent animal study comparing resuscitation techniques in a lethal hemorrhage model. Standard fluid resuscitation was compared with vasopressin infusion and saline placebo. All the animals in the vasopressin group survived with good neurologic outcome, and none survived in the other 2 groups. Heart rate, blood pressure and cardiac output were better maintained in the vasopressin group. In addition, blood loss was far greater in the standard fluid resuscitation group. Further study is warranted in human beings, but this study suggests another use for vasopressin in trauma and resuscitation.

Yu et al (Abstract 16–3) performed another animal study that highlights the importance of adequate chest compressions and quick evaluations of the ECG for defibrillation prescriptions. The study was to mimic the time delays of automated external defibrillators (AEDs) but it shows the importance of sufficient coronary perfusion pressure for an adequate amount of time before attempts at defibrillation. This has been noted in other papers.[12] The take-home points are (1) chest compressions continuously whenever possible and perhaps before defibrillation attempts in prolonged arrest (>4 minutes) and (2) quick looks with the defibrillator. For those of us involved in the purchase of automated external defibrillatory, analysis and capacitor charge times should be in the analysis.

Nolan et al (Abstract 16–7) in an advisory statement give some guidance into therapeutic options, namely hypothermia, after VF cardiac arrest followed by spontaneous circulation and coma. It gives clear guidance based on the available literature and should be read by all who take care of these patients after resuscitation.

Sumann et al (Abstract 16–8) in a case report reviews much of what has been discussed above. The report describes a near-drowning victim with prolonged cardiac arrest who was severely hypothermic and unresponsive to boluses of epinephrine. Spontaneous circulation occurred after a single bolus of vasopressin. The final outcome was poor, but this report reminds us to add vasosopressin early if epinephrine is failing. I have seen similar responses to vaso pressin in the ICU after prolonged unsuccessful CPR.

We as anesthesiologists are often called to assist with resuscitation in the ED, ICU, and on the floor. Techniques and protocols for resuscitation are evolving rapidly. Epinephrine in high dose appears to not offer any value as noted in a recent meta-analysis which included more than 6000 patients. Vasopressin has promise, at least in selected situations such as asystole and hemorrhagic shock. Yet, we must remember that a more fundamental controversy still exists. The mainstay of resuscitation for decades, epinephrine, has never been shown to be more beneficial than placebo. Published guidelines lag behind the literature as well as local protocols. An example of this is the recent adoption of chest compressions without ventilation (mouth to mouth) during cardiac arrest in many areas of the country. The papers discussed, many of which were performed by anesthesiologists, outline some of the issues we all need to be aware of.

M. F. Trankina, MD

References

1. Argenziano M, Chen JM, Choudhri AF, et al: Management of vasodilatory shock after cardiac surgery: Identification of predisposing factors and use of a novel pressor agent. *J Thorac Cardiovasc Surg* 116:973-980, 1998.
2. Gold JA, Cullinane S, Chen J, et al: Vasopressin as an alternative to norepinephrine in the treatment of milrinone-induced hypotension. *Crit Care Med* 28:249-252, 2000.
3. Morales DL, Gregg D, Helman DN, et al: Arginine vasopressin in the treatment of 50 patients with postcardiotomy vasodilatory shock. *Ann Thorac Surg* 69:102-106, 2002.
4. Morris DC, Dereczyk BE, Grzybowski M, et al: Vasopressin can increase coronary perfusion pressure during human cardiopulmonary resuscitation. *Acad Emerg Med* 4:878-883, 1997.
5. Medina P, Acuna A, Martinez-Leon JB, et al: Arginine vasopressin enhances sympathetic constriction through the V1 vasopressin receptor in human saphenous vein. *Circulation* 97:865-970, 1998.
6. Sellke FW, Quillen JE: Altered effects of vasopressin on the coronary circulation after ischemia. *J Thorac Cardiovasc Surg* 1992;104:357-363, 1992.
7. Jett GK, Arcidi JM, Jr, Dorsey LM, et al: Vasoactive drug effects on blood flow in internal mammary artery and saphenous vein grafts. *J Thorac Cardiovasc Surg* 94:2-11, 1987.
8. Shapira OM, Xu A, Vita JA, et al: Nitroglycerin is superior to diltiazem as a coronary bypass conduit vasodilator. *J Thorac Cardiovasc Surg* 117:906-911, 1999.
9. Zabeeda D, Medalion B, Jackobshvilli S, et al: Comparison of systemic vasodilators: Effects on flow in internal mammary and radial arteries. *Ann Thorac Surg* 71:138-141, 2001.
10. Lindner KH, Strohmenger HU, Ensinger H, et al: Stress hormone response during and after cardiopulmonary resuscitation. *Anesthesiology* 77:662-668, 2002.

11. Stiell IG, Hebert PC, Wells GA, et al: Vasopressin versus epinephrine for inhospital cardiac arrest: A randomised controlled trial. *Lancet* 358:105-109, 2001.
12. Niemann JT, Cairns CB, Sharma J, et al: Treatment of prolonged ventricular fibrillation. Immediate countershock versus high-dose epinephrine and CPR preceding countershock. *Circulation* 85:281-287, 1992.

17 Medical Education and Simulation

The UCSF Academy of Medical Educators
Cooke M, Irby DM, Debas HT (Univ of California, San Francisco)
Acad Med 78:666-672, 2003   17–1

Background.—The mission of the Academy of Medical Education at the University of California, San Francisco (UCSF) is to foster excellence in teaching, support and reward medical teachers and educators, and promote innovation in curricula. Established in 2000 in response to a critical need to reinvigorate the undergraduate medical curriculum of UCSF, the Academy of Medical Education is a membership organization that has been well received thus far. The criteria for membership, selection process, benefits, programs and activities, and early accomplishments were outlined.

Criteria, Selection Process, and Benefits.—Five categories of educational activity were identified, including direct teaching, curriculum development and assessment of learner performance, advising and mentoring, educational administration and leadership, and educational research. Membership is based on outstanding performance in any 1 of the 5 in the 5 years preceding the candidate's application. The term of membership is 5 years but is renewable. A selection committee screens applications, from which are chosen those qualifying for an outside review by a panel of national experts in medication education, the educator's portfolio, or faculty development. Then the selection committee makes the final choices. Members are expected to continue to perform at their outstanding level of excellence, participate in activities supporting the mission of the academy, and submit a 1-page form outlining his or her educational activities and educational service, on which renewal will be based. Members are eligible to receive salary support, which is distributed through the program's innovations-funding program, a project-driven internal grant-making initiative available to nonacademy members as well. Selection identifies the faculty member as an outstanding teacher who is often then sought by colleagues for advice and gives an advantage regarding promotions. Partially endowed chairs have also been established to reward key educators.

Programs, Activities, and Impact.—In the 6 projects funded from 2001 to 2002 and 14 projects in 2002 to 2003, 76% of the funds expended were in faculty salary supporting release time for creative work in education, with a special emphasis on program development. The faculty development working group has endeavored to enhance faculty members' understanding of the educator's portfolio and encouraging its use, initiated a mentoring program for junior faculty members built on peer observations of teaching, and made efforts to strengthen the scholarship of members' work. As curricular priorities have been identified, the academy has worked in cooperation with faculty curriculum oversight committees and the Office of Medical Education to direct appropriate energy without stifling creativity. Faculty members have had the opportunity to establish themselves as scholars nationally as well as within their community.

Conclusions.—After just 3 years, the Academy of Medical Educators has proved itself an active force in reinventing the undergraduate medical curricula at UCSF. Future developments await rethinking the emphasis on undergraduate medical education to the exclusion of residents; energizing an endowment sufficient to maintain or expand the innovations-funding program; and developing the ability to motivate the voluntary donation of thousands of faculty teaching hours to support medical education. Currently it is enhancing the status of medical education and teachers.

▶ This is an important article. Endeavors such as this may change the status of medical education and provide an enhanced career pathway for innovations in the teaching of medical students.

M. Wood, MD, FRCA

Effectiveness of Medical Resident Education in Mechanical Ventilation
Cox CE, Carson SS, Ely EW, et al (Univ of North Carolina at Chapel Hill; Vanderbilt Univ, Nashville, Tenn; Duke Univ, Durham, NC; et al)
Am J Respir Crit Care Med 167:32-38, 2003   17–2

Background.—Mortality can be reduced and health care costs minimized if the correct methods of mechanical ventilation management are employed. With the aging of the population, the management of patients requiring mechanical ventilation becomes a special concern in that the incidence of acute respiratory failure that requires mechanical ventilation increases almost 10-fold from age 55 to age 85 years. The trend is for more generalists to be directing the care of these patients, so residency training programs must address the vital elements of managing mechanical ventilation patients appropriately.

A written mechanical ventilation test and questionnaire were developed to measure the knowledge needed to provide effective care to ventilated patients, to describe the perceptions of residents and residency program directors concerning the adequacy of this knowledge, and to assess characteristics of residents and residency programs that are associated with higher levels of mechanical ventilator knowledge and satisfaction during training.

Methods.—The 19-item case-based test and survey were administered to resident physicians at 31 internal medicine residency programs in the United States. Three hundred forty-seven senior residents were contacted. The test comprised 4 case vignettes featuring patients with frequently encountered potential indications for the use of mechanical ventilation. Multiple-choice questions followed the case presentations.

Results.—Seventy-five percent of the residents (259 of 347) completed the tests, and 29 of 31 program directors (94%) returned questionnaires. For senior residents, the mean test score was 74% correct, with a range of 37% to 100%. Fewer than half of the questions were correctly answered by 10% of the residents, and over one third answered fewer than 70% correctly. Incorrect answers were given by significant percentages of the residents on important questions such as choosing an appropriate tidal volume setting for a patient with acute respiratory distress syndrome (48%), deciding when a patient was ready for a weaning trial (38%), and identifying indications for noninvasive ventilation (27%). Eighty-six percent of residents properly diagnosed serious tension pneumothorax and were able to distinguish between an obstructed endotracheal tube and tension pneumothorax, using information from the ventilator.

Training programs with better test scores tended to have closed rather than open ICU organization, more senior residents in their program, and more attending physicians on staff. Residents with higher test scores showed perceived adequacy of ventilator knowledge, had an awareness of learning objectives, and had graduated from a medical school in the United States. Resident satisfaction showed strong links to awareness of learning objectives, perceived adequacy of ventilator skills, and the belief that time for instruction was adequate. The program directors largely (92%) believed their residents were adequately knowledgeable concerning mechanical ventilation by graduation, but only 44% of the residents held this belief. Only 57% of the program directors agreed or strongly agreed that learning mechanical ventilation was a significant aspect of medical practice.

Conclusion.—The evidence-based knowledge needed to provide effective care for patients needing mechanical ventilation is not always given in the training of senior internal medicine residents. Residency programs require improved means for evaluating educational effectiveness and learning objectives specific to mechanical ventilator use to improve the educational outcomes in this area.

▶ An insightful study involving high tier internal medicine programs that we can glean a lot from. I have given this test to my residents for the past 6 months and have had similar results, even though residents in anesthesiology have a much greater familiarity with mechanical ventilation than the average internal medicine resident. The recurring deficit among my residents is circumstances in which the application of noninvasive positive pressure ventilation may be useful. With the efforts to push the concept of the perioperative physician and to increase our presence in the area of critical care medicine, focused learning must be placed in this area, especially on common medical-surgical clinical scenarios encountered outside of the operating room. This exam can be viewed on the online supplement at www.atsjournals.org.

J. D. Lang, Jr, MD

A Worldwide Survey of the Use of Simulation in Anesthesia

Morgan PJ, Cleave-Hogg D (Univ of Toronto)
Can J Anesth 49:659-662, 2002   17–3

Background.—There has been a significant expansion in the use of simulation technology in medical education in recent years. The simulator provides opportunities for standardized, reproducible critical events in a safe and realistic environment. However, there are few indications as to the extent of high-fidelity simulation use worldwide. The purpose of this study was to gather information regarding the use of simulation technology throughout the world in education, evaluation, and research in anesthesia.

Methods.—A search was conducted of the World Wide Web, and 158 sites with simulation centers were located. A 57-item questionnaire was mailed to these sites requesting information about patient demographics, personnel, education use, and research involvement. This study was concerned only with medical school data.

Results.—Two web sites were used to generate the list of simulation centers. A total of 60 responses were received (38%), and 41 of these responses came from medical schools. Of the centers that responded, 67% were involved in undergraduate education and 85% were involved in postgraduate education. Few centers were involved in evaluation or competency assessments. Participation in ongoing research was indicated by 61% of centers, and an additional 25% indicated an interest in international collaboration. The use of simulation technology in medical schools is, for the most part, supported by university or university department–based funding. The most common problem identified by respondents was a lack of financial and human resources.

Conclusion.—The simulator appears to be underutilized as a performance assessment tool in anesthesia. This underutilization may be a result of a lack of research in this area; a lack of standardized, valid, and reliable tests; and the fact that most centers have only recently acquired simulation technology. Thus, there is a need for additional research in this area.

▶ Unlike the situation in the airline industry, we don't use simulations in testing competence. What the authors found is that simulation is largely used to teach medical students and postgraduates but not in assessing competence. They also found that most of the funding for such simulation comes from universities or university departments and not from either user fees or grants. This article may be an important one for a research journal club, as it brings out the question of why hasn't there been research in competency education. Like most good studies, this one stimulates more questions than it answers. The authors should be congratulated for their interesting presentation and comments.

M. F. Roizen, MD

The Use of Advanced Simulation in the Training of Anesthesiologists to Treat Chemical Warfare Casualties
Berkenstadt H, Ziv A, Barsuk D, et al (Chaim Sheba Med Ctr, Tel Hashomer, Israel; Tel Aviv Univ, Israel)
Anesth Analg 96:1739-1742, 2003   17–4

Background.—Exposure to volatile nerve agents from chemical attack as a result of warfare or terrorist attack on a civilian population may result in mass casualties, an unfamiliar scenario for most medical practitioners, including anesthesiologists. Training anesthesiologists to address and treat victims of nerve gas intoxication in a mass-casualty scenario is a complicated task because of the unfamiliarity of the medical and physical conditions and because there is a need to train in realistic conditions in which medical teams are expected to be physically protected from secondary contamination and to decontaminate the patients before definitive medical treatment can be provided. A simulation-based training program for anesthesiologists in the treatment of chemical warfare casualties was described.

Methods.—Training was conducted at the Israeli Center for Medical Simulation and included 25 anesthesiologists working with teams of surgeons and intensive care and postanesthesia nurses. In 1 area of a virtual hospital, anesthesiologists were trained in initial airway and breathing resuscitation before decontamination while wearing full protective gear. In another area of the virtual hospital, anesthesiologists were trained in the treatment of critically injured patients with combined conventional and chemical injuries or severe intoxication. Intubation simulators of newborn, pediatric, and adult patients, advanced full-scale simulators, and actors simulating patients were used.

Results.—Initial airway, breathing, and antidotal treatment were performed successfully with and without full protective gear. Although the gas mask did not interfere with orotracheal intubation, it was found to limit effective communication among the medical team. Chemical-protective gloves were found to be the sole limiting factor in performance of tasks such as fixing the orotracheal tube. Nearly all of the participants (22 of 25, or 88%) found that the simulated cases represented realistic problems in the scenario, and all 25 participants reported that this simulation-based training was superior to the previous traditional training they had received.

Conclusion.—Advanced simulation is an effective method for training anesthesiologists to treat victims of nerve gas intoxication and to provide insight into the limitations of providing medical care in the setting of a mass-casualty scenario involving chemical warfare.

▶ While not perfect, the use of simulation is proving to be a significant enhancement for high-risk scenarios. In this case, the limitations observed may lead to significant breakthroughs that can have far-reaching repercussions. Simulation training has now become commonplace in most anesthesiology departments, for both operating room and ICU scenarios.

J. D. Lang, Jr , MD

Subject Index

A

adenotonsillectomy in, urgent, risk
factors for postoperative
respiratory morbidity after, 18
analgesia in, patient-controlled epidural,
242
anesthesia in, caudal, 77
aprotinin during craniofacial surgery in,
86
cardiopulmonary bypass in, adverse
events after protamine after, 90
catheters in, traditional *vs.* new needle
retractable IV, 76
circumcision in, EMLA cream *vs.* dorsal
penile nerve block for analgesia
after, 74
craniosynostosis repair in, sagittal,
comparison of 2 surgical techniques
for, 8
heart surgery in
antibiotic prophylaxis regimens in, 88
congenital, intraoperative
transesophageal echocardiography
in, 66
infant (*see* Infant)
in intensive care unit with prolonged
stay, nature of conflict in care of,
142
newborn (*see* Newborn)
nitric oxide in, adverse effect in child
with 5,10-
methylenetetrahydrofolate, 80
respiratory distress syndrome in, severe
acute, bovine surfactant in, 128
scoliosis in, autologous blood donation
for, 85
spinal fusion surgery in, predictors of
red cell transfusion in, 83
Chloroprocaine
neurotoxicity, sodium bisulfite as
scapegoat for (in rat), 224
Cholecystectomy
laparoscopic, in elderly, 299
Circadian
rhythms, adjustment to nocturnal
period, massage therapy by
mothers enhances, in full-term
infants, 73
Circumcision
analgesia after, EMLA cream *vs.* dorsal
penile nerve block for, in children,
74
Claims
medicolegal, in vascular surgery, 169
Cleansing
hand, during postanesthesia care, 153

Clinic
preoperative assessment, alterations in,
effect on number and yield of
cardiology consultants, 27
Clinical
productivity
in anesthesiology groups, comparison
of, 1
hourly, of anesthesiologists, effects of
surgical case duration and type of
surgery on, 2
trials, 283
Clonidine
epidural, combined with spinal
bupivacaine, effect on postoperative
outcome after lumbar laminectomy,
233
in prevention of perioperative
cardiovascular complications, 15
CO_2
absorbents containing strong base, use
of Amsorb to detect dehydration
of, 53
noninvasive partial CO_2 rebreathing
cardiac output *vs.* continuous
thermodilution cardiac output in
patients undergoing aortic
reconstruction surgery, 51
Coagulation
of crystalloid or colloid, IV, effects in
patients undergoing peripheral
vascular surgery, 71
Colloid
IV, coagulation of, effects in patients
undergoing peripheral vascular
surgery, 71
Colonoscopy
outpatient, conscious analgesia/sedation
with remifentanil/propofol *vs.* total
IV anesthesia with
fentanyl/midazolam/propofol for,
293
Coma
post-anoxic, serum neuron-specific
enolase predicts outcome in, 103
Complications
in anesthesia, 163
Compression
aortocaval, in pregnancy, 202
myelopathy, cervical, laminectomy for,
intraoperative neurophysiologic
detection of iatrogenic C5 nerve
root injury during, 110
precordial, interrupted, during
automated defibrillation, adverse
outcomes of (in pig), 303

Author Index

A

Abdi S, 246
Abel MD, 171
Abodeely A, 233
Abouleish AE, 1, 2
Abramovitz S, 214
Ahn S-H, 262
Aiken LH, 13
Andreae MH, 218
Angelini M, 7
Araujo-Preza CE, 137
Arcand G, 47
Ashraf Z, 245
Avidan MS, 212
Aya AGM, 209

B

Bach FW, 269
Bajwa ZH, 245
Balestrieri PJ, 213
Balki M, 105
Bamber JH, 202
Bärlocher CB, 250
Barnett GH, 108
Barsuk D, 317
Barzilai B, 113
Baumgarten M, 38
Beattie S, 15
Béchir M, 55
Beilin B, 227
Beilin Y, 214
Bellomo R, 118
Benhamou D, 184
Bensard DD, 145
Bergman BD, 241
Berkenstadt H, 317
Berman MF, 10
Bernath M-A, 66
Bessler H, 227
Bettex DA, 66
Biegon A, 95
Bingener J, 299
Birmingham PK, 242
Birnbach DJ, 178
Blott M, 212
Bodenham A, 50
Boehnke T, 133
Bollen AW, 224
Bolton J, 244
Bone M, 265
Botteri M, 22
Boucher M, 219
Bove EL, 88
Boxer LK, 67

Braverman AC, 113
Breen TW, 181
Brill S, 268
Brown KA, 18
Bruppacher H, 82
Bryssine B, 221
Buchman SR, 86
Buclin T, 44
Buggy DJ, 265
Buie D, 281
Bujold E, 219
Bullock MFM, 167
Burgener D, 135
Burke AP, 56
Burns JP, 142
Buttermann GR, 252

C

Calkins CM, 145
Camann WR, 177
Cameron AG, 218
Camorcia M, 187
Campbell DC, 181
Campbell WB, 169
Cannesson M, 221
Capogna G, 187
Carlson P, 225
Carman TL, 108
Carpenter M, 206
Carson SS, 314
Caruso DM, 131
Castillo D, 223
Castillo J, 112
Catling S, 204
Cederholm I, 273
Cepeda MS, 38
Chan HT, 85
Chan L, 99
Chan VW, 47
Chapman MD, 4
Chatfield DA, 97
Chenevard R, 55
Cheung RB, 13
Chinkes DL, 140
Choi KC, 180
Choi WY, 74
Chouinard P, 47
Chow BFM, 85
Church EJ, 172
Ciu M, 266
Claridge JA, 158
Clarke SP, 13
Cleave-Hogg D, 316
Cohane GH, 291
Cohen SE, 186

Cohen SP, 246, 255
Coley KC, 9
Columb MO, 184, 185, 186, 187
Contini P, 157
Cooke M, 313
Cooper A, 115
Cooper DW, 206
Coppejans HC, 220
Coratti A, 7
Corbin AE, 259
Coté CJ, 76
Cox CE, 314
Critchley P, 265
Curry R, 277

D

Dalgic H, 216
DaPos SV, 9
Das S, 42
Dauri M, 238
Dàvalos A, 112
David LR, 8
Davies J, 196
Davis N, 33
De Backer D, 130
Debaene B, 168
Debas HT, 313
De Bast Y, 130
Deibert E, 113
De Jonghe B, 141
Dela F, 136
Dennewitz MB, 159
Derby R, 251
Derdak S, 125
D'Errico CC, 86
Deutsch R, 95
Dexter F, 79
Dilly M-P, 168
Dimick JB, 67
Dindo D, 30
Dogru K, 216
Dorn C, 261
Doud T, 276
Douglas MJ, 219
Drasner K, 224
Dresner M, 202
Drewe J, 294
Dunn AS, 148
Dworkin RH, 259
Dyer RA, 210